NUTRITIONAL SUPPLEMENTS IN SPORT, EXERCISE AND HEALTH

Nutritional Supplements in Sport, Exercise and Health is the most up-to-date and authoritative guide to dietary supplements, ergogenic aids and sports nutrition foods currently available. Consisting of over 140 evidence-based review articles written by world-leading research scientists and practitioners, the book aims to dispel the misinformation that surrounds supplements and supplementation, offering a useful, balanced and unbiased resource.

The reviews are set out in an A–Z format and include: definitions alongside related products; applicable food sources; where appropriate, practical recommendations such as dosage and timing, possible nutrient interactions requiring the avoidance of other nutrients, and any known potential side effects; and full research citations. The volume as a whole addresses the key issues of efficacy, safety, legality and ethics, and includes additional reviews on the WADA code, inadvertent doping and stacking.

Combining the most up-to-date scientific evidence with consideration of practical issues, this book is an essential reference for any healthcare professional working in sport and exercise, any student or researcher working in sport and exercise science, sports medicine, health science or nutrition, and for all coaches and support teams working with athletes.

Linda M. Castell is a Visiting Research Fellow at Green Templeton College, University of Oxford, UK. In 1990, she joined Professor Eric Newsholme's Cellular Nutrition Research Group (CNRG) at Oxford, working on amino acids and immunology; and, after his retirement in 1996, she took over directing the CNRG. She has published several chapters and 30 full papers. She initiated the A–Z series on nutritional supplements for athletes in the *British Journal of Sports Medicine* (2009–2013).

Samantha J. Stear (Nottingham) is a consultant with a PhD in Biomedical Science and more than 25 years' experience in the health, nutrition, sport and exercise sectors. Sam established the English Institute of Sport's Performance Nutrition Service and has individually worked with Olympic medallists and world record holders. Sam has published three books, more than 50 papers and more than 150 consumer magazine articles.

Louise M. Burke is a sports dietitian with more than 35 years of experience, serving for the past 25 years as Head of Sports Nutrition at the Australian Institute of Sport, and more recently as a Chair in Sports Nutrition, at the Australian Catholic University in Melbourne, Australia. Louise has published more than 20 books and more than 200 papers.

NUTRITIONAL SUPPLEMENTS IN SPORT, EXERCISE AND HEALTH

An A–Z guide

Edited by
Linda M. Castell,
Samantha J. Stear
and Louise M. Burke

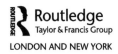

Routledge
Taylor & Francis Group

LONDON AND NEW YORK

First published 2015
by Routledge
2 Park Square, Milton Park, Abingdon, Oxon OX14 4RN

and by Routledge
711 Third Avenue, New York, NY 10017

Routledge is an imprint of the Taylor & Francis Group, an informa business

British Library Cataloguing-in-Publication Data
A catalogue record for this book is available from the British Library

Library of Congress Cataloging in Publication Data
Nutritional supplements in sport, exercise and health : an A-Z guide / edited by Linda M. Castell, Samantha J. Stear, and Louise M. Burke.
    p. ; cm.
Includes bibliographical references and index.
I. Castell, Linda M., editor. II. Stear, Samantha J., editor. III. Burke, Louise, 1959–, editor.
[DNLM: 1. Dietary Supplements. 2. Sports Nutritional Physiological Phenomena. 3. Exercise. QT 263]
RM301
615.1–dc23   2014040633

ISBN: 978-1-138-77763-7 (hbk)
ISBN: 978-1-138-77764-4 (pbk)
ISBN: 978-1-315-77250-9 (ebk)

Typeset in Bembo
by HWA Text and Data Management, London

CONTENTS

FIGURES

CONTRIBUTORS

Stephen J. Bailey PhD, Sport and Health Sciences, University of Exeter, Exeter, UK.

Arash Bandegan PhD, Exercise Nutrition Research Laboratory, Western University, London, ON, Canada.

Richard Baskerville MB BS FRCS, Green Templeton College, University of Oxford, Oxford, UK.

David Bentley PhD, The University of Adelaide, Adelaide, Australia.

Michael F. Bergeron PhD, Sanford Sports Science Institute, University of South Dakota, Sioux Falls, SD, USA.

Stéphane Bermon MD, Monaco Institute of Sports Medicine and Surgery, Monaco.

Eva Blomstrand PhD, Astrand Laboratory, Swedish School of Sport and Health Sciences, Stockholm, Sweden.

Sarah L. Booth PhD, Jean Mayer USDA Human Nutrition Research Center on Aging at Tufts University, Boston, MA, USA.

James R. Borchers MD MPH, Division of Sports Medicine, Ohio State University, Columbus, OH, USA.

Hans Braun MSc, Center for Preventive Doping Research, German Sport University of Cologne, Cologne, Germany.

Gregory A. Brown PhD FACSM, Department of Kinesiology and Sports Science, University of Nebraska, Kearney, NE, USA.

Richard Budgett OBE FFSEM FRCP, Medical and Scientific Department, International Olympic Committee, Lausanne, Switzerland.

Nicholas A. Burd PhD, Department of Kinesiology and Community Health, University of Illinois at Urbana-Champaign, Urbana, IL, USA.

Louise M. Burke OAM PhD RD, Australian Institute of Sport, Canberra and Australian Catholic University, Melbourne, Australia.

José A.L. Calbet PhD, Department of Physical Education and Research Institute of Biomedical and Health Sciences, University of Las Palmas de Gran Canaria, Canary Island, Spain.

Philip C. Calder DPhil PhD, Faculty of Medicine, University of Southampton, Southampton, UK.

Linda M. Castell MSc MA Status, Green Templeton College, University of Oxford, Oxford, UK.

Sarah Chantler MSc RD, Shelly Meltzer & Associates, Sports Science Institute of South Africa, Cape Town, S. Africa.

Kieran Clarke PhD, Department of Physiology, Anatomy and Genetics, University of Oxford, Oxford, UK.

James Collins MSc, Arsenal Football Club, London, UK.

Pete J. Cox DPhil MD, Department of Physiology, Anatomy and Genetics, University of Oxford, Oxford, UK.

Siobhan Crawshay MSc RD, Australian Institute of Sport, Canberra, Australia.

Rui Curi PhD, Institute of Biomedical Sciences, University of Sao Paolo, Sao Paolo, Brazil.

Kevin Currell PhD, English Institute of Sport, Loughborough University, Loughborough, UK.

Wim Derave PhD, Department of Movement and Sports Sciences, Ghent University, Ghent, Belgium.

Patricia A. Deuster PhD, Department of Military and Emergency Medicine, USUHS, Bethesda, MD, USA.

Nancy M. DiMarco PhD RDN LDN CSSD, Institute for Women's Health, Texas Woman's University, Denton, TX, USA.

Christine E. Dziedzic MSc RD APD, Canadian Sport Institute Ontario, Toronto, Canada.

Björn Ekblom PhD, Astrand Laboratory, Swedish School of Sport and Health Sciences, Stockholm, Sweden.

Mark Ellison MSc, English Institute of Sport, Sheffield, UK.

Edzard Ernst MD PhD, University of Exeter, Exeter, UK.

Inge Everaert PhD, Department of Movement and Sports Sciences, Ghent University, Ghent, Belgium.

Hans Geyer PhD, Center for Preventive Doping Research, German Sport University of Cologne, Cologne, Germany.

Martin J. Gibala PhD, Department of Kinesiology, McMaster University, Hamilton, ON, Canada.

Michael Gleeson PhD, School of Sport, Exercise and Health Sciences, Loughborough University, Loughborough, UK.

Richard J. Godfrey PhD, Department of Life Sciences, Brunel University, Uxbridge, London, UK.

Carmel Goodman MD PhD, Western Australian Institute of Sport, Mount Claremont, Australia.

Paul L. Greenhaff PhD, School of Life Sciences, The Medical School, University of Nottingham, Nottingham, UK.

Stephen Gurr BHlthSci APD, Orthopaedic and Sports Medicine Hospital, ASPETAR, Doha, Qatar.

Satoshi Haramizu PhD, Kao Corporation Biological Science Laboratories, Tochigi, Japan.

Roger C. Harris PhD, Junipa Limited, Newmarket, UK.

Ylva Hellsten MSc RD, Department of Exercise and Sports Sciences, University of Copenhagen, Copenhagen, Denmark.

Adrian B. Hodgson PhD, LR Suntory, London, UK.

Linda K. Houtkooper PhD RDN, Department of Nutritional Sciences, College of Agriculture and Life Sciences, University of Arizona, Tucson, AZ, USA.

Juha J. Hulmi PhD, Department of Biology of Physical Activity, University of Jyvaskyla, Jyvaskyla, Finland.

Kate Jackson MD, Arthritis Research UK Centre for Sport, Botnar Research Centre, University of Oxford, Oxford, UK.

Nikki A. Jeacocke BND APD, Australian Institute of Sport, Canberra, Australia.

Asker Jeukendrup PhD, Gatorade Sports Science Institute, Barrington, IL, USA and Loughborough University, Loughborough, UK.

Andrew M. Jones PhD, Sport and Health Sciences, University of Exeter, Exeter, UK.

Christopher C. Kaeding MD, Department of Orthopaedics, Dept. of Athletics, Ohio State University, Columbus, OH, USA.

Andreas N. Kavazis PhD, Muscle Biochemistry Laboratory, School of Kinesiology, Auburn University, Auburn, AL, USA.

Mhairi Keil MSc, English Institute of Sport, Lilleshall National Sport Centre, Newport, Shropshire, UK.

Douglas S. King PhD, Department of Kinesiology, Iowa State University, Ames, IA, USA.

Mauricio Krause PhD, Department of Physiology, Federal University of Rio Grande do Sul, RS, Brazil.

D. Enette Larson-Meyer PhD RD, Department of Family and Consumer Services, Laramie, University of Wyoming, WY, USA.

Markus Laupheimer MD MBA MSc, Centre for Excellence in Musculoskeletal and Sports Medicine, BUPA Basinghall, BMI The London Independent Hospital, London, UK.

Peter W.R. Lemon PhD, Exercise Nutrition Research Laboratory, Western University, London, ON, Canada.

Nathan A. Lewis MSc RD, English Institute of Sport, Sports Training Village, University of Bath, Bath, UK.

Martin R. Lindley PhD, School of Sport, Exercise and Health Sciences, Loughborough University, Loughborough, UK.

Ano Lobb MPH, Master of Health Care Delivery Science Program, Dartmouth College, Hanover, NH, USA.

Joseph Lockey BM BCh, Green Templeton College, University of Oxford, Oxford, UK.

Bronwen Lundy MSc APD, Australian Institute of Sport, Belconnen, ACT, Australia.

Melinda M. Manore PhD RD CSSD, Nutrition Department, Oregon State University, Corvallis, OR, USA.

Ronald J. Maughan PhD, School of Sport, Exercise and Health Sciences, Loughborough University, Loughborough, UK.

Michael J. McNamee BA MA MA PhD FECSS, College of Engineering, Swansea University, Swansea, UK.

Lars R. McNaughton PhD, Department of Sport and Physical Activity, Edge Hill University, Ormskirk, UK.

Romain Meeusen PhD, Department of Human Physiology, Vrije Universiteit Brussel, Brussels, Belgium.

Shelly Meltzer MSc RD, Sports Science Institute of South Africa, Cape Town, S. Africa.

Geoffrey W. Melville PhD, School of Science and Health, University of Western Sydney, Penwrith, NSW, Australia.

Antti A. Mero PhD, Department of Biology of Physical Activity, University of Jyvaskyla, Jyvaskyla, Finland.

Adrian W. Midgley PhD, Department of Sport and Physical Activity, Edge Hill University Ormskirk, UK.

James C. Miller PhD, Air Force Research Laboratory (Retired), Brooks City Base, San Antonio, TX, USA.

Nigel Mitchell MSc RD, National Cycling Centre, Manchester, UK.

Daniel R. Moore PhD, Faculty of Kinesiology and Physical Education, University of Toronto, Toronto, ON, Canada.

Frank C. Mooren MD, Department of Sports Medicine, Justus-Liebig-University, Giessen, Germany.

Michael J. Naylor MSc, England Institute of Sport, St Mary's University College, Twickenham, UK.

Philip Newsholme DPhil, School of Biomedical Sciences, Faculty of Health Sciences, Curtin University, Perth, Australia.

David C. Nieman PhD, School of Biomedical Sciences, Human Performance Laboratory, Appalachian State University, NC, USA.

Tuomo Ojala MSc, Department of Biology of Physical Activity, University of Jyvaskyla, Jyvaskyla, Finland.

Jeni Pearce MSc RD, High Performance Sport New Zealand, Auckland, New Zealand.

Peter Peeling PhD, School of Sports Science, Exercise and Health, The University of Western Australia, Crawley, Australia.

Jacques R. Poortmans PhD, Faculté des Sciences de la Motricité, Université Libre du Bruxelles, Brussels, Belgium.

Alex D. Popple MSc, High Performance Sport New Zealand, Cambridge, New Zealand.

John C. Quindry PhD, School of Kinesiology, Auburn University, AL, USA.

Ros Quinlivan MB BS MD, MRC Centre for Neuromuscular Disease, National Hospital for Neurology and Neurosurgery, London, UK.

Mayur K. Ranchordas D Prof, Academy of Sport and Physical Activity, Sheffield Hallam University, Sheffield, UK.

Eric S. Rawson PhD, Department of Exercise Science, Bloomsburg University, Bloomsburg, PA, USA.

Michael B. Reid PhD, College of Health and Human Performance, University of Florida, Gainesville, FL, USA.

Bart Roelands PhD, Department of Human Physiology, Vrije Universiteit Brussel, Brussels, Belgium.

Peter J. Rogers PhD, School of Experimental Psychology, University of Bristol, Bristol, UK.

Craig Sale PhD, Sport, Health & Performance Enhancement Research Group, Nottingham Trent University, Nottingham, UK.

David S. Senchina PhD, Biology Department, Drake University, Des Moines, IA, USA.

Greg Shaw MSc APD, Australian Institute of Sport, Canberra, Australia.

Cecilia Shing PhD, School of Health Sciences, University of Tasmania, Launceston, Australia.

Susan M. Shirreffs PhD, GlaxoSmithKline, Brentford, UK.

Jason C. Siegler PhD, School of Science and Health, University of Western Sydney, Penwrith, NSW, Australia.

Gary Slater PhD APD, School of Health & Sports Sciences, University of the Sunshine Coast, Queensland, Australia.

Karlien Smit RD, Shelly Meltzer & Associates, Sports Science Institute of South Africa, Cape Town, S. Africa.

Lawrence L. Spriet PhD, Department of Human Health and Nutritional Sciences, University of Guelph, Guelph, ON, Canada.

Samantha J. Stear (Nottingham) PhD MBA, Performance Influencers, Northstar-at-Tahoe, CA, USA.

Francis B. Stephens PhD, School of Life Sciences, The Medical School, University of Nottingham, Nottingham, UK.

François Trudeau PhD, Département des Sciences de l'Activité Physique, Université du Québec à Trois-Rivières, Quebec, Canada.

Luc van Loon PhD, Maastricht University, Maastricht, the Netherlands.

Stephan van Vliet PhD, Division of Nutritional Sciences, University of Illinois at Urbana-Champaign, Urbana, IL, USA.

Alan Vernec MD, World Anti-Doping Agency, Montreal, Quebec, Canada.

Matthew Vukovich PhD, Dept of Health & Nutritional Sciences, South Dakota State University, Brookings, SD, USA.

Malcolm Watford DPhil, School of Environmental and Biological Sciences, Rutgers University, New Brunswick, NJ, USA.

Nicholas P. West PhD, Griffith Health Institute, Griffith University, Australia.

Robert R. Wolfe PhD, Center for Translational Research in Aging and Longevity, A&M University, Texas, TX, USA.

Takanobu Yamamoto PhD, Department of Psychology, Tezukayama University, Nara, Japan.

Adam Zemski BNutrDiet BCom APD, Australian Institute of Sport, Canberra, Australia.

PREFACE

Many supplement and sports foods compete for the minds and wallets of athletes, creating the need for clear and accessible resources that can assist these athletes to make informed decisions about their use (or not) of these products. There are many reviews on supplementation and exercise/sports performance, some of which are very good. Our aim is not to replicate these but to provide a series of concise yet comprehensive overviews, including opinion from experts in the field. The original individual nutritional supplement reviews, written by kowledgeable contributors from across the globe, are published as a series in the *BJSM* (2009–2013). That series covered in excess of 100 supplements, with particular emphasis on those commonly used by athletes, recreational and elite. For this book, the original reviews have been updated and expanded, where appropriate, according to the latest available information and scientific evidence. In addition, due to the evolving nature of the supplement world, some additional topics have been reviewed for inclusion in this book. Furthermore, in the concluding chapter, alongside authoritative input from the individual authors, we have attempted to standardise the level of efficacy for all the ingredients, supplements and products reviewed within the book in terms of sports and/or health performance with respect to the level of peer-reviewed scientific evidence currently available. In turn, from this efficacy index, we have taken this a stage further in order to categorise and summarise the huge amount of information contained within this book.

Throughout this book, our main aim has been to demystify some of the many ingredients/supplements on the market in order to provide a useful, reliable, balanced, unbiased resource, in particular for healthcare professionals specialising in, or studying, sport and exercise. The book will also be useful for other healthcare professionals and scientists, such as physicians, physiotherapists, psychologists, physiologists, dietitians/nutritionists and students with an interest in/studying sport and exercise medicine/nutrition. It is also hoped that the reviews will provide a useful and practical resource for coaches, athletes (from recreational to elite) and enthusiasts of sport and exercise who are interested in supplements for sports performance and/or health.

The reviews are set out in alphabetical order and cover complete products or the individual substances that make up the many poly-ingredient supplements on the market. Each review has been written by contributors from academia/research and/or a practical standpoint. The reviews are succinct yet comprehensive and include: definitions alongside related products; applicable food sources; and, where appropriate, practical recommendations such as dosage and timing, and possible nutrient interactions requiring the avoidance of other nutrients alongside any known potential side effects. Some key research citations for each topic (or comment on the lack of them) are provided in the reference list and further reading list, found at the end of the book, for those who wish to investigate further.

The vital issues of efficacy, safety and legality/ethics associated with the ingredients/supplements are addressed in the introductory chapter. Safety concerns include both the possibility of taking a toxic dose of a compound either through indiscriminate supplement use or the belief that 'if a little is good, more is better' alongside any medical concerns that may conflict with sports nutrition goals or advice. An additional consideration in the safety of supplements, particularly due to the lack of regulation, is the issue of purity of products and the risk of consuming contaminants that are either directly harmful or banned by the Anti-Doping Codes under which competitive sport is organised. The ethical/legality issues of sport can be contravened either by deliberate use of over-the-counter compounds that are prohibited by such codes (e.g. prohormones and stimulants) or by inadvertent ingestion of these products due to contamination, faking or doping issues. The serious issue of inadvertent doping is stressed throughout the reviews with additional expert commentary being provided in the introduction chapter on the WADA code and inadvertent doping to enhance knowledge in this critical area. The 'In Practice' chapter delves deeper into the practical aspects surrounding nutritional supplements and includes an important commentary on the ethics of supplementation.

There are still vulnerable athletes around the world failing doping tests, possibly due to inadvertent doping, but nevertheless having their sporting career terminated prematurely, alongside so much misinformation in books, magazines and on the internet regarding nutritional supplements. Therefore, a book consisting of comprehensive evidence-based reviews is timely. The reviews combine both the peer-reviewed scientific research which is all-too-often lacking in popular books on the market along with different and more practical information that is absent in average scientific reviews.

We are extremely grateful to our authors, not only for their wonderful contributions to this book, but also for their support and commitment throughout. We are grateful to the *British Journal of Sports Medicine* for giving us permission to reproduce the A–Z Series of Nutritional Supplements published in the journal from 2009–2013. All of us hope that this book *Nutritional Supplements in Sport, Exercise and Health: An A–Z Guide* will provide a useful resource to everyone working, studying or involved in sport, exercise and health across the globe.

Linda M. Castell, Samantha J. Stear and Louise M. Burke

FOREWORD

After the success of the *BJSM* A–Z Series on Nutritional Supplements this comprehensive review provides reliable, balanced and unbiased information for athletes and their support staff. The subject of supplements is of crucial importance, and position statements on supplements have been published over the last 20 years by the IOC, National Olympic Committees (NOCs), National Anti-Doping Organisations (NADOs) and others, but there has been an unmet need for a comprehensive and authoritative review such as this.

The review includes all the material from the A–Z Series on Nutritional Supplements, together with some new topics, a detailed introduction with usage charts and an important contribution by WADA; in addition there is an 'In Practice' chapter that contains key practical aspects in terms of supplement consideration and usage. In the concluding chapter, the Editors, with authoritative input from the individual authors, have taken on the impressive task of attempting to standardise the level of efficacy for the 140+ supplements/ products reviewed within this book. Consequently, the Editors provide very useful efficacy index categories to summarise the findings from the book's supplement reviews, in terms of sports and/or health performance with respect to the level of peer-reviewed scientific evidence currently available.

The use and potential for abuse of supplements in sport have been of concern to all those involved in supporting athletes for many years. Of primary concern is the health of the athlete. Performance issues are secondary and performance will only be helped if optimum health is maintained. The ergogenic effects of many supplements are controversial, and good evidence for efficacy is rare.

Athletes are uniquely vulnerable to claims regarding dietary supplements, sports nutrition foods and ergogenic aids. They are concerned that their competitors will steal an advantage. This A–Z guide on nutritional supplements is a very valuable reference for doctors and all support staff, enabling them to counsel athletes from a position of knowledge and decide whether a particular athlete really needs a supplement. Is it effective? Is it safe? What are the risks of contamination? All those involved with athletes need to know the answers to these questions and when to seek expert advice from a qualified sports nutrition professional. By giving an overview of the evidence, presenting the views of experts in the field and providing practical advice, these reviews will enable support staff to protect the health of athletes and help them to optimise safely both health and performance. The Series Editors and the *BJSM* are to be congratulated for having taken on the original task of publishing the A–Z series. The follow-up to this book *Nutritional Supplements in Sport, Exercise and Health: An A–Z Guide* that the Series Editors subsequently embarked upon will be a tremendous resource for all those involved in sport, exercise and health.

Dr Richard Budgett OBE
*Medical and Scientific Department,
International Olympic Committee, Lausanne, Switzerland*

INTRODUCTION

Samantha J. Stear, Hans Braun and Kevin Currell

The use of nutritional supplements for sport, exercise and health goals is widespread. 'Dietary/Nutritional supplements, functional foods, nutraceuticals, sports/performance-boosting supplements, ergogenic aids … ' are just some of the terms used interchangeably within both scientific publications and the sporting arena, to describe and sometimes entice the unwary to spend money on products that claim to enhance their health and/or sports performance.

The term 'dietary supplement' (DS) implies that it is something which supplements the diet, whether it is, strictly speaking, nutritional or not. The Oxford English Dictionary definition of a supplement is 'Something added to supply a deficiency'. However, this definition is inconsistent with the majority of DS usage, with many supplements, or their individual ingredients, being nutrients or food chemicals for which the body does not have an estimated or theoretical requirement. Thus, there are clearly other factors that underpin their use by athletes.

According to the U.S. Food and Drug Administration (FDA),

> A dietary supplement is a product (other than tobacco) that is intended to supplement the diet and bears or contains one or more of the following dietary ingredients: a vitamin, a mineral, a herb or other botanical, an amino acid, a dietary substance for use by humans to supplement the diet by increasing its total daily intake, or a concentrate, metabolite, constituent, extract, or combination of these ingredients.

This differs slightly from the definition of the European Food Safety Authority (EFSA) which uses the term food supplement.

> A Food Supplement is a concentrated source of nutrients or other substances with a nutritional or physiological effect whose purpose is to supplement the normal diet. They are marketed in 'dose' form i.e. as pills, tablets, capsules, liquids in measured doses etc.

Furthermore, EFSA states that

> Supplements may be used to correct nutritional deficiencies or maintain an adequate intake of certain nutrients. However, in some cases excessive intake of vitamins and minerals may be harmful or cause unwanted side effects; therefore, information on maximum levels are necessary to ensure their safe use in food supplements.

The European Commission has established coherent rules to help ensure that food supplements are safe and properly labelled. In the EU, food supplements are regulated as foods and the legislation (Directive 2002/46/EC: www.efsa. europe.eu) focuses on vitamins and minerals used as ingredients of food supplements. Nutrients other than vitamins and minerals, or other substances with a nutritional or physiological effect, are being considered for regulation at a later stage when adequate and appropriate scientific data about them becomes available. Until then, national rules concerning nutrients or other substances with nutritional or physiological effects may be applicable.

The regulatory environment is under constant progressive change, with legislation differing across countries. Although the dietary supplement (DS) category is subject to strict regulations, it has historically suffered from poor policing of claims. In general, the food industry firmly adheres to country-specific legislation, but this is not always seen to be the case for some DS manufacturers who appear to 'sit outside' the food industry. Increasingly strict monitoring by regulatory bodies in USA, Europe, Asia and Oceania, will hopefully improve the situation.

The consequence of the current situation is that international sporting authorities including the IOC and the World Anti-Doping Agency (WADA), advise athletes not to take supplements due to the associated risks. They also provide resources to help the sporting community make informed choices by better understanding the risks involved. Other leading sports authorities and organizations (e.g. FIFA, ACSM) also recommend that 'athletes should ensure they have a good diet before contemplating supplement use'.

In the USA, the medical division of the US Olympic Committee (USOC) provides supplementation guidelines for athletes, coaches and healthcare professionals based on the goal of providing safe intakes of individual nutrients to promote healthful training regimens and recovery periods. In conclusion the USOC states that

The use of supplements is appropriate only in conjunction with a good diet. Dietary evaluation should be made by a qualified health professional and food intake patterns should be adjusted if necessary to promote optimal health. If a thorough dietary evaluation is not possible and cursory review of the athlete's dietary habits indicates possible reason for concern, prophylactic supplementation may be desirable.

UK Sport's resource 'Sports Supplements and the Associated Risks' takes this a stage further in its conclusion stating that 'whilst a healthy, balanced diet remains the best way to achieve sufficient levels of vitamins, minerals and other nutrients, some supplements do have a place in high performance sport for some athletes'. The Australian Institute of Sport (AIS) ran a publicly transparent Sports Supplement Programme for the athletes within its care from 2000–2013, involving an integrated series of activities around education (www.ausport.gov. au/ais/supplements), provision of products to athletes and applied research (see 'In Practice' chapter).

However, across the world, many athletes, even at the elite level, have a low level of nutritional knowledge, not unlike the general population. Furthermore, very few athletes have access to a qualified dietetic/nutritional professional for dietary evaluation and nutritional counselling. A varied, well-balanced diet that meets the energy demands of training should provide adequate amounts of all the essential nutrients. However, sometimes this is not possible, and in some situations, obtaining sufficient amounts from the diet is often not straightforward. Consequently, many athletes take dietary supplements in the hope that it will compensate for poor food choices as well as making up for vital nutrients that they feel are potentially lacking in their diet.

Prevalence of dietary supplements (DS)

Surveys show that nearly half of all athletes use supplements, with their popularity varying widely between different sports and between athletes of differing ages, performance levels and cultural backgrounds. In some sports, particularly strength and power sports, supplement usage is so common that it is perceived as the norm. However, it should be noted that it is difficult to compare across surveys, as most make up their own definition of the products to be included in their investigation. Most surveys do not include sports foods (e.g. drinks, bars, powders, etc.) and may therefore underestimate the true intake of products we have considered in our more inclusive review terms in this book, and at the same time this may also alter the identification of 'most popular' products.

According to a TGI (Target Group Index, 2012 Product Book) survey, vitamins and other supplement use of the adult population differs between countries (www.tgisurveys.com). Supplement use seems to be lowest in Thailand (3%), Argentina (8%) and Spain (9%), moderate in France (28%), Germany (32%),

Great Britain (34%) and Russia (38%), and highest in USA (56%), Serbia (56%) and Denmark (72%). A meta-analysis of 51 studies on supplements, involving more than 10,000 athletes at all levels and participating in 15 sports, albeit with differing definitions of which products were included in the investigations, found that the mean prevalence of supplement use among all subjects was 46%, with a large variance between individual sports that ranged from 6% to 100% (Sobal and Marquardt, 1994).

Studies on UK athletes found similar supplement use. One study found that 59% of UK athletes used at least one supplement (Petroczi and Naughton, 2008), with another showing 62% DS usage in British junior national track and field athletes (Nieper, 2005). A study of DS usage in 286 GB Olympic athletes, competing at the 2004 Athens Olympics, found 53% declared taking supplements on their medical preparation forms, with DS usage being more common in female (59.3%) than male (48.5%) athletes (Stear et al., 2006).

A higher dietary supplement (DS) usage can be expected with increasing age and the performance level of the athlete, with DS usage by elite athletes exceeding that of college athletes, which, in turn, exceeds that of high school athletes. There is good evidence that DS use increases with age both in elite athletes (Maughan et al., 2007) and in the general population. A difference in DS usage between genders has only been found in a few studies.

Furthermore, not only is supplement usage common, but all too often the recommended doses are exceeded. Sometimes this is simply an attempt to outdo what the athlete believes their opponent is taking. However, there is a common misunderstanding that, for example, taking twice the dose will work twice as well. But more does not necessarily mean better; indeed, in the case of some supplements, such as the fat-soluble vitamins (A, D, E and K) and iron, more can be toxic. Therefore, caution is not only advised in terms of taking supplements per se, but also that excessive intakes of some DS may do more harm than good.

Common dietary supplements (DS)

Dietary supplements (DS) come in many forms and guises. The list of supplements and ergogenic aids used within the exercise and sporting environment is exhaustive. Figure 1 uses a 'tag cloud' to illustrate some of the most popular DS used in the sport and exercise arena in terms of general efficacy. Here the largest font size (e.g. carbohydrate, electrolytes and protein) represent the most efficacious down to the smallest font size (e.g. bee pollen, glandulars and yucca) representing the least efficacious, according to current information.

Among 32 studies reviewed in 1994, albeit gain with differing definitions of products investigated, multivitamins were the most popular dietary supplements (DS), followed by vitamin C, iron and B vitamins (Sobal and Marquardt, 1994). This seems to continue to be the trend. The 2004 study of DS usage in 286 GB Olympic athletes, found that vitamin C (65% of supplement users) was

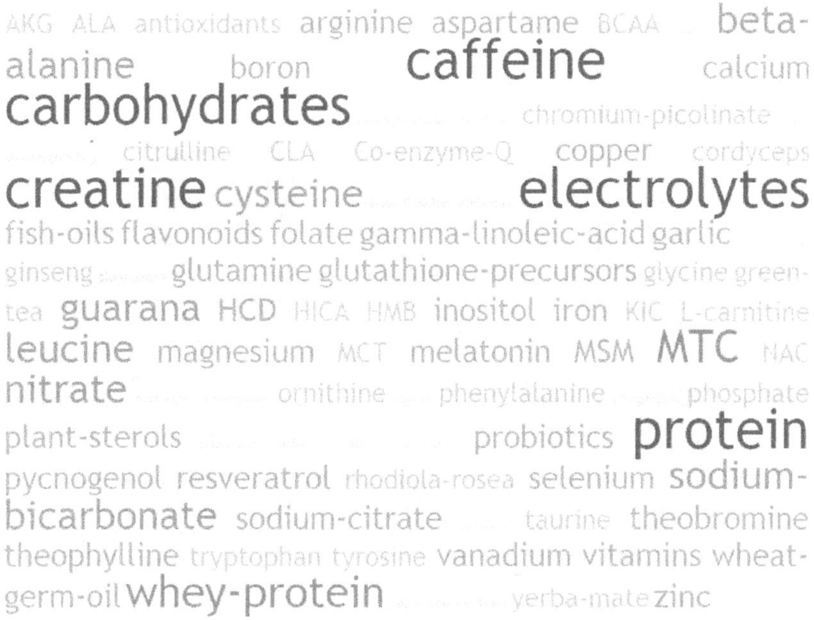

AKG ALA antioxidants arginine aspartame BCAA beta-alanine boron caffeine calcium carbohydrates chromium-picolinate citrulline CLA Co-enzyme-Q copper cordyceps creatine cysteine electrolytes fish-oils flavonoids folate gamma-linoleic-acid garlic ginseng glutamine glutathione-precursors glycine green-tea guarana HCD HICA HMB inositol iron KIC L-carnitine leucine magnesium MCT melatonin MSM MTC NAC nitrate ornithine phenylalanine phosphate plant-sterols probiotics protein pycnogenol resveratrol rhodiola-rosea selenium sodium-bicarbonate sodium-citrate taurine theobromine theophylline tryptophan tyrosine vanadium vitamins wheat-germ-oil whey-protein yerba-mate zinc

FIGURE 1 Tag cloud of popular sports nutrition supplements (reproduced with permission: copyright © 2014 Samantha Stear)

the most common DS declared by athletes, followed by multivitamins and minerals, iron, protein supplements, vitamin E, Selenium and Zinc (Stear *et al.*, 2006). A further, larger study that analysed questionnaires from 874 UK athletes, where ~60% (520 athletes) declared DS use (Petroczi and Naughton, 2008), found that the most common DS were multivitamins (73%) and vitamin C (71%), followed by creatine (36%), whey protein (32%), echinacea (31%), iron (30%), caffeine (24%), magnesium (11%) and ginseng (less than 11%). A study of 113 German Olympic athletes in 2009 found magnesium to be the most popular (81%), followed by vitamin C (59%), multivitamins (52%), iron (50%), zinc (42%), while ergogenic aids such as creatine (20%) and caffeine (6%) were rarely used (Braun *et al.*, 2009b). Further, examination of the popularity of magnesium found it to vary widely between countries, with it being one of the most common DS in Germany, Portugal and Poland (~80% usage), but less popular in the UK and Norway (~10% usage).

Therefore DS usage patterns not only vary across countries, age (and, to a lesser extent, gender), athletic level and sport, but also types of DS. For example, fish oils constitute over 40% of the market of other supplements in the UK, but under 3% in Spain and in Italy. Probiotics account for 44% of the market in Italy and only 1% in the UK. Herbal products (e.g. ginkgo, ginseng, St John's Wort, echinacea and garlic) make up 75% of the market in the Netherlands, 40% in

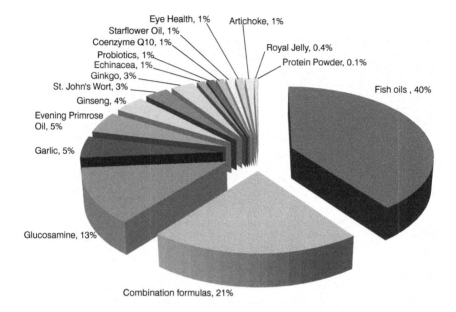

FIGURE 2 An example of popular dietary supplements bought in the UK

Data source: http://ec.europa.eu/food/food/labellingnutrition/supplements/documents/2008.

France and 16% in the UK. Figure 2 provides an example and range of popular DS bought in the UK.

The popularity of certain types of DS demonstrates that athletes may often be more motivated by health rather than the ergogenic benefits of some DS. However, some 'sports foods', such as carbohydrate-electrolyte sports drinks, have become so commonplace in the sporting and exercise environment that athletes no longer perceive these as DS and hence the recording of their usage amongst studies may be inconsistent, resulting in further inaccuracies in studies.

Rationale for dietary supplements (DS)

Athletes should always consider the issues of efficacy, safety and legality/ethics associated with dietary supplement (DS) products prior to considering their use. Unfortunately, all too frequently, specific information is limited. Studies examining the performance-enhancing effects of the vast array of supplements are relatively few, especially investigations which are relevant to real-life sports events and elite athletes. Furthermore, studies involving specialised sub-populations, such as Paralympic athletes, are particularly rare. Subsequently decisions regarding efficacy must often be extrapolated from the best available research rather than from clear-cut evidence.

Common reasons to justify the use of DS by athletes include:

- to prevent or treat a perceived nutrient deficiency, particularly when requirements for a nutrient are increased (believed or real) by their exercise programme;
- to provide a more convenient form of nutrients in situations where everyday foods are not practical – particularly to address nutritional needs/ goals around an exercise session;
- to provide a direct ergogenic (performance-enhancing) effect;
- because they believe every top athlete is consuming it and they can't afford to miss out.

Interestingly, studies have also found that large numbers of athletes who report using supplements do so just because others (e.g. colleagues, coaches) recommended them. Among the many support staff working with athletes, coaches seem to be an important source of information on DS. While adult athletes also report health professionals (physicians, physiotherapists, dietitians/ nutritionists) as influential, young athletes state their parents as being an important source of information on DS.

Other influential factors include marketing and advertising of supplements, which are dependent on the sport and/or media where they are published (such as muscle-increasing supplements in bodybuilding magazines). Based on all these findings, it seems necessary to educate not only athletes but also coaches, parents and health professionals about the use of supplements together with the associated risks and benefits.

Even if the key rationale behind DS use cannot be identified among studies, it seems that health and performance-related reasons are the most popular. However, this might be different according to type of product (vitamins vs. carbohydrates), time of use (daily use vs. competition), age or gender. Importantly, the decision to use supplements is not always a rational one. Even when athletes are informed that the appropriate diet is sufficient, or that the nutrient status of their body's stores is normal (for example, iron stores), they often still continue to take DS perhaps as a form of 'just in case' insurance.

Consequently, in the concluding chapter of this book, we have taken the current information presented in the supplement reviews throughout the book, and attempted to standardise the level of efficacy in terms of sports and/or health performance.

Problems with dietary supplements (DS)

Despite the fact that information regarding the efficacy of dietary supplements (DS) is sometimes lacking, athletes often use DS with an expectation of performance and/or health benefits. DS cannot simply be classified into two groups of useful and not useful or risky vs. beneficial. In fact, it is a question of individual circumstances and response to a supplement. However, before athletes consider using a DS, they should ensure their diet is optimised as well as sport specific if appropriate. Furthermore, it is also crucially important to understand the potential risks involved with DS usage. Although it is not possible to offer a general risk assessment on DS use, the following sections, including some invited expert commentary, aim to help identify and assess the potential risks that, in turn, can be balanced with any potential benefits.

Safety issues

DS use is pervasive in athletes and the general population, with vitamins and minerals being particularly popular. Recently, there has also been an increase in the fortification of foods, with drinks, yoghurts, cereals and many 'sports foods' now being fortified with micronutrients. So it's important to consider whether this fortification could in turn be detrimental. Indeed, prolonged use of any single vitamin or mineral supplement, in the absence of a clinically diagnosed deficiency, may not only do more harm than good, but may also interfere with the balance and interaction of other micronutrients. See the 'In Practice' chapter for an authoritative commentary on 'stacking' which addresses the issues of taking multiple supplements alongside fortified food and drinks.

Decisions regarding safety need to include the possibility of taking a 'toxic' dose of a compound either through indiscriminate supplement use or the belief that 'if a little is good, more is better'. Furthermore, safety issues should also take into account any medical concerns that may conflict with sports nutrition goals or advice. For example: recommended protein requirements are reduced in diabetes; hypertension may have implications for sodium intake; and some medical conditions may contra-indicate the use of caffeine. Supplement dosages for special groups such as wheelchair athletes may also need to be altered because of decreased active muscle mass.

Institutions such as the USA's Institute of Medicine's Food and Nutrition Board (FNB), the European Food Standard Agency (EFSA) and the UK Expert Group on Vitamins and Minerals (EVM) have recently summarized their opinions on the safety of vitamin and mineral intakes, particularly from supplementation or fortification. Consequently, tolerable 'upper intake levels' (UL) or 'safe upper levels' (SUL) for vitamins and minerals have been established. The UL is defined by EFSA as the 'maximum level of total chronic daily intake of a nutrient (from all sources) judged to be unlikely to pose a risk of adverse health effects to humans'. Furthermore, as intakes increase above the UL, the risks of adverse health effects also increase. However, it is important to note that the ULs provided are not based on precise measurements and are more an approximation dependent on the availability and quality of data. Critics of the UL cite several limitations including: lack of well-designed human studies; lack of exposure and intake data in epidemiological studies; over-interpretation and usefulness of epidemiological data with regard to safety; lack of data in children; insufficient data on the variability of the sensitivity of individuals to adverse effects; and its dependency on various factors such as age, gender, body weight, lean body mass and genetics. Furthermore, specific UL and SUL for athletes or active people are not available.

There are also health risks associated with poor manufacturing practice and possible contamination. A growing number of reports show products containing harmful impurities like glass, lead or animal faeces. Other reports show that products may not contain an adequate dose of the labelled ingredients. Furthermore, the FDA regularly reports on products found to contain effective amounts of prescriptive drugs, which could lead to detrimental side effects.

Contamination and inadvertent doping

A further consideration in the safety of supplements is the issue of purity of products and the risk of consuming contaminants that are either directly harmful or banned by the anti-doping codes under which elite sport is organised. An overview of The World Anti-Doping Agency (WADA) is provided by Alan Vernec.

THE WORLD ANTI-DOPING AGENCY

Alan Vernec

Athletes have a long history of using substances in an attempt to gain an advantage in sporting competitions. The ancient Greeks and Romans used herbs, fungi, poppy seeds and stimulants such as strychnine in order to boost performance (Papagelopoulos *et al.*, 2004). In the modern era, this practice continued mostly with the use of stimulants and narcotics. Sports federations took notice and in 1928 the International Association of Athletics Federations (IAAF) became the first federation to prohibit the use of performance-enhancing drugs (PEDs), although there would be no testing in sport for another 40 years (Vettenniemi, 2010).

Amphetamine use was involved in the deaths of cyclists Knud Jensen and Tommy Simpson in the 1960 Olympic Games and the 1967 Tour de France respectively: this spurred the development of the International Olympic Commission's (IOC) Medical Commission, which published the first IOC Prohibited List in 1967. This became the *de facto* Prohibited List for Olympic Sport Federations. The 'Festina affair' (1998 Tour de France), where a team trainer's car was found to contain a panoply of PEDs, was the catalyst to create a new organisation to harmonise, coordinate and promote the fight against doping in sport in all its forms (Catlin *et al.*, 2008). The IOC convened the first World Conference in Doping in Sport in 1999, which resulted in the formation of the World Anti-Doping Agency (WADA).

WADA is a unique, independent body representing equally sport and the governments of the world. The World Anti-Doping Code is the core document on which anti-doping programmes are modelled. The first version of the Code came into effect in January 2004. There are presently over 600 signatories, including almost all the world's sport federations. The Code applies to Athletes, as defined by their national anti-doping organisations (NADOs) or international federations. Who is considered an athlete for anti-doping purposes may vary widely and a NADO may still test recreational athletes but not apply all elements of the Code, for example, the requirement for whereabouts or advanced therapeutic use exemptions. Athletes may be subjected to sanctions based on possession or trafficking of prohibited substances and not simply due to a positive doping test. However, it is important to be aware that criminal legislation exists in certain countries (e.g. for narcotics) which may be in addition to, or completely separate from, anti-doping sanctions.

WADA also took over the role of publishing the Prohibited List (List), revised annually since 2004. The List has expanded considerably from the original IOC Prohibited List of the 1960s and contains numerous classes of substances as well as prohibited methods such as blood manipulation. A substance (or method) is considered for inclusion if it meets any two of the following criteria: (1) potential for performance enhancement; (2) detrimental to the athlete's health and (3) contrary to the spirit of sport. The deliberations on whether to include substances in the List are a highly interactive and consultative process which includes stakeholders and experts. It is impractical to list all known and possible compounds; thus, most of the prohibited classes contain an important clause stating: '… and other substances with similar chemical structure or similar biological effect(s)' (World Anti-Doping Agency, 2013a).

Some substances have permitted routes of administration, (e.g. glucocorticosteroids are allowed by inhalation or topically). A few substances are permitted but only to a certain threshold level (e.g. pseudoephedrine). The List is divided into substances prohibited in competition only (e.g. stimulants), and those prohibited at all times (e.g. anabolic steroids and erythropoietin). It is irrelevant whether the prohibited substance is synthetic or from botanical sources or whether it is considered a pharmaceutical product or a dietary supplement.

'Strict Liability' means that every athlete is responsible for the substances found in their bodily specimen during a doping control sample analysis. The first line of defence for many cheating athletes has been to claim that the positive test resulted from a tainted dietary supplement. Many of these same athletes later confessed to deliberate ingestion of a prohibited substance. The athlete's responsibility to explain how a prohibited substance entered his/her body (Strict Liability) has existed for many years, being initially implemented by the IOC. It has withstood the scrutiny of the Court of Arbitration in Sport and civil courts, and is a balance between protecting all athletes by ensuring fair, clean sport and the rights of individual athletes.

For an athlete confronted with an anti-doping rule violation, section 10.5 of the Code (World Anti-Doping Agency, 2013b) allows for no sanction, or reduced sanctions, if the athlete can demonstrate no fault or no significant fault. As far as supplements are concerned, simply stating the unknowing ingestion of a tainted dietary supplement is not sufficient – an athlete would have to demonstrate clearly that every reasonable precaution was taken to avoid ingestion of a prohibited substance.

An athlete taking a spiked supplement with intent to dope may claim that he/she did not realise the product contained a prohibited substance. It is difficult to know the intent: nevertheless, the athlete will benefit from the ergogenic effect of the prohibited substance and have an unfair advantage over their competitor. There are many cautionary tales of athletes taking energy boosting supplements before or during the games and subsequently being sanctioned. Many dietary supplements that promise to enhance performance either contain a prohibited substance or are an example of false advertising.

The reality is that a significant percentage (5–20%) of supplements contain prohibited substances, either by inadvertent contamination or deliberate adulteration, during the production process. This phenomenon has been demonstrated repeatedly (Schänzer, 2002; Geyer et al., 2004b, 2008; Maughan, 2005), and sporting federations as well as anti-doping organisations continue to impress this warning upon athletes. For example, several athletes have been recently sanctioned over the stimulant methylhexaneamine (MHA), explicitly prohibited since 2009. This was considered to be a dietary supplement from geranium oil, despite the fact that several studies, including a very recent one (Elsohly et al., 2012), demonstrated that its presence in supplements was not from geranium oil but due to the addition of synthetic MHA. Whether natural or synthetic, athletes need to avoid these types of products.

Many athletes continue to take supplements to try and improve recovery from training or to gain a performance edge in competition or are advised that supplements are necessary for health maintenance. Dietary supplement use by high-level athletes is estimated at 65–95% (Ronsen et al., 1999; Baylis et al., 2001; Kim et al., 2010). Supplement commercialization is a multibillion dollar industry where many claims are made with little scientific evidence; regulation for purity or side effects is still lacking in many countries. Members of the athletes' entourage often push substances without sufficiently understanding physiology or nutrition. There are a very limited number of dietary supplements which are permitted and considered ergogenic (Maughan et al., 2011; Suzic Lazic et al., 2011). Athletes need to focus on proper training, optimal recovery practices and wholesome nutrition regimens before they even consider supplements. Some education programmes appear to be resulting in decreased supplement use among Olympic athletes (Heikkinen *et al.*, 2011).

If an athlete truly believes he/she should take a dietary supplement, everything should be done to minimise the risk:

1. Do not rely on advice from friends, fellow athletes or coaches but undergo a proper evaluation by a qualified physician and/or sports nutrition professional familiar with sport and anti-doping rules. It is quite likely that dietary supplements are not necessary and nutrient deficiencies may be corrected from food sources.
2. Avoid any product for which claims are made of performance enhancement, or any exaggerated claims, or for which the words: 'stimulant, energy or muscle booster, enhancer, legal or alternate steroid, extreme, blast, weight loss' are used. Even if no prohibited substance is listed on the label, the product may be spiked with one.
3. Herbal stimulants and prohormones are especially high risk. Use of the terms herbal or natural does not in any way mean that the product does not contain a prohibited substance.
4. Some companies offer guarantees of purity or are certified by other companies that do quality control. Verify the third-party testing system reputation and remember there are no absolute guarantees.
5. Avoid any company that states their products are WADA approved. WADA or its accredited laboratories never test supplements or any products when not part of a doping control process. WADA cannot recommend any company or quality control system. In order to guarantee purity, each product batch would have to be tested for all prohibited substances.
6. Avoid products containing multiple ingredients as there is a higher risk of contamination. Vitamins and minerals (often classified as supplements) should be from reputable pharmaceutical companies and should not be mixed with other products.
7. Seek guidance from your anti-doping organisation about recent information on contaminated or dangerous products in your part of the world (e.g. USA Anti-Doping Agency High Risk List).

Although athletes must exhibit utmost caution when using supplements due to risk of contamination, governmental authorities also have a duty to endeavour to ensure proper regulation and quality control within the supplement industry. Some initiatives are trying to improve this situation. According to Article 10, UNESCO International Convention against Doping in Sport, governments must encourage producers and distributors of dietary or nutritional supplements to establish marketing best practices, including accurate labelling, quality assurance and avoidance of false marketing. In a survey (UNESCO Conference of Parties 2011), only 43% of governments responded that they implemented extensive or substantial measures to address these issues (UNESCO, 2011).

Furthermore, a more systematic approach is needed for analysing risks and benefits of dietary supplements (Cellini *et al.*, 2013). The real risks to health of ingesting potentially dangerous substances contained in poorly regulated supplements are occasionally lost in the discussion of inadvertent doping (Gee *et al.*, 2012; Katz, 2013).

Anti-doping regulations were developed over many years to promote fairness in sport and to protect the health of the athlete. Athletes are keen to improve their performance and nutrition may play an integral part in their overall plan. However, when athletes embark upon using performance-enhancing supplements, the risks often outweigh the benefits. Improved regulation of the dietary supplement industry would go a long way towards reducing the risks, but the onus remains on the athlete to make the right choices.

As published in *Br J Sports Med Series*, October 2013

As highlighted in the overview on WADA, elite athletes remain solely responsible for any prohibited substances found in their system (Strict Liability). Therefore, the ethical/legal issues of sport can be contravened either by deliberate use of over-the-counter compounds that are prohibited by such codes (e.g. prohormones and stimulants) or by inadvertent intake of these products when they are hidden in supplements. Consequently, one of the key factors that elite athletes need to consider in negotiating the complex world of supplements and sports foods is whether the consumption of these products could lead to an inadvertent case of doping. Dietary supplements (DS) frequently contain one or more different products, some of which are banned by WADA (www.wada-ama.org).

Following a wave of Nandrolone findings in doping offences in the late 90s, several studies have sought to explore the extent of supplement contamination. These studies have shown that many DS are mislabelled or do not reflect the true ingredients, demonstrating insufficient quality control in the production process. Therefore, concern was raised regarding the potential for contamination from doping substances that were not declared on the label but would lead to a positive doping test.

In 2000–2001, following several positive doping cases, many of which were connected with prohormones in DS, the International Olympic Committee (IOC) funded a comprehensive study at the Centre of Preventive Doping Research in Cologne, Germany, to independently analyse 634 non-hormonal nutritional supplements purchased across 13 different countries (Geyer *et al.*, 2004b; see Figure 3).

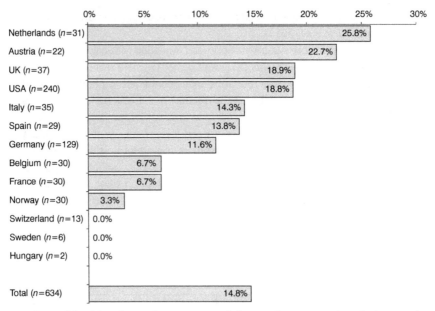

FIGURE 3 Nutritional supplements containing prohormones, in relation to the total number of supplements purchased in different countries

Data source: Geyer *et al.*, *Int J Sports Med* (2004) 25: 124–9.

This pivotal research confirmed the contamination issue, with 15% (94 products) of the non-hormonal nutritional supplements being found to contain undeclared anabolic androgenic steroids banned by WADA: 37 products analysed from the UK showed 7 products (18.9%) contaminated. Altogether, 289 samples (21% positives) were from companies that were known to sell steroids/prohormones, but perhaps more worrying 345 samples (9.6% positives) came from companies which did not sell steroids/prohormones. On the basis of the low and varying concentration (0.01–190μg/g) of the prohormones, the authors interpreted this as cross-contamination and not as intentional administration. Reasons for the cross-contamination were most likely that companies manufacturing prohormones also produced other supplements without sufficient cleaning of production lines, or the transport containers from raw material suppliers were unclean.

These findings resulted in warnings for athletes and federations upon supplement use and the risk of inadvertent doping cases. With the Anabolic Steroid Act 2004, the sale or possession of all prohormones is banned in the USA, and the problem of contamination with prohormones has slightly improved.

However, the problem has shifted, and results of the IOC Cologne study continue to be confirmed, illustrating that the issues of contamination are still around. In 2007, HFL Sport Science (a WADA experienced laboratory, part of the Quotient Bioscience group) in the UK analysed 58 supplements purchased through standard retail outlets in the USA and found that 25% were contaminated with prohibited steroids and 11% were contaminated with prohibited stimulants (personal communication Catherine Judkins, HFL Sport Science). In 2008, HFL Sport Science followed this up with the analysis of 152 products purchased from standard retail outlets in the UK and found that over 10% were contaminated with steroids and/or stimulants (personal communication Catherine Judkins, HFL Sport Science).

This emerging hazard of contaminated supplements resulting in inadvertent ingestion of substances that are banned by WADA is a continuous serious concern for elite athletes. This problem was first brought to scientific recognition in the research highlighted above by Hans Geyer and his colleagues (Geyer *et al.*, 2004b), and the following expert commentary, by Hans Geyer and Hans Braun, provides an update of the current situation of a recent review by this team (Geyer *et al.*, 2008, 2011).

INADVERTENT DOPING

Hans Geyer and Hans Braun

In the past years an increasing number of dietary supplements, containing undeclared doping substances, have been detected. The consumption of these supplements can lead to inadvertent doping cases. Although warnings about the risk of inadvertent doping have been communicated, recent studies show that athletes' knowledge of the problem is inadequate (Braun *et al.*, 2009a). Furthermore, it seems that the risk has been growing due to the increased availability of pharmaceutical substances via the internet, which are admixed by criminal manufacturers to their arguably non-effective supplement products.

Dietary supplements containing stimulants

The main candidates from the dietary supplement market for inadvertent doping with stimulants are products containing ephedrine and analogues, sibutramine and methylhexaneamine. Such products are mainly advertised as fat burner or mood enhancer and their use may lead to positive doping results in competition. The risk of inadvertent doping with such supplements is based on different reasons.

In the case of supplements containing ephedrines, the natural sources of ephedrine such as Ma Huang or ephedra sinica are frequently mentioned on the label rather than the names of the active ingredients ephedrine, pseudoephedrine, methylephedrine, etc. Despite extensive education of athletes regarding unclear labelling, or the variety of names by which banned substances may be referred to, many athletes still fall into this doping trap.

In case of supplements enriched with sibutramine, this ingredient is not declared on the label and the consumer is only provided with the information that the product contains 'pure herbal ingredients' that are advertised to have considerable weight-loss capabilities. Sibutramine can be found in therapeutic or even supra-therapeutic doses in slimming capsules, powders and even slimming teas (Jung *et al.*, 2006; Koehler *et al.*, 2007; Vidal and Quandte, 2006). Sibutramine is a synthetic anorectic drug, only approved as pharmaceutical preparation and only available on prescription. Because of its enormous side effects (stroke and heart attack risk for patients with a history of cardiovascular disease), the European Medicines Agency (EMEA) recommended in January 2010 that this drug be withdrawn from the market. Sibutramine has been on the list of prohibited substances from the World Anti-Doping Agency (WADA) since 2006.

Since 2008/2009, there has been a high risk for inadvertent doping with the stimulant methylhexaneamine, which was added to the WADA Prohibited List in 2009 (Thevis *et al.*, 2010). The issue of inadvertent doping arises from the fact that numerous different names for methylhexaneamine can be found on the labels, such as dimethylamylamine, dimethylpentylamine, pentylamine, geranamine, forthane, 2-amino-4-methylhexane, etc. On WADA's 2011 Prohibited List, only the names methylhexaneamine and dimethylpentylamine are mentioned in the group of stimulants, which complicates the identification of the substance as a prohibited compound. In some supplements, geranium root extract or geranium oil is mentioned as an alleged natural source of methylhexaneamine. However, recent investigations have shown that geranium oil does not contain methylhexaneamine (Lisi *et al.*, 2011) or only extremely small amounts (Fleming *et al.*, 2012), which means that synthesized methylhexaneamine must have been added. Despite warnings by different national anti-doping agencies in 2009 and 2010, numerous elite athletes in competition have been found to have a positive test for methylhexaneamine. In the years 2010–2012 methylhexaneamine was the most frequently detected stimulant in elite sports (WADA, 2014a).

Another stimulant which can be found in adulterated nutritional supplements is oxilofrine (also known as methylsynephrine, hydroxyephrine and oxyephrine). In 2013 and 2014 several products were detected containing oxilofrine, which was not declared on the label. The oxilofrine-containing supplements were advertised as slimming products and neuroenhancers (ASADA, 2014a; NADA, 2013).

Dietary supplements containing prohibited anabolic agents

Dietary supplements contaminated with prohormones

The extent of the contamination of dietary supplements with anabolic agents was evaluated in 2001 and 2002. A well-publicised study showed that about

15% of a sample of non-hormonal supplements such as vitamins, minerals, proteins, creatine, etc. contained anabolic androgenic steroids (mainly prohormones) that were not declared on the label (Geyer *et al.*, 2004b). The reason for the contamination was most probably the fact that manufacturers of prohormones (legally marketed as dietary supplements in the USA until 2004) also manufactured other supplements on the production line without sufficient cleaning. Another source of cross-contamination could have been the unclean transport containers from raw material suppliers of prohormones. The amount of detected prohormones, especially prohormones of nandrolone, could produce positive doping cases.

Faked dietary supplements contaminated with 'classic' anabolic steroids

Since 2002, dietary supplements have appeared on the market, which are probably intentionally spiked with high amounts (more than 1 mg/g) of 'classic' anabolic steroids, not declared or declared with non-approved or fancy names on the label. Among these, steroids including stanozolol, metandienone, dehydrochloromethyltestosterone, oxandrolone, have been identified. All these steroids are orally effective drugs based on their 17-alkyl group. These dietary supplements are advertised as leading to enormous enhancement of strength and lean body mass. The concentrations of the anabolic androgenic steroids are in the therapeutic or supra-therapeutic range per serving leading to positive doping cases detectable for several days and weeks respectively, depending on the type of steroid administered.

Because the manufacturers of these faked products also prepare other nutritional supplements on the same production line, the risk of cross-contaminations with such 'classic' anabolic androgenic steroids is very high. Such contaminations have been found in fizzy tablets of vitamin C, magnesium, and multivitamins produced for Spanish and German supermarkets containing, for example, small amounts of stanozolol and metandienone with the potential to produce a positive doping response.

Since 2002, so-called 'designer steroids' can also be found on the dietary supplement market. These steroids are neither listed as ingredients in any currently available medication nor do their names appear in the WADA list of prohibited substances. Most of these 'designer steroids' have been synthesized in the 1960s and were tested only in animal studies for their anabolic and androgenic effects. Nowadays these steroidal agents are produced exclusively for the nutritional supplement market and are advertised for their anabolic or aromatase inhibiting capacities. With regard to the effects and side effects of these steroids for humans, there is limited or no knowledge. In most cases the labelling of these products contains non-approved or fancy names of the steroids. More than 40 of such designer steroids have been detected. The detection of metabolites of such a steroid in an athlete's urine sample is likely to lead to a positive doping case.

Dietary supplements with clenbuterol

According to our knowledge, until now only two cases have been detected in which dietary supplements have contained therapeutic, 30µg per tablet (Parr *et al.*, 2008), and supra-therapeutic (2mg/capsule) doses of the β2-agonist clenbuterol (Parr *et al.*, personal communication 2010). In the supra-therapeutically dosed product clenbuterol was not declared on the label. Both supplements were advertised as weight loss products. Because of the extremely high concentration of clenbuterol in the second product (100-fold more than the therapeutic dose), severe side effects could occur: in addition, a high risk of cross-contamination of other products with clenbuterol is likely. Because WADA has classified clenbuterol as an anabolic agent, its detection in doping control may lead to severe sanctions.

Dietary supplements containing prohibited peptide hormones

In 2009 and 2010 dietary supplements containing the prohibited growth hormone-releasing peptide-2 (GHRP-2) were detected (Kohler *et al.*, 2010; Thomas *et al.*, 2010). The products were advertised to produce anabolic, fat-reducing and anti-catabolic effects and to improve regeneration. One product, in an ampoule of a drinking solution, contained an orally active concentration of GHPR-2. Such a product may lead to inadvertent doping cases because the name GHPR-2 is not specifically listed on the WADA prohibited list and is unknown by the majority of the sports community. However, GHRP-2 belongs as a releasing factor to the prohibited substance group S2 on the WADA list.

Emerging drugs

In 2009 and 2010 the first prohibited Selective Androgen Receptor Modulators (SARMs) and the gene doping substances AICAR and GW1516 were detected on the black market (Kohler *et al.*, 2010; Thevis *et al.*, 2011). All these substances are still in clinical trials and have not yet been approved as medications. According to our experience we expect that these substances will appear very soon on the dietary supplement market, with advertising that the SARM products will achieve anabolic effects while the gene doping substances will enhance endurance. If these substances are added to other supplement products without being declared on the label, new sources of risk for inadvertent doping will be created.

What can athletes do?

According to our experience, the risk of inadvertent doping is predominantly connected to dietary supplements aggressively marketed for their physiological effects, e.g. muscle gain and fat loss, but cannot be confined exclusively to such products. Therefore, athletes should in general carefully consider the risks and benefits of dietary supplements. If use seems to be essential, athletes should purchase dietary supplements only from low risk sources. Such sources are established in some countries such as Germany (www.colognelist.com), the Netherlands (http://antidoping.nl/nzvt), the UK (www.hfl.co.uk) and the USA (www.nsf.org/certified/dietary), where databases list dietary supplements from companies whose products undergo frequent quality controls concerning the presence of doping agents. However, these sources cannot guarantee that dietary supplements are free of risk, but offer a risk minimization. Dietary supplements produced by pharmaceutical companies might represent an alternative as such products have not yet been found to be contaminated with doping substances (Geyer et al., 2004a).

Health issues

As discussed in the review on inadvertent doping, DS have been detected with high amounts of classic anabolic steroids or stimulants. For example the drug sibutramine, classified by WADA as a prohibited substance in competition, has been found in slimming products (e.g. capsules or tea). Not only was the drug not declared on the label, but the products declared only 'natural' ingredients. Furthermore, in addition to sibutramine causing a positive doping test, there are also potential side effects such as increased heart rate or blood pressure.

Furthermore, DS with high amounts of anabolic steroids (e.g. stanozolol, boldenone, oxandrolone) were likely to have been intentionally faked with steroids, but not labelled correctly, due to steroids not being allowed in DS. Again not only is the consumption of such products an issue for anti-doping, but the high amounts (< 1mg/g) of steroids found in these products can also result in serious side effects such as abnormal liver function, menstrual disorders, virilisation, psychological or psychiatric disorders.

As the manufacturers of such products also produce other DS, the risk of cross-contamination is very high. Therefore it is not surprising that, in 2005, vitamin C, multi-vitamins and magnesium tablets containing metandienone or stanozolol were confiscated, with suggestions the contamination came through badly cleaned production lines (Geyer et al., 2006). Again this is not just an issue for anti-doping, but also has potential health risks for young people, females and pregnant women.

Finally, DS have also recently been found with new designer steroids, which are neither listed in the WADA list nor as ingredients in any available medication. Furthermore, little knowledge exists surrounding the effects and side effects of these new steroids. Once again, since manufacturers of these products also produce other DS, a cross-contamination with 'new' steroids can be expected with further potential of detrimental health issues and inadvertent positive doping cases.

The assumption has generally been that the presence of WADA-prohibited substances is the result of inadvertent contamination of raw materials and/ or cross-contamination within the manufacturing or packaging process rather than deliberate adulteration of the products in an attempt to increase the supplement's effectiveness. Consequently, the amounts of steroids detected have been extremely variable, even within a single batch, but have generally been very small. However, very low levels of contamination (measured in parts per billion) can cause positive drug tests in an elite athlete. These levels are much lower than acceptable impurity levels (typically around 0.01%) in good manufacturing practice regulations. It is important to note that, although this minimal amount of contamination could produce dire consequences for an athlete competing under the WADA code, this amount, in most cases, is unlikely to cause detrimental health issues for the general consumer. However, daily food product withdrawals and recalls due to mislabelling and undeclared allergens plus issues with impurities and contamination from medicine residues, insects and small pieces of metal and plastic, demonstrate that inadvertent contamination is not just an issue for sports nutrition products.

The inadequate regulation of dietary supplements means there is no way for consumers to know what many supplements actually contain or how pure the product and its ingredients are. Manufacturers with good quality controls and testing for banned substances are better able to control the risk. The inception of the WADA code and the implications of strict liability mean that an athlete is held responsible for whatever is in his/her body, irrespective of how it got there.

Therefore, athletes who compete under the WADA code should be extremely cautious about using supplements and always work with a qualified professional on risk minimisation of supplement use. To help prevent athletes from inadvertent doping, they should use only supplements from low risk sources. Such sources are established in some countries such as Germany, the Netherlands, the UK and the USA, where the databases list DS from companies which perform quality control and screening for WADA substances. However, these databases are still unable to guarantee that the DS is free from risk, but simply offer this minimization of risk.

There are cases in which a doping infringement can be traced back to supplement use and for which the athlete has undertaken some strategies to reduce this risk. For example, the athlete has received written advice from a supplement manufacturer that their product does not contain banned substances but, following a positive doping test, a sealed container of the dietary supplement has been examined and found to contain the banned ingredient. Unfortunately, strict liability applies to these situations and, even if an athlete has been successful in having the terms of their ban from sport reduced, a doping infringement will still be recorded against their name. The loss of a career, livelihood and reputation are stakes that an athlete must take into account when using dietary supplements.

Consumers of DS should be aware that if a product offers enormous benefit on performance, increased muscle mass or weight loss, it might be faked or contaminated with a prescriptive drug or even illegal substance, which can cause a positive doping case or serious side-effects that may be detrimental to health.

Evaluation of supplements

When deciding on the efficacy of a supplement it is important to first consider the level of scientific evidence available to support the supplement's efficacy. The traditional view of evidence is based on four levels (Figure 4).

On assessing whether there is sufficient evidence to support considering using a supplement, the research should be at level III or IV. Caution should always be taken when considering a supplement if the research is only at levels I aor II.

Coupled with the level of evidence, there are also other aspects surrounding the individual research studies from which the evidence is taken that need to be considered (Figure 5).

Recent advances in technology have resulted in an increase in the amount of in vitro research being conducted, and subsequently further claims regarding

Level I	Anecdotal evidence or expert opinion	These are common in the supplement marketplace, particularly when high-profile athletes promote the use of a particular supplement
Level II	Case series or observational studies	Less common in the supplement research literature
Level III	Randomised control trials (RCT)	The most common type of research undertaken in the supplement literature. However, it is key that the research is of suitable quality (Figure 5)
Level IV	Systematic reviews and meta-analysis	The highest level of evidence to show efficacy of a supplement. However, these are rare and may not always be available, especially for newer supplements which appear on the market

FIGURE 4   Levels of evidence

Factor	Consideration
Participants	Are they similar to the athletes you want to use the supplement with? Consider age, gender and training status.
Control of the studied supplement	Was the supplement tested for the amount of the declared substance (adequate dose, poor manufacturing) and/or substances probably not declared on the label (contamination/fake), of which both might have an effect on the study results?
Type of performance test	Is the test valid and reliable?
Control of the study	Is the study well controlled? Do they account for factors such as diet, training, sleep and gender issues such as controlling for stage of menstrual cycle?
Design of the study	Is the study placebo-controlled and double-blinded? Are there enough participants to provide statistical power? Does the design mimic the conditions under which a sport/exercise activity is conducted in real life? Is the supplement given acutely or chronically?
Funding source	Is the research funded by an organisation with a vested interest in the outcome of the research?

FIGURE 5 Factors to consider when assessing research on supplements

Does the supplement get broken down in the mouth?
Does the supplement interact with receptors in the mouth?
How is the supplement absorbed in the gastrointestinal (GI) system?
Once absorbed does it get to the site of action?
Is the amount absorbed enough to provide a performance-enhancing effect?
Is the amount which reaches the site of action enough to provide a performance-enhancing effect?
Are there other confounding factors to consider?

FIGURE 6 Supplement bioavailability

supplements being made. This in vitro evidence is important to consider and should not be dismissed. However, quite often when looking at the body as a whole, the supplement may work differently in vivo as to what may happen in vitro. Therefore, aspects regarding the supplement's potential bioavailability and effectiveness also need to be considered (Figure 6).

Measuring sports performance

Ideally, the considerations of using supplements should be based on sound scientific evidence, which conclusively provides support for a performance- or health-enhancing effect. However, measuring sports performance in particular in a scientific controlled manner is difficult and open to debate (Currell and Jeukendrup, 2008b; Hopkins et al., 1991). Consequently, validity, reliability and sensitivity all need to be considered when evaluating sports performance research (Figure 7).

Furthermore, in linear based sports, such as running and cycling, there has been much discussion about how best to measure performance, e.g. time to exhaustion (TTE) versus time trial.

'Time to exhaustion' (TTE), the traditional mode to measure performance, is a steady state TTE trial that was originally derived from animal studies. TTE trials provide a useful way within which to control many external variables. However, they have limited validity in terms of actual sports performance as no sporting event aim is to perform to exhaustion. There is a counter-argument to this view in that in many events, there are scenarios in which one athlete (e.g. a runner or cyclist) sets the pace at the front of the race while the other competitors strive to hold on to this speed for as long as possible to stay in contention. This race tactic provides some sympathy for the application of the TTE to sports performance. However, exercising at a single and externally determined pace/speed/power output eliminates the role of pacing (self-chosen and often varying speed/intensity/power output) as a key aspect of sports performance. TTE trials tend to have a high coefficient of variation (CV), with values greater than 10% frequently reported in the literature, although this can be reduced by various tactics such as familiarising the subject.

'Time trials', conversely, are more representative of sports performance and therefore are a more ecologically valid measure of performance. In competitive

Validity	Is the protocol measuring the type of performance desired?
Reliability	Can the test be repeated with only a small variance in performance?
Sensitivity	Is the test able to detect a change in performance which has both practical and statistical significance?

FIGURE 7   Evaluating sports performance research

Factor	Rationale
Subject preparation	Training and sleep over the day(s) leading into the trial should be standardised, as should diet over the hours and day(s) pre-trial
Familiarisation	Reliability increases with increased exposure to the protocol
Verbal encouragement	If this was not standardised then this could affect the performance outcome
Music	Music affects performance and ideally should not be available during a performance trial
Feedback	Minimal feedback should be provided so as to not influence performance in subsequent trials
Measurements	Taking physiological measures during performance may disrupt performance

FIGURE 8 Factors to control when measuring performance

athletes who are familiarised to the task, they also tend to have a lower CV with values between 1–5% generally being reported in the literature.

For sports which are more complicated and where performance is determined by a complex mixture of movement patterns, skill execution, decision making and interaction with competitors (e.g. team and racket sports), it is important to ensure that the characteristics measured in a study actually influence the match outcome (e.g. goals scored or points won). Furthermore, whilst measuring sports performance there are other key factors, including the testing environment, that also need to be considered and controlled for as appropriate (Figure 8).

True performance effects versus risk

In order to find a true performance effect of a supplement it is important to determine the size of the smallest worthwhile effect which will lead to a difference in the outcome of an event or sport. The difference between coming first and second in a race is often much less than 1% of the overall time of the race. This is such a small difference that it can frequently not be detected by traditional methods of performance testing and statistical analysis. These small differences between winning and losing are important when considering using a supplement. Quite often a coach and athlete will be unconcerned with statistical significance if they believe that there may be a chance of improving performance. Some sports scientists have tried to address the need for a different statistical determination of the effects of an intervention on sports performance, using magnitude-based inferences, which compare the true likely effect of the intervention to the daily variability of performance in a sport (Batterham and Hopkins, 2006; Hopkins et al., 2009).

Factor	Rationale
Cost	Quite often supplements can be costly, particularly those which are for chronic use
Doping	Will there be any inadvertent positive doping test using the supplement?
Interaction with other supplements	While some supplements work in synergy together, others may interact to provide negative outcomes
Adaptation to training	Some supplements can interfere with the natural adaptation to training
General diet	Supplements should not be used as a method to support a poor diet. Athletes may want to use supplements to avoid having to eat appropriately
Performance	Some supplements which have side effects such as weight gain may not be appropriate in some sports

FIGURE 9 Additional factors regarding supplement use

When there does appear to be sufficient evidence to show a possible benefit to performance it is absolutely critical that any side effects together with the alongside potential negative aspects of using the supplement are also considered. If there are any known effects which could be detrimental to the athletes' health these must be explored and controlled for.

Figure 9 summarises some of the other key factors, including the aforementioned issue of inadvertent doping, that should be considered alongside potential negative health effects.

Placebo effect

Finally the placebo effect must also be considered. Although supplement use amongst athletes is extremely prevalent, many do not have an evidence-based proven effect on health or sports performance. In contrast, athletes explore through their own experiences and so it is not surprising that some athletes claim to have success or feel good with certain supplements. This can result from one of two things:

1   Individual athletes respond differently according to the use of supplements (responder and non-responder effect). [See 'In Practice' chapter.]
2   The belief that a product increases performance by stimulating performance reserves.

In competition, and training, psychological variables such as motivation or expectancy are important factors in achieving maximum performance. Since there is an interaction between mind and body it is not surprising that athletes

1. Inform supplement/receive supplement
2. Inform supplement/receive placebo
3. Inform placebo/receive supplement
4. Inform placebo/receive placebo

FIGURE 10. Latin-square design to investigate the placebo effect of supplements

and coaches sometimes report a positive effect from using supplements. If this effect is based on a 'positive outcome resulting from the belief that a beneficial treatment has been received', it can be classified as a 'placebo' effect. Although this placebo effect has been acknowledged in medicine for more than 50 years, it is a relatively new consideration and area of research in sports performance.

Several authors suggest that investigations into the placebo effect of DS in sports performance should use a Latin-square design, using four conditions (1–4) to investigate the placebo effect of supplements (Figure 10).

One of the first placebo studies (Maganaris et al., 2000) was undertaken on 11 weightlifters. They were told they would receive a placebo fast-acting anabolic steroid, which led to a mean improvement of 3.5–5.2% in maximal weight lifted at different tests. In the subsequent second experimental trial, six athletes were correctly informed about the placebo. Those athletes reduced their performance into the range of baseline levels, while the remaining five athletes maintained their improvement.

Another 'placebo' study (Porcari et al., 2006) reported a significant difference on a 5km run using super-oxygenated water versus placebo. However, the improvements over baseline levels were higher for the less accomplished runners compared to the experienced runners. Furthermore, the less-experienced runners reported that they felt better and asked where they could buy the product, while the experienced runners did not believe that the product worked. The observed differences in perception suggest a relationship between performance level and placebo response, which also needs to be considered when interpreting other studies surrounding the efficacy of supplements. Therefore, depending on the research design, the interpretation is somewhat limited by the training status of the subjects.

While most studies investigate a positive belief in a treatment, Beedie et al. (2007) found a negative influence on sports performance if subjects were told that the treatment would have a negative effect on sprinting performance. Based on this proposition, the authors speculated that a negative belief in a legitimate supplement might reduce the expected beneficial effects on performance.

Foad et al. (2008) studied the psychological and pharmacological effects of caffeine in cycling performance. The authors supported their data with the ergogenic effect of caffeine use. Surprisingly the effect was higher when athletes were told that they did not receive caffeine, versus telling them that they had received caffeine. Additionally, a negative placebo effect was found in the trial 'inform no treatment/ give no treatment' (Foad *et al.*, 2008).

Therefore, it seems that a placebo effect in relation to the use of supplements on sport performance does exist, with current findings suggesting:

- a relationship between performance status and placebo response might exist;
- a positive belief in a product can increase performance, while a negative belief can decrease performance;
- the placebo effect observed is different if an active substance is given and belief is manipulated versus a study in which only the belief is manipulated.

Since a placebo effect does exist, research studies investigating supplements should include randomized double-blind treatments. However, some scientists speculate that the placebo effect can be seen more within studies than in the real world (Beedie and Foad, 2009), due to the fact that subjects might not perform at volitional maximum in performance research, but will do so more readily in competition. This suggests that personality might influence placebo response or that placebo response is different according to personality. Therefore, researchers, athletes and coaches are advised to be cautious in translating observations from the laboratory into the real world, not just those from placebo studies.

About the book

There are many reviews on supplementation in athletes, some of which are very good. Our aim is not to replicate these but to provide a series of concise yet comprehensive overviews, including opinion from experts in the field. Our main aim is simply to demystify some of the many supplements on the market in order to provide a useful resource for athletes, sport and exercise enthusiasts, along with allied professionals such as nutritionists, coaches, physiotherapists and doctors. Some research citations for each topic are provided in the reference list, found at the end of the book, for those who wish to investigate further. When feasible, practical advice will be given in regard to dosage and timing. Needless to say, this advice will be based upon the best available sources at the time. Notwithstanding, the authors, editors and publishers cannot be held responsible for advice on the purity of the supplement or the failure of any specific dose to improve performance.

We previously ran a similar series of reviews, the 'A–Z of Supplements: Dietary Supplements, Sports Nutrition Foods and Ergogenic Aids for Health and Performance' in the *British Journal of Sports Medicine* (*BJSM*) on a monthly basis from 2009–2013 (Castell *et al.*, 2009). Across the four years we covered a vast range of the supplements that are commonly used by athletes, totalling 124 topics. The list of the original topics covered, the author and *BJSM* reference for these earlier reviews are provided in Figure 11 (p. 30).

For this book, all the original reviews have been updated and expanded, where appropriate, according to the latest available information and scientific evidence. In addition, due to the evolving nature of the supplement world, some additional topics have been reviewed for individual inclusion in this book, including: D-Aspartic acid (DAA); chlorogenic acid; DMAA (methylhexanamine/ dimethylamylamine); ginger; glucuronolactone; HICA, inositol; Jack3D; ketones; α-lipoic acid; OxyElite Pro; papain/protease; D-pinitol; and sodium.

As can be seen from the combined lists, some of these are complete products, while others will be the individual substances that make up the many poly-ingredient supplements on the market. Furthermore, some topics, such as Chinese herbs and weight loss supplements, review multiple ingredients and the various combinations of ingredients within these supplement categories.

With such a vast range of supplements and ingredients marketed for sport, exercise and health, we simply will not be able to cover them all and for some it will be just a brief mention or cross-reference. All reviews are cross-referenced to allow for those supplements which are popularly known to athletes by more than one name. Furthermore, aligned with the purpose of this book, the reviews will deal specifically with the effects of these supplements on exercise and sport-related health and performance issues rather than general health or clinical issues.

Alongside the additional topics, and updated reviews for the book, the concluding chapter also provides an efficacy index, where appropriate, for the supplements reviewed.

Efficacy index

There are numerous methods by which it is possible to classify supplements including their efficacy. Due to the vast array of supplements it is often felt useful to provide practitioners working alongside athletes, in particular, with guidance such as a classification framework based on a standardised ranking methodology, for example, efficacy. Many of the Olympic Training Centres and Institutes of Sports across the world have devised their own supplement frameworks for this purpose.

It is both scientifically and practically difficult to attempt to devise a summary table for such a vast array of ingredients and supplements. In the efficacy index for this book, the level of evidence as per the standardised four categories, Levels I–IV (Figure 4), is considered first.

For this book's efficacy index, with the evidence level in mind, the strength of the direction of effect on sports performance and/or health is then considered. The direction of the effect is then ranked from 1–7 accordingly, ranging from strongly positive (1) to fairly positive (2) for a beneficial effect, to fairly negative (4), strongly negative (5), with a mid-way ranking (3) given for those supplements where the evidence has produced mixed results, a mixed effect or no effect. In some instances, where there are known issues, for example banned by WADA, FDA, or toxicity concerns, the supplement/product is assigned to the (6) 'Caution' category, with explanatory remarks provided in the comments column. Plus, as the majority of supplements have either supporting evidence for an effect on sports performance or for health, and not both, then the final ranking (7) is used for not applicable.

Furthermore, in light of the discussion in the previous section regarding factors to consider when assessing research on supplements (see Figures 5–9), a comments column is also provided as part of the efficacy index table, where any key factors or issues with the research and/or supplement can be highlighted. For example, issues surrounding toxicology, safety, side effects, nutrient-interactions, dosage and timing can be highlighted in the comments column so that these are considered alongside the level of evidence and effect of sports performance and/or health. However, it is also worth noting that the level of evidence may not be as substantial, for example, for safety issues, and indeed some ingredients/supplements may be acceptable from a safety perspective but still have a negative impact on sports performance. All factors and aspects surrounding the supplement and the evidence need to be taken into consideration.

Consequently, we, the authors and editors alike, have taken the current evidence-based information presented in the supplement reviews throughout this book, and have attempted to standardise the level of efficacy in terms of sports and/or health performance. The summary tables for the efficacy index alongside key commentary are provided in the concluding chapter of the book.

However, it is important to note that, in consideration of current scientific research and increasing innovation and development in the sports nutrition arena, all supplement frameworks, including the book's own efficacy index, are working documents that are only accurate to the date of the most recent publication.

Furthermore, athletes should always consider the issues of efficacy, safety and legality/ethics associated with supplements prior to considering using any supplement. Unfortunately, all too frequently, specific information is limited. Furthermore, due to poor manufacturing practice, some supplements do not contain (a) an adequate dose of the labelled ingredients but do contain (b) impurities like glass, lead or animal faeces. Moreover, the FDA regularly reports on products found to contain effective amounts of prescription drugs, which could lead to detrimental side effects. As also discussed in this chapter, another potential health risk is from contamination or fake supplements which can cause a positive doping test for those athletes competing under the WADA code. Therefore, athletes competing under the WADA code need to be extremely cautious about using supplements and are advised always to work with a qualified professional to minimise the risks of supplement use.

FIGURE 11 Topics covered in BJSM series: A–Z of supplements

Supplement/product	Author(s)	BJSM part	British Journal of Sports Medicine reference
Amino acids	L.M. Castell	2	Brown,G.A., Vukovich M.D., King, D.S., Wolfe R.R., Newsholme E.A., Trudeau F., Curi,R., Burke L.M., Stear S.J., Castell L.M. (2009). BJSM reviews: A–Z of supplements: dietary supplements, sports nutrition foods and ergogenic aids for health and performance Part 2: Amino acids, androstenedione, arginine, asparagine and aspartate. *Br J Sports Med* 43(11): 807–810.
Arginine	R.R. Wolfe and E.A. Newsholme	2	
Aspartate and Asparagine	F. Trudeau and R. Curi	2	
Androstenedione	G.A. Brown, M.D. Vukovich and D.S. King	2	
Antioxidants	S.K. Powers, A.N. Kavazis and W.B. Nelson	3	Powers S.K., Kavazis A.N., Nelson W.B., Ernst E., Stear S.J., Burke L.M., Castell L.M. (2009). BJSM reviews: A–Z of nutritional supplements: dietary supplements, sports nutrition foods and ergogenic aids for health and performance Part 3: Antioxidants and arnica. *Br J Sports Med* 43(12): 890–892.
Arnica	E. Ernst	3	
Aspartame	P.J. Rogers	4	Rogers P.J., Blomstrand E., Gurr S., Mitchell N., Stephens F.B, Greenhaff P.L., Burke L.M., Stear S.J., Castell L.M., (2009). BJSM reviews: A–Z of nutritional supplements: dietary supplements, sports nutrition foods and ergogenic aids for health and performance Part 4: Aspartame, branched chain amino acids, bee pollen, boron, carnitine. *Br J Sports Med* 43(14): 1088–1090.
Branched-chain amino acids	E. Blomstrand	4	
Bee pollen	S. Gurr	4	
Boron	N. Mitchell	4	
L-Carnitine	F.B. Stephens and P.L. Greenhaff	4	
Buffers: β-alanine and carnosine	R.C. Harris	5	McNaughton L.R., Harris R.C., Burke L.M., Stear S.J., Castell L.M. (2010). BJSM reviews: A–Z of nutritional supplements: dietary supplements, sports nutrition foods and ergogenic aids for health and performance Part 5: Buffers: sodium bicarbonate and sodium citrate; β-alanine and carnosine. *Br J Sports Med* 44(1): 77–78.
Buffers: Sodium bicarbonate and Sodium citrate	L.R. McNaughton	5	

Supplement/product	Author(s)	BJSM part	British Journal of Sports Medicine reference
Caffeine	L.L. Spriet and L.M. Burke	6	Spriet, L.L., Stear, S.J., Burke, L.M., Castell, L.M. (2010). BJSM reviews: A–Z of nutritional supplements: dietary supplements, sports nutrition foods and ergogenic aids for health and performance Part 6: Caffeine. Br J Sports Med 44: 297–298
Calcium and bone health	L. Houtkooper and M. Manore	7	Houtkopper L., Manore M., Senchina D., Stear S.J., Burke L.M., Castell L.M. (2010). BJSM reviews: A–Z of nutritional supplements: dietary supplements, sports nutrition foods and ergogenic aids for health and performance Part 7: calcium and bone health, Vitamin D, and Chinese herbs. Br J Sports Med 44(3): 389–391.
Chinese herbs	D.S. Senchina	7	
Carbohydrate	R.J. Maughan and L.M. Burke	8	Maughan R.J., Burke L.M., Stear S.J., Castell L.M. (2010). BJSM reviews: A–Z of nutritional supplements: dietary supplements, sports nutrition foods and ergogenic aids for health and performance Part 8: Carbohydrate. Br J Sports Med 44(4): 468–470.
Choline Bitartrate plus Acetylcholine	J. Pearce	9	Pearce J., Borchers J.R., Kaeding C.C., Rawson E.S., Shaw G., Burke L.M., Stear S.J., Castell L.M. (2010). BJSM reviews: A–Z of nutritional supplements: dietary supplements, sports nutrition foods and ergogenic aids for health and performance Part 9: Choline bitartrate plus acetylcholine, chondroitinn/glucosamine, chromium picolinate and cissus quadrangularis. Br J Sports Med 44: 609–611.
Chondroitin/ Glucosamine	J.R. Borchers C.C. Kaeding	9	
Chromium Picolinate	E.S. Rawson	9	
Cissus Quadrangularis	G. Shaw	9	
Citrulline	N. Jeacocke	10	Jeacocke N., Ekblom B., Shing C., Calder P.C., Lewis N. Stear S.J., Burke L.M., Castell L.M. (2010). BJSM reviews: A–Z of nutritional supplements: dietary supplements, sports nutrition foods and ergogenic aids for health and performance Part 10: Citrulline, coenzyme Q10, colostrum, conjugated linoleic acid, copper. Br J Sports Med 44: 688–690.
Co-Enzyme Q10	B. Ekblom	10	
Colostrum	C. Shing	10	
Conjugated linoleic acid	P.C. Calder	10	
Copper	N. Lewis	10	

Supplement/product	Author(s)	BJSM part	British Journal of Sports Medicine reference
Creatine	J.R. Poortmans1 and E.S. Rawson2	11	Poortmans J.R., Rawson E.S., Burke L.M., Stear S.J., Castell L.M. (2010). BJSM reviews: A–Z of nutritional supplements: dietary supplements, sports nutrition foods and ergogenic aids for health and performance Part 11: Creatine. *Br J Sports Med* 44: 765–766
Cysteine and Cystine	K. Currell1 and A. Syed	12	Currell K., Syed A., Dziedzic C.E., king D.S., Spriet L.L., Collins J., Castell L.M., Stear S.J., Burke L.M. (2010). BJSM reviews: A–Z of nutritional supplements: dietary supplements, sports nutrition foods and ergogenic aids for health and performance Part 12: Cysteine & cystine, cytochrome C, dehydroepiandrosterone, dihydroxyacetone phosphate & pyruvate, dimethylglycine. *Br J Sports Med* 44(12): 905–907
Cytochrome C	C.E. Dziedzic	12	
Dehydroepi-androsterone (DHEA)	D.S. King	12	
Dihydroxy-acetone phosphate (DHAP) and Pyruvate	L.L. Spriet	12	
Dimethylglycine (DMG)	J. Collins	12	
Electrolytes	M.F. Bergeron	13	Bergeron M.F., Senchina D.S., Burke L.M., Stear S.J., Castell L.M. (2010). BJSM reviews: A–Z of nutritional supplements: dietary supplements, sports nutrition foods and ergogenic aids for health and performance Part 13: Electrolytes, ephedra, echinacea. *Br J Sports Med* 44: 985–986.
Ephedra and Echinacea	D.S. Senchina	13	
Fatty Acids	P.C. Calder	14	Calder P.C., Lindley M.R., Burke L.M., Stear S.J., Castell L.M. (2010). BJSM reviews: A–Z of nutritional supplements: dietary supplements, sports nutrition foods and ergogenic aids for health and performance Part 14: Fatty acids and fish oils. *Br J Sports Med* 44: 1065–7.
Fish Oils	P.C. Calder and M.R. Lindley	14	

Supplement/product	Author(s)	BJSM part	British Journal of Sports Medicine reference
Flavonoids	D.C. Nieman	15	Nieman D.C., Stear S.J., Burke L.M., Castell L.M. (2010). BJSM reviews: A–Z of nutritional supplements: dietary supplements, sports nutrition foods and ergogenic aids for health and performance Part 15: Flavonoids. *Br J Sports Med* 44: 1202–1205
Folate	M. Manore	16	Manore M, Meeusen R., Roelands B., Moran S., Popple A.D., Naylor M.J, Burke L.M., Stear S.J., Castell L.M. (2011). BJSM reviews: A–Z of nutritional supplements: dietary supplements, sports nutrition foods and ergogenic aids for health and performance Part 16: Folate, γ-aminobutyric acid, gamma-oryzanol and ferulic acid, γ-hydroxybutyrate and γ-butyrolactone. *Br J Sports Med* 45: 73–74.
γ-aminobutyric acid (GABA)	R. Meeusen and B. Roelands	16	
Gamma-oryzanol and Ferulic acid	S. Moran	16	
γ-hydroxy-butyrate and γ-butyrolactone	A.D. Popple and M.J. Naylor	16	
Ginkgo	D.S. Senchina	17	Senchina D.S., Bermon S.,Stear S.J., Burke L.M., Castell L.M. (2011). BJSM reviews: A–Z of nutritional supplements: dietary supplements, sports nutrition foods and ergogenic aids for health and performance Part 17: Gingko, ginseng, green tea, garlic and glandulars. *Br J Sports Med* 45: 150–151
Ginseng	D.S. Senchina	17	
Green Tea	D.S. Senchina	17	
Garlic	S. Bermon	17	
Glandulars	S.J. Stear	17	
Glutathione and Glutamate	P. Newsholme and M. Krause	18	Newsholme P.Krause M., Newsholme E.A., Burke L.M., Stear S.J., Castell L.M. (2011). BJSM reviews: A–Z of nutritional supplements: dietary supplements, sports nutrition foods and ergogenic aids for health and performance Part 18: Glutamine, glutathione and glutamate. *Br J Sports Med* 45: 230–232.
Glutamine	L.M. Castell, P. Newsholme and E.A. Newsholme	18	

Supplement/product	Author(s)	BJSM part	British Journal of Sports Medicine reference
Glycerol	L.M. Burke	19	Lobb, A., Ellison M., Burke L.M., Stear S.J., Castell L.M. (2011). BJSM reviews: A–Z of nutritional supplements: dietary supplements, sports nutrition foods and ergogenic aids for health and performance Part 19: GlycLoxycut. *Br J Sports Med* 45: 456–458.
Guarana	S.J. Stear	19	
Hydroxycut	A. Lobb and M. Ellison	19	
Glycine	K. Currell	20	Currell K., Derave W., Everaert I, McNaughton L., Slater G.,Burke L.M., Stear S.J., Castell L.M. (2011). BJSM reviews: A–Z of nutritional supplements: dietary supplements, sports nutrition foods and ergogenic aids for health and performance Part 20: GlycLning peptides, HMB and Le.*Br J Sports Med* 45: 530–532.
Histidine-containing dipeptides	W. Derave and I. Everaert	20	
HMB	G. Slater	20	
Inosine	L.R. McNaughton	20	
Iron	C. Goodman and P. Peeling	21	Goodman C., Peeling P., Ranchordas M.K, Burke L.M., Stear S.J., Castell L.M. (2011). BJSM reviews: A–Z of nutritional supplements: dietary supplements, sports nutrition foods and ergogenic aids for health and performance Part 21: Iron, α-ketoisocaproate and α-ketoisocaproate. *Br J Sports Med* 45: 677–679.
α-ketoglutarate	M.K. Ranchordas	21	
α-ketoisocaproate	M.K. Ranchordas	21	
Inadvertent doping	H. Geyer and H. Braun	22	Geyer, H., Braun, H., Burke, L.M., Stear, S.J., Castell L.M. (2011). BJSM reviews: A–Z of nutritional supplements: dietary supplements, sports nutrition foods and ergogenic aids for health and performance Part 22: Inadvertent doping. *Br J Sports Med* 45: 752–754.
Leucine	E. Blomstrand	23	Ranchordas M.K, Blomstrand E., Calder P.C., Burke L.M., Stear S.J., Castell L.M. (2011). BJSM reviews: A–Z of nutritional supplements: dietary supplements, sports nutrition foods and ergogenic aids for health and performance Part 23: Leucine, lecithin, linoleic and linolenic acid. *Br J Sports Med* 45: 830–831.
Lecithin	M.K. Ranchordas	23	
Linoleic and linolenic acid	P.C. Calder	23	

Supplement/product	Author(s)	BJSM part	British Journal of Sports Medicine reference
Leptin	J.A. L. Caldet	24	Calbet J.A., Mooren F.C, Burke L.M., Stear S.J., Castell L.M. (2011). BJSM reviews: A–Z of nutritional supplements: dietary supplements, sports nutrition foods and ergogenic aids for health and performance Part 24: Leptin, magnesium and medium chain triglycerides. *Br J Sports Med* 45: 1005–1007.
Magnesium	F.C. Mooren	24	
Medium chain triglycerides (MCTs)	L.M. Burke	24	
Melamine	D.S. Senchina	25	Lundy B., Miller J.C., Jackson K., Senchina D.S., Burke L.M., Stear S.J., Castell L.M. (2011). BJSM reviews: A–Z of nutritional supplements: dietary supplements, sports nutrition foods and ergogenic aids for health and performance Part 25: Melamine, melatonin and methylsulphonylmethane. *Br J Sports Med* 45: 1077–1078.
Melatonin	B. Lundy and J.C. Miller	25	
Methyl-sulphonylethane (MSM)	K. Jackson	25	
Methionine	N.A. Burd	26	Burd N.A., Jeukendrup A., Reid M.B., Burke L.M., Stear S.J., Castell L.M. (2011). BJSM reviews: A–Z of nutritional supplements: dietary supplements, sports nutrition foods and ergogenic aids for health and performance Part 26: Methionine, multiple transportable carbohydrates and N-acetylcysteine. *Br J Sports Med* 45: 1163–1164.
Multiple transportable carbohydrates	A.E. Jeukendrup	26	
N-acetylcysteine (NAC)	M.B. Reid	26	
Nitrates	A.M. Jones	27	Jones A.M., Haramizu S., Ranchordas M.K., Burke L.M., Stear S.J., Castell L.M. (2011). BJSM reviews: A–Z of nutritional supplements: dietary supplements, sports nutrition foods and ergogenic aids for health and performance Part 27: Nitrates, nootkatone, octacosanol and policosanol. *Br J Sports Med* 45: 1246–1248.
Nootkatone	S. Haramizu	27	
Octacosanol and Policosanol	M.K. Ranchordas	27	
Peptides	N.A. Burd	47	Burd, N.A., Stear S.J., Burke L.M., Castell L.M. (2013). BJSM reviews: A–Z of nutritional supplements: dietary supplements, sports nutrition foods and ergogenic aids for health and performance Part 47: Peptides. *Br J Sports Med* 47:993–934.

Supplement/product	Author(s)	BJSM part	British Journal of Sports Medicine reference
Ornithine	K. Currell	28	Currell K, Moore D.R, Peeling P., Burke L.M., Stear S.J., Castell L.M. (2012). BJSM reviews: A–Z of nutritional supplements: dietary supplements, sports nutrition foods and ergogenic aids for health and performance Part 28: Ornithine, phenylalanine, phosphate and pangamic acid. *Br J Sports Med* 46: 75–76.
Phenylalanine	D.R. Moore	28	
Phosphate	P. Peeling	28	
Pangamic acid	L.M. Burke	28	
Phlogenzym and Wobenzym	M.K. Ranchordas	29	Ranchordas M.K., Burd N.A, Senchina D.S. Burke L.M., Stear S.J., Castell L.M. (2012). BJSM reviews: A–Z of nutritional supplements: dietary supplements, sports nutrition foods and ergogenic aids for health and performance Part 29: Phlogenzym and wobenzym, phosphatidylserine and plant stanols. *Br J Sports Med* 46:155–156.
Phosphatidyl-serine	N.A. Burd	29	
Plant sterols	D.S. Senchina	29	
Potassium	N. DiMarco	30	DiMarco N.M., West N.P, Burke L.M., Stear S.J., Castell L.M. (2012). BJSM reviews: A–Z of nutritional supplements: dietary supplements, sports nutrition foods and ergogenic aids for health and performance Part 30: Potassium and prebiotics. *Br J Sports Med* 46: 299–300.
Prebiotics	N.P. West	30	
Probiotics	M. Gleeson	31	Gleeson M., Siegler J.C., Burke L.M., Stear S.J., Castell L.M. (2012). BJSM reviews: A–Z of nutritional supplements: dietary supplements, sports nutrition foods and ergogenic aids for health and performance Part 31: Probiotics and pycnogenol. *Br J Sports Med* 46: 377–378.
Pycnogenol	J. Siegler	31	
Proline	M. Watford and L.M. Castell	32	Breen L., Phillips S.M., Watford M., Burke L.M., Stear S.J., Castell L.M. (2012). BJSM reviews: A–Z of nutritional supplements: dietary supplements, sports nutrition foods and ergogenic aids for health and performance Part 32: Protein and proline. *Br J Sports Med* 46: 454–456.
Protein	L. Breen and S.M. Phillips	32	

Supplement/product	Author(s)	BJSM part	British Journal of Sports Medicine reference
Quercetin	D.C. Nieman	33	Nieman D.C, Laupheimer M.W., Ranchordas M.K., Burke L.M., Stear S.J., Castell L.M. (2012). BJSM reviews: A–Z of nutritional supplements: dietary supplements, sports nutrition foods and ergogenic aids for health and performance Part 33: Quercitin, resveratol and rhodiola rosea.. *Br J Sports Med* 46: 618–620.
Resveratrol	M. Laupheimer	33	
Rhodiola rosea	M.K. Ranchordas	33	
Prohormones	D.S. King and R. Baskerville	34	King D.S., Baskerville R., Hellsten Y., Senchina D.S., Burke L.M., Stear S.J., Castell L.M. (2012). BJSM reviews: A–Z of nutritional supplements: dietary supplements, sports nutrition foods and ergogenic aids for health and performance Part 34: Prohormones, ribose, royal jelly and similax. *Br J Sports Med* 46: 689–690.
Ribose	Y. Hellsten	34	
Royal Jelly	L.M. Castell	34	
Smilax (Sarsaparilla)	D.S. Senchina	34	
Selenium	N. Lewis	35	Lewis N.,Keil M., Ranchordas M.K., Burke L.M., Stear S.J., Castell L.M. (2012). BJSM reviews: A–Z of nutritional supplements: dietary supplements, sports nutrition foods and ergogenic aids for health and performance Part 35: Selenium, serine and sibutramine. *Br J Sports Med* 46: 767–768.
Serine	M. Keil	35	
Sibutramine	M.K. Ranchordas	35	
Spirulina	A.J. Zemski	36	Zemski A.J.,Quinlivan R.M., Gibala M., Burke L.M., Stear S.J., Castell L.M. (2012). BJSM reviews: A–Z of nutritional supplements: dietary supplements, sports nutrition foods and ergogenic aids for health and performance Part 36: Spirulina, succinate, sucrose. *Br J Sports Med* 46: 893–894.
Succinate	M.J. Gibala	36	
Sucrose	R. Quinlivan	36	
Stacking	J. Pearce and L. Norton	37	Pearce J., Norton L., Senchina D.S., Spriet L.L., Burke L.M., Stear S.J., Castell L.M. (2012). BJSM reviews: A–Z of nutritional supplements: dietary supplements, sports nutrition foods and ergogenic aids for health and performance Part 37: Stacking, taurine, theobromine and theophylline. *Br J Sports Med* 46: 954–956.
Taurine	L.L. Spriet	37	
Theobromine and theophylline	D.S. Senchina	37	

Supplement/product	Author(s)	BJSM part	British Journal of Sports Medicine reference
Threonine	N. Cernak	38	Cemak N., Yamamoto T., Meeusen R., Burke L.M., Stear S.J., Castell L.M. (2012). BJSM reviews: A–Z of nutritional supplements: dietary supplements, sports nutrition foods and ergogenic aids for health and performance Part 38: Threonine, tryptophan and tyrosine. *Br J Sports Med* 46: 1027–1028.
Tryptophan	T. Yamamoto and L.M. Castell	38	
Tyrosine	R. Meeusen	38	
Vitamins A, C, and E	D.S. Senchina	39	Senchina D.S., Burke L.M., Stear S.J., Castell L.M. (2012). BJSM reviews: A–Z of nutritional supplements: dietary supplements, sports nutrition foods and ergogenic aids for health and performance Part 39: Vitamin A, C and E. *Br J Sports Med* 46: 1145–1146.
Vitamin D	D.E. Larson-Meyer	40	Larson-Meyer D.E., Burke L.M., Stear S.J., Castell L.M. (2013). BJSM reviews: A–Z of nutritional supplements: dietary supplements, sports nutrition foods and ergogenic aids for health and performance Part 40: Vitamin D. *Br J Sports Med* 47:118–120.
Vitamin B	M.K. Ranchordas	41	Ranchordas M.K., Lundy B., Burke L.M., Stear S.J., Castell L.M. (2013). BJSM reviews: A–Z of nutritional supplements: dietary supplements, sports nutrition foods and ergogenic aids for health and performance Part 41: Vitamin B and K. *Br J Sports Med* 47: 185–186.
Vitamin K	B. Lundy	41	
Valine	A.B. Hodson	42	Hodgson A.B., Baskerville R., Burke L.M., Stear S.J., Castell L.M. (2013). BJSM reviews: A–Z of nutritional supplements: dietary supplements, sports nutrition foods and ergogenic aids for health and performance Part 42: Valine, vanadium and water (oxygenated). *Br J Sports Med* 47: 247–248.
Vanadium	R. Baskerville	42	
Water (oxygenated)	L.M. Burke	42	

Supplement/product	Author(s)	BJSM part	British Journal of Sports Medicine reference
WADA	A. Vernec	48	Vernec, A., Stear S.J., Burke L.M., Castell L.M. (2013). BJSM reviews: A–Z of nutritional supplements: dietary supplements, sports nutrition foods and ergogenic aids for health and performance Part 48: The World Anti Doping Agency. *Br J Sports Med* 47: 998–1000.
Wheat germ oil	M.K. Ranchordas and S.J. Stear	43	Ranchordas M.K., Stear S.J., Burd N.A., Godfrey R.J., Senchina D.S., Burke L.M., Castell L.M. (2013). BJSM reviews: A–Z of nutritional supplements: dietary supplements, sports nutrition foods and ergogenic aids for health and performance Part 43: Wheat germ oil, whey protein and wolfberry. *Br J Sports Med* 47: 659–660.
Whey protein	N.A. Burd	43	
Wolfberry (goji berry)	R.J. Godfrey and D.S. Senchina	43	
Weight loss supplements	D.S. Senchina and S.J. Stear	44	Senchina D.S., Stear S.J., Burke L.M., Castell L.M. (2013). BJSM reviews: A–Z of nutritional supplements: dietary supplements, sports nutrition foods and ergogenic aids for health and performance Part 44: Weight loss strategies and herbal weight loss supplements.*Br J Sports Med* 47: 595–598.
Yerba maté	S.J. Stear	45	Godfrey R.J., Laupheimer M., Stear S.J., Burke L.M., Castell L.M. (2013). BJSM reviews: A–Z of nutritional supplements: dietary supplements, sports nutrition foods and ergogenic aids for health and performance Part 45: Yerba mate, yohimbine and yucca. *Br J Sports Med* 47: 659–660.
Yohimbine	R.J. Godfrey	45	
Yucca	M. Laupheimer	45	
ZMA	A.B. Hodson	46	Deuster P.A., Hodgson A.B., Stear S.J., Burke L.M., Castell L.M. (2013). BJSM reviews: A–Z of nutritional supplements: dietary supplements, sports nutrition foods and ergogenic aids for health and performance Part 46: Zinc and ZMA. *Br J Sports Med* 47:089–810.
Zinc	P.A. Deuster	46	

Nutritional Supplements in Sport, Exercise and Health

An A–Z Guide

AMINO ACIDS

Arash Bandegan, Linda M. Castell and
Peter W.R. Lemon

Amino acids (AA) contain both amine and carboxyl functional groups. Most are the building blocks for protein and are absorbed into the bloodstream following digestion of ingested animal and/or vegetable protein sources. However, not all proteins in the diet have the same nutritional value because each contains different proportions of the essential (or indispensable) AA. The essential and non-essential (or dispensable) AA terminology (see Figure 12) refers to whether or not a specific AA can be synthesised by the body at a rate sufficient to meet the normal requirements for protein synthesis. When sufficient essential AA are present, the protein is considered 'first-class' or 'complete', e.g. dairy products, eggs, fish and meat. In contrast, plant proteins are described as 'second-class' or 'incomplete' proteins and must be combined to equal 'complete' proteins. Specifically, if combinations of grains plus legumes (peas, beans and peanuts), grains plus nuts or seeds, and/or legumes plus nuts or seeds are consumed throughout the day, adequate amounts of the essential AA are available and protein synthesis is normal (these are often called complementary proteins). Otherwise, growth and/or tissue repair is impaired. As a result, strict vegetarians need to plan their diet carefully to ensure their daily ingestion of plant foods provides them with adequate quantities of each essential AA. Further, several AA (known as conditionally indispensable) including arginine, cysteine, glutamine, proline, tyrosine and perhaps others, can become essential under conditions of stress, e.g. trauma, exercise, etc.

Several studies have measured changes in total plasma AA with exercise in an attempt to understand whether exercise alters AA requirements; however, this information is of limited value because both intracellular (Wolfe, 2002) and extracellular (Bohe *et al.*, 2003) AA are the more relevant precursor pools for protein synthesis. Although debated for decades (Lemon and Nagle, 1981), it is likely that exercise increases dietary AA requirements (Philips and van Loon, 2011). The confusion on this issue is due, at least in part, to several complicating factors including age, gender, protein quality, overall dietary energy, time since last meal, type of exercise training, etc. Recent consensus indicates that AA needs are increased with regular exercise (both endurance and strength) suggesting that protein intakes as high as ~150–200% of current recommendations might be necessary for those involved in regular exercise training (Phillips and van Loon, 2011).

Furthermore, the quality of protein is important as milk protein induces a greater muscle protein synthesis (vs. some plant proteins; Wilkinson *et al.*, 2007).

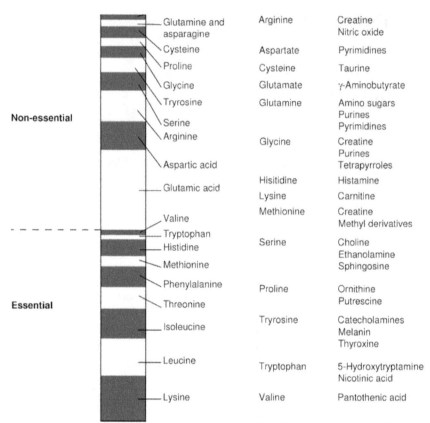

FIGURE 12 The amino acid composition of myosin, one of the two major proteins in muscle and therefore in lean meat, and the biosynthetic role of some of these amino acids. Reproduced with permission from E.A. Newsholme, L.M. Castell. In: R. Maughan (ed.) (2000) *Nutrition in Sport*, Ch. 11. Oxford: Blackwell Science.

Also, the peak response is greater with faster-digesting protein (whey) compared with a slower-digesting protein (casein) (Pennings *et al.*, 2011; Tang *et al.*, 2009), due to the associated rapid aminoacidaemia (West *et al.*, 2011a). Fortunately, it appears that only the essential AA are needed to achieve an increased muscle protein synthesis. Consequently, those who need to be energy conscious may opt to consume sufficient essential AA rather than a whole protein source. Further, some of these essential AA, especially leucine, appear to be key signallers of muscle protein synthesis (Xu *et al.*, 2014; Norton *et al.*, 2012) so for those attempting to increase/preserve muscle mass-specific AA supplementation may be most important.

Although the timing of any protein or AA ingestion related to exercise plays a role (Lemon *et al.*, 2002), the total quantity consumed in a day may be most important (Schoenfeld *et al.*, 2013). In the case of strength training an intake of ~20–25g of a high quality protein source within one hour following exercise appears to produce the maximum rate of muscle protein synthesis, at least in acute studies with young adults, whereas the amount to induce the same response in older adults is 35–40g (Moore *et al.*, 2012; Kakigi *et al.*, 2014; Pennings *et al.*, 2012; Yang *et al.*, 2012a). Also, it has been suggested that ingestion pattern (evenly spaced intakes throughout the day of ~20–30g protein per meal; 3 times/day) might be the best approach to maximize muscle protein synthesis (Moore *et al.*, 2012; Areta *et al.*, 2013; Mamerow *et al.*, 2014). However, these studies may not reflect net protein anabolism because protein breakdown must be considered (Deutz and Wolfe, 2013). Further, it has been shown that these acute increased muscle protein synthesis measurements after a bout of strength exercise do not correlate well with long-term hypertrophy (Mitchell *et al.*, 2014), indicating that other factors are involved. Clearly, therefore, the adaptations to strength training are more complicated. For example, desensitization with training may create a need for a greater AA intake for the same response (Bucci *et al.*, 1990; Fogelholm *et al.*, 1993a; Lambert *et al.*, 1993). Consequently, long-term training studies (months or even years) are needed to confirm AA or protein intake recommendations for physically active individuals.

Finally, whenever individual AA are consumed, concerns arise because an imbalance with other AA is possible. Therefore, caution is recommended until these dietary recommendations can be confirmed. Amino acids that have been researched individually or in combination as an ingredient of a supplement will each be the focus of separate articles in this book.

Competing interests   None

γ-AMINOBUTYRIC ACID (GABA)

Romain Meeusen and Bart Roelands

γ-aminobutyric acid (GABA) is synthesized through the decarboxylation of glutamate by the enzyme glutamatic acid decarboxylase. Glutamate is the main excitatory neurotransmitter, and GABA is the major inhibitory neurotransmitter in the mature brain. GABA acts primarily by activating CL^- channels called $GABA_A$ receptors, and by eliciting metabotropic G-protein mediated responses by $GABA_B$ receptors (Kornau, 2006; Möhler, 2006). GABA is considered to act as a natural tranquilizer and anti-epileptic agent in the brain.

$GABA_A$ receptors are the site of action of benzodiazepines, barbiturates and anaesthetics (Whiting et al., 2001) and known to mediate sedation. $GABA_B$ agonists may be useful for the treatment of pain and drug dependence (Kornau, 2006). Baclofen, the first synthetic $GABA_B$ receptor agonist, is used clinically for the treatment of spasticity and skeletal muscle rigidity (Bowery, 1993). $GABA_B$ antagonists on the other hand have shown antidepressant and cognition-enhancing effects (Cryan and Kaupmann, 2005; Kornau, 2006). Furthermore, recent data (Banuelos et al., 2014) suggest that the age-related dysregulation of GABAergic signalling in the prefrontal cortex may play a crucial role in impaired working memory, making $GABA_B$ a potential target to provide a therapeutic benefit for age-related impairments in cognitive function.

In rats, baclofen has shown to prolong time to fatigue, possibly because of a boost in glycogen due to the effect of IL-6 release in the muscle (Abdelmalki et al., 1997). In humans, on the other hand, Collomp et al. (1985) found no effect on performance after administration of lorazepam (a benzodiazepine drug). Recently it was shown that GABA ingestion at rest increases immunoreactive growth hormone (irGH) and immunofunctional GH secretion (ifGH), which may enhance the skeletal muscle response to resistance training. Moreover, when GABA ingestion was combined with exercise, concentrations of irGH and ifGH rose even higher (Powers et al., 2007). Although some effects have been found, specifically for the response to resistance training, much more research regarding the effects of GABAergic manipulations on exercise performance is needed to elucidate the role of GABA.

Competing interests None

ANDROSTENEDIONE ('ANDRO' OR 'DIONE')

Gregory A. Brown, Matthew D. Vukovich and Douglas S. King

Androstenedione ('Andro' or 'DIONE'), an androgenic steroid hormone that is a precursor to testosterone, was marketed in the late 1990s and early 2000s as a 'natural' alternative to anabolic steroid use. Androstenedione was purported to raise blood testosterone levels and subsequently promote muscle size and strength.

A review of the research on androstenedione supplementation published between 1999 and 2006 (Brown *et al.*, 2006) concluded that it does not support the efficacy or safety of this product. In young men, a single dose of 100–200mg Andro does not increase blood testosterone levels or stimulate muscle protein synthesis, and chronic intake of 100mg Andro (three times per day for eight weeks or twice per day for 12 weeks) does not augment increases in muscle size and strength during resistance training. Although a single dose of 300mg Andro may raise blood testosterone levels slightly (~15%) in young men, it is unlikely that this increase in testosterone would increase muscle size or strength. In women and middle-aged men, Andro intake raises blood testosterone levels, although an anabolic effect of androstenedione has not been demonstrated in either population.

Chronic supplementation with Andro may pose significant health risks. High density lipoprotein cholesterol is reduced with chronic Andro intake, corresponding to a 10–15% increase in cardiovascular disease risk. Andro intake raises blood dihydrotestosterone and oestrogen levels, which have been linked to benign prostate hypertrophy, baldness, increased risk of cardiovascular disease, various forms of cancer, and gynaecomastia in men. High blood levels of androstenedione may increase the risk for prostate cancer and pancreatic cancer as well as cause neural/behavioural changes such as increased hostility.

Androstenedione was explicitly included as an illegal androgenic hormone in the 2004 revision of the United States Anabolic Steroid Control Act, and has subsequently largely disappeared from the market and research. However, other hormones of structural similarity with other names can be found in nutritional supplements marketed towards weightlifters and body builders, and these products are largely of unknown safety or efficacy. In summary, androstenedione has not been demonstrated to produce either anabolic or ergogenic effects in supplement form at supraphysiological doses. There is also strong evidence of dose and time-related widespread adverse effects resulting in several negative health consequences. Androstenedione is classified as an androgenic/anabolic steroid and included on the WADA Prohibited List (WADA, 2014a).

Competing interests   None

ANTIOXIDANTS

Andreas N. Kavazis and John C. Quindry

Over the last 30+ years a wealth of scientific evidence has clearly demonstrated that physical exercise results in elevated free radical production in active skeletal muscle. Understanding free radical generation during exercise is important because 1) excess free radical production during exercise can result in oxidative stress, and 2) free radicals can contribute to muscular fatigue during exercise (Powers and Jackson, 2008). This collective knowledge has motivated many athletes to use dietary antioxidant supplements as a means to prevent exercise-induced free radical stress and/or muscular fatigue. To date, however, the scientific evidence to support effective use of dietary antioxidants to prevent oxidative stress or muscular fatigue is equivocal. To understand whether supplementation with dietary antioxidants is efficacious in athletic applications, one must first address the following two questions: 1) is exercise-induced oxidative stress a bad occurrence? and 2) can dietary antioxidant supplement use prevent or prolong fatigue during exercise? This review summarises current understanding of exercise-induced oxidative stress with the purpose of addressing a perceived need to consume dietary antioxidants by many athletes and physically active individuals. The review begins with an overview of key terms and concepts related to free radical biology and antioxidants.

Free radical biology and antioxidants – key terms

Free radicals are molecules that contain one or more unpaired electrons in the outer orbital. Free radicals are formed by either losing or gaining an electron in reactions with other molecules (Halliwell and Gutteridge, 2007). Because most of the free radicals of importance to biological organisms are oxygen-centred, the term reactive oxygen species (ROS) is used to include radicals and non-radicals, and reactive derivatives of oxygen (e.g. hydrogen peroxide). Reactive oxygen species are chemically unstable and can damage important cellular constituents including proteins, lipids and DNA. ROS-mediated damage is termed 'oxidative damage' and results in cellular dysfunction.

Coined in 1985, 'oxidative stress' is a collective term that describes a prooxidant:antioxidant imbalance that favours oxidants (Powers and Jackson, 2008). In theory, oxidative stress can be caused by ROS over-production or antioxidant depletion. Independent of cause, a scientific hallmark of oxidative stress is the appearance of oxidative damage biomarkers (e.g. oxidized proteins and/or lipids). Oxidative stress is commonly quantified by the observance of increased oxidative damage markers and/or the decrease in antioxidant content within blood or muscle tissue.

Fundamental question 1: is exercise-induced oxidative stress a bad occurrence?

The notion that exercise-induced oxidative stress could be a bad occurrence seems at clear odds with undeniable evidence that regular participation in exercise or physical activity is a potent lifestyle factor for improved morbidity and mortality outcomes. While chronic oxidative stress is a cornerstone of most disease states, exercise-induced oxidative stress is a transient occurrence. Specifically, recent data suggest that the exercise-induced spike in ROS production is short-lived by biological design, in that many of the tell-tale adaptive responses to exercise training require a spike in ROS (Powers and Jackson, 2008).

If exercise-induced ROS are central to beneficial adaptations, the next logical question is what factor(s) keeps oxidative stress in check, preventing exercise from inducing pathology? Cells throughout the body have several systems in place to counteract ROS production during exercise. For example, myofibres contain a network of enzymatic and non-enzymatic antioxidant defence mechanisms used to attenuate oxidative damage. In the context of this review, an antioxidant will be defined as any substance that delays or prevents oxidative damage to a target molecule (Powers and Jackson, 2008). Enzymatic and non-enzymatic antioxidants work in concert with dietary antioxidants (e.g. vitamin C and vitamin E) serving to 'replenish the antioxidant machine'. Cooperative interaction between dietary and endogenous antioxidants has fuelled the notion that antioxidant supplementation is needed to boost the muscle fibres' ability to scavenge ROS and protect against exercise-induced oxidative stress and fatigue. Based on current understanding, however, it is presumptuous to assume that dietary antioxidant supplementation beyond recommended daily allowance (RDA) is needed to fortify antioxidant defences in athletes.

Fundamental question 2: can dietary antioxidant supplement use prevent or prolong fatigue during exercise?

Muscle fatigue is defined as an acute reduction in the ability of a muscle to generate force. Exercise-induced muscle fatigue is a multi-faceted process and the specific causes of fatigue vary. Growing evidence indicates that ROS production is among the most important contributors to muscular fatigue during prolonged submaximal exercise (i.e. events lasting >30 minutes). Interestingly, levels of ROS production in contracting skeletal muscle represent a 'double-edged sword'. Low levels of ROS in active skeletal muscle are required to achieve optimum force production, while high ROS levels induce oxidative damage to muscle proteins that can diminish muscle force production. Findings from well-controlled animal studies indicate that scavenging ROS via exogenous antioxidants protects skeletal muscle against oxidative damage and delays fatigue during prolonged submaximal exercise. By contrast, antioxidant scavengers are ineffective in delaying muscle fatigue in animals performing high-intensity exercise (Powers and Jackson, 2008).

Following on from these findings in animal studies, the next important question is, do ROS also contribute to exercise-induced muscular fatigue in humans? The answer to this question remains under debate. However, preliminary conclusions can be drawn from numerous human studies in which supplementation with the antioxidant N-acetylcysteine has been shown to delay muscle fatigue during submaximal exercise including submaximal electrical stimulation of human limb muscle, cycle exercise and repetitive handgrip contractions (Powers and Jackson, 2008). The proposed pathway by which N-acetylcysteine delays fatigue involves support of glutathione resynthesis via an enhancement of muscle cysteine and glutathione availability. In less complex terms, glutathione is thought to be one of the most important non-enzymatic antioxidants in the antioxidant network (see section on GSH). It should be noted, however, that human studies have failed to show a benefit of N-acetylcysteine supplementation during intense exercise which approached VO_{2max} (Powers and Jackson, 2008). More importantly, optimism regarding the use of N-acetylcysteine as an ergogenic aid is severely challenged by the fact that its use in humans is associated with numerous side effects that are likely to counter any performance advantages due to antioxidant fortification (see section on NAC). The evidence that commonly used antioxidant supplements (e.g. beta carotene, vitamin E and/or vitamin C) improve human exercise performance by reducing muscular fatigue is less promising (Powers et al., 2004). In summary, there is some evidence that supplementation with N-acetylcysteine may be able to increase performance during prolonged exercise in humans, but there is limited support for performance benefits from supplementation with vitamin C, vitamin E, or beta carotene (see section on vitamins A, C andE).

Does exercise increase the need for dietary antioxidants?

Regardless of whether antioxidants delay muscular fatigue, advocates of antioxidant supplementation for athletes argue that rigorous exercise training results in increased ROS production in skeletal muscle. Therefore, they maintain that antioxidant supplements are required to protect skeletal muscle fibres against oxidative stress. While this logic appears reasonable, numerous arguments oppose a conclusion of an established need for antioxidant supplementation in athletes. First, there is currently no clear evidence that exercise-induced ROS production in skeletal muscle is detrimental to human health. Second, regular exercise training promotes natural fortification of enzymatic and non-enzymatic antioxidants in muscle fibres. The increase in endogenous antioxidants in exercised muscle appears to be sufficient to protect against exercise-induced oxidative stress. As such, for athletes who consume an appropriate energy intake from nutrient-dense food choices, scientific consensus holds that antioxidant supplementation is unnecessary. Given this understanding, the one plausible circumstance in which supplemental dietary antioxidants may be warranted is individual cases of nutrient deficiencies (e.g. antioxidant status below the normal range for good health). This exception to our broader understanding of exercise and oxidative stress is sometimes supported by investigations of the dietary practices of athletes.

The next important question that may be posed by athletes who are eager to gain an advantage over their competitors is whether dietary antioxidants should be consumed on the off-chance that nutrient deficiencies exist. Herein are perhaps the two strongest arguments against the case for antioxidant supplementation in athletes and physically active individuals. There is emerging evidence that antioxidant supplementation mitigates important exercise-induced adaptations in skeletal muscle. This recent discovery supports the well-established understanding that exercise-induced ROS production is a potent cellular signal promoting the expression of numerous skeletal muscle proteins including antioxidant enzymes, mitochondrial proteins and heat shock proteins (Powers et al., 2010a). Thus, while antioxidant supplementation won't prevent exercise adaptations, there is evidence that the magnitude of the exercise adaptations is lessened in the presence of dietary antioxidant supplements.

A recent illustration of this effect was provided by the observation that 11 weeks of daily supplementation with 1,000mg vitamin C and 235mg vitamin E blunted the endurance training-induced increase in mitochondrial biogenesis needed for improving muscular endurance (Paulsen et al., 2014). This report confirms the outcomes of the two frequently cited studies which first demonstrated that chronic supplementation with vitamins E and C attenuated the training adaptation to exercise (Gomez-Cabrera et al., 2008; Ristow et al., 2009). Furthermore, although N-acetylcysteine supplementation may acutely delay muscle fatigue during submaximal exercise (as discussed above), it also disrupts the exercise-induced inflammatory response and repair capability within skeletal muscle by blunting activation of redox-sensitive signalling pathways (Michailidis et al., 2013). See section on vitamins A, C and E.

A second key argument against antioxidant supplementation in athletes is that existing research does not support the notion that antioxidant supplementation benefits human health. A meta-analysis of 68 randomized antioxidant supplement trials (total of 232,606 human participants) reported that, independent of dose, dietary supplementation with beta carotene, vitamin A and vitamin E does not improve health outcomes and appears to be associated with increased mortality (Bjelakovic et al., 2007). Given these findings, the authors wisely concluded a need to understand better the roles of vitamin C and selenium supplementation on human mortality before recommendations can be made.

Summary

The question of whether or not athletes should use antioxidant supplements remains an important and highly debated topic of interest to the health, fitness and athletic communities (Powers *et al.*, 2009). Arguments for and against antioxidant supplementation persist and, in order to gain a better understanding on this topic, additional research is required. However, it is clear that physical exercise results in a transient oxidative stress that is a cornerstone of the adaptive stimulus to exercise. Consumption of supplemental dietary antioxidants attenuates exercise-induced oxidative stress, but also mitigates the benefits of ROS-induced adaptations to exercise training. Therefore, scientists from exercise and nutritional disciplines should join with practitioners to educate athletes about the current scientific understanding regarding antioxidant supplements and exercise-induced oxidative stress. Education efforts should be strategic and be ever mindful of consumer demand for pill-based solutions to complex problems like performance enhancement.

Competing interests   None

ARGININE

Robert R. Wolfe and Eric A. Newsholme*

Arginine is a conditionally essential amino acid ($C_6H_{14}N_4O_2$). It is found in a wide variety of protein-rich foods, including both animal and plant sources. Arginine is an amino acid that serves functions of relevance to athletes. It is not only required for protein synthesis but also plays a role in regulating protein synthesis (Zhang *et al.*, 2008). In addition, arginine is a precursor for the production of the messenger molecule nitric oxide, an important vasodilator and also for creatine. Arginine can remove ammonia from the blood, which may be important in recovery from hard training. Finally, the ingestion of arginine can stimulate the secretion of growth hormone and the recovery of muscles after exercise.

Supplementation with arginine could be expected to enhance the response to training but may be particularly important to aid recovery from severe training sessions. Under normal conditions blood flow during aerobic exercise is sufficient and arginine supplementation has no beneficial effect (Liu *et al.*, 2009). However, blood flow through tendon connective tissue is normally poor and may not provide nutrients sufficiently rapidly for cells to repair stressed or damaged tendons during training. Arginine supplementation increases blood flow due to the provision of nitric oxide (Nagaya *et al.*, 2001). Recovery is dependent upon the activity of the tendon cells, which must be provided with oxygen and nutrients.

The ability of arginine to stimulate creatine synthesis and growth hormone secretion could enhance muscle gain from resistance training. Studies have shown varying results, perhaps because the dose of ingested arginine is often insufficient (Wagenmakers, 1999). Effects of arginine supplementation on strength gains during training may be related to the naturally occurring level of arginine. Beneficial effects of arginine supplementation on muscle strength may be minimal in young, healthy men who are already eating plenty of protein. If further research is undertaken, it might be prudent to focus on groups who wish to improve muscle strength without increasing the amount of muscle and therefore body weight (e.g. lightweight rowers, boxers, endurance runners).

Competing interests None

---

* Tribute to Professor Eric Arthur Newsholme can be found after Glutamine review.

ARNICA

Edzard Ernst

Arnica Montana is a herbaceous plant, native to many regions of Europe. Its flowering heads have been used for medicinal purposes for millennia. Arnica extracts contain sesquiterpene lactones, volatile oils and flavonoids. They are said to have anti-inflammatory and anti-microbial activity. The former property has rendered arnica preparations popular remedies for sports injuries. There are two fundamentally different types of arnica preparations: herbal and homeopathic.

Herbal arnica is administered topically, because arnica can be neurotoxic when given orally (Venkatramani *et al.*, 2013). Unfortunately, only a few trials testing herbal arnica are currently available. A recent randomized clinical trial (RCT) of topical arnica used after intense eccentric exercise failed to demonstrate an effect on performance or blood markers (Pumpa *et al.*, 2014). Another RCT even suggested that, rather than decreasing pain, arnica would increase delayed onset muscle soreness (DOMS) (Adkison *et al.*, 2010). A further RCT of topical arnica suggested this preparation to be not inferior to ibuprofen when treating pain caused by osteoarthritis of the hands (Widrig *et al.*, 2007). Finally, an RCT suggested that topical arnica reduced bruising more effectively than placebo (Leu *et al.*, 2010).

Homeopathic arnica preparations are typically highly diluted, often to the extent that they don't contain a single molecule of the original arnica extract. Thus they are safe for oral administration. Homeopathic arnica has been tested in several clinical trials, most frequently as a treatment of DOMS. The results of these studies are contradictory. Two independent systematic reviews are available concluding that the effectiveness of homeopathic arnica is unproven (Ernst and Pittler, 1998; Lüdtke and Hacke, 2005). An RCT which was published after these systematic reviews also failed to demonstrate any effect of homeopathic arnica (Plezbert and Burke, 2005), while another trial seemed to show a small positive effect on DOMS (Tveiten and Bruset, 2003). An RCT suggested that arnica D4, a homeopathic potency that still does contain active molecules, might promote postoperative wound healing (Karow *et al.*, 2008). However, the evidence whether homeopathic arnica is beneficial for patients after surgery is highly contradictory (Brinkhaus *et al.*, 2006) and our own study of both low and high dilution homeopathic arnica failed to show effectiveness of either preparation (Stevinson *et al.*, 2003). Despite this inconclusive evidence, the Medicines and Healthcare Products Regulatory Agency (MHRA) issued a licence for a homeopathic arnica preparation for the treatment of minor injuries. In conclusion, there is little compelling evidence that herbal or homeopathic arnica preparations have a role in sports medicine.

Competing interests   None

ASPARTAME

Peter J. Rogers

Aspartame ($C_{14}H_{18}N_2O_5$) is an example of an intense or non-nutritive sweetener and an ingredient of many thousands of drink and food products consumed worldwide. It is a methyl ester of a dipeptide composed of the amino acids aspartic acid and phenylalanine, which are constituents of all protein-containing foods. Aspartame is about 180 times sweeter than sucrose with, for most individuals, minimal bitterness and a good quality of sweet taste. Being composed of amino acids it has an energy value of 4 kcal/g; however at the concentrations needed to sweeten foods and drinks its nutritive value is negligible. In products it may be blended with one or more other intense sweeteners (e.g. acesulfame K and sucralose) and/or with sugars, including sucrose, fructose and glucose.

The safety of aspartame has been the subject of much, often ill-informed, debate. After ingestion, aspartame is broken down to its constituent amino acids and methanol, and some further minor products. Even at high dietary intakes of aspartame, the amount of methanol produced is too small to be harmful. Because high intakes of phenylalanine are undesirable for those born with phenylketonuria (Acosta and Elsas, 1999), products with aspartame may contain information such as 'contains a source of phenylalanine'. A recent comprehensive review concluded that 'The weight of existing evidence is that aspartame is safe at current levels of consumption as a nonnutritive sweetener' (Magnuson *et al.*, 2007).

By replacing sugars in products, intense sweeteners can potentially aid control of energy intake and weight, but the extent of any benefit would appear to be dependent on the context of use (Mattes and Popkin, 2009). The clearest evidence concerns the use of intense sweeteners, including aspartame, to replace sugar in drinks. Results show that this results in lower overall energy intake and lower body weight or reduced weight gain (de la Hunty *et al.*, 2006). Drinks sweetened with aspartame do not increase energy intake compared with water (Daniels and Popkin, 2010). Additionally, aspartame reduces appetite independent of its sweet taste in the mouth. This is demonstrated by studies in which aspartame was consumed in capsules (Rogers *et al.*, 1990). The physiological basis of this effect, which is not shared by other intense sweeteners, is currently unknown.

Aspartame, and other intense sweeteners, are used in sport drinks to allow adjustment of nutrient profile and tonicity, whilst maintaining a pleasant level of sweetness. The flavour and sweetness of such products are important for motivating consumption, and thereby achieving desired levels of hydration and nutrient intake.

Competing interests None

ASPARTATE AND ASPARAGINE

François Trudeau and Rui Curi

Aspartate (ASP) is a non-essential amino acid ($C_4H_7NO_4$) which is found in the L- or the D- form. The normal daily requirement of L-aspartate in humans is ~2g. It is found mainly in meat, fish, seafood (0.6–2.6g/100g), cheese (1.2–2.9g/100g) and eggs (1.3–1.5g/100g) and less so in plant sources (USDA, 2009). The main purported ergogenic effects of ASP supplementation are attenuation of exercise-induced hyperammonaemia and increased exercise endurance. The D-aspartate enantiomer and N-methyl-D-aspartate (NMDA) are thought to increase testosterone secretion.

L-aspartate: Support for an ergogenic effect of L-aspartate supplementation can be found in six rat studies which showed increased time to exhaustion from 14.5% to 111%. However, this is counterbalanced by one dog and six rat studies which failed to find a positive effect on endurance exercise (Trudeau, 2008). This 2008 review of the available literature on humans identified that the first study of L-aspartate supplementation reported a 50.5% increase in time to exhaustion (Ahlborg *et al.*, 1965). It also noted that two further studies reported increased exercise capacity in the order of 14–16%, while another five studies reported the absence of effects on endurance exercise (Trudeau, 2008). No correlation was found between the dosage of ASP and changes in exercise capacity. Neither were the claims of glycogen-sparing, reduced hyperammonaemia or higher rate of free fatty acid oxidation as a result of L-aspartate supplementation confirmed by the literature.

In rats, the combination of asparagine ($C_4H_8N_2O_3$) and L-aspartate supplementation has been shown to result in a significant reduction in blood lactate levels, a decreased degradation of skeletal muscle and liver glycogen content and an increase in exercise endurance (Lancha *et al.*, 1995; Marquezi *et al.*, 2003). However, a study performed in triathletes failed to find evidence of glycogen sparing or enhanced capacity for high-intensity (90% VO_{2max}) exercise (Parisi *et al.*, 2007).

D-aspartate: Studies of a 28-day resistance training programme, supplemented with either NMDA (Willoughby *et al.*, 2014) or D-aspartate (Willoughby and Leutholtz, 2013) failed to find evidence of an enhancement of hormonal profile (testosterone, luteinizing hormone or oestradiol), or muscle strength and mass.

Competing interests None

D-ASPARTIC ACID (D-AA)

Jason C. Siegler and Geoffrey W. Melville

D-aspartic acid (D-AA) is an α-amino acid and is one of the two isoforms of aspartic acid. In mammals it is found in tissues and cells of the central nervous and endocrine systems (D'Aniello, 2007; Furuchi and Homma, 2005). D-AA is believed to stimulate the production and release of testosterone through multiple pathways of the hypothalamic-pituitary-gonadal axis. Supplementation of d-aspartic acid has been reported to increase luteinizing hormone and total testosterone levels in male IVF patients, whereas *in vitro* animal studies have demonstrated increased levels of testosterone, luteinizing hormone, progesterone and growth hormone (D'Aniello *et al.*, 1996, 2000).

D-AA is widely available as a sports supplement, marketed as a testosterone booster for increasing strength and inducing hypertrophy. Currently there is very little scientific evidence available in healthy human populations (Topo *et al.*, 2009; Willoughby and Leutholtz, 2013). Only one study has investigated its efficacy in athletes, but failed to show increases in total and free testosterone levels or strength and hypertrophy gains, following 3g/day D-AA for one month in resistance-trained males (Willoughby and Leutholtz, 2013). Further research is needed to determine if D-AA is a viable option for increasing testosterone in athletes, and whether any such increases translate into strength or hypertrophic gains.

Competing interests   None

BEE POLLEN

Stephen Gurr

Bee pollen is a mixture collected by bees of pollen granules from the stamens of flowers and flower nectar. It is commercially available in granule, capsule or tablet preparations. These contain a wide and varying array of nutrients, including saccharides, amino acids, vitamins and minerals, as well as possible contaminants.

Despite a long history in traditional medicine as a 'superfood', there is little evidence to support the range of health claims for bee pollen. Interest in its ergogenic properties stems from anecdotal reports and testimonies from successful athletes (Williams *et al.*, 1985). However, the few available studies from the 70s and 80s involving athletes and bee pollen supplementation (3–12-week protocols following manufacturers' recommended doses) have found minimal effects on: haemoglobin concentrations (Steben and Boudreaux, 1978), strength and aerobic capacity (Maughan and Evans, 1982), perceived exertion (Woodhouse *et al.*, 1987), time trial performance (Steben and Boudreaux, 1978), or repeated high-intensity exercise (Woodhouse *et al.*, 1987). One study (Maughan and Evans, 1982) did note fewer days lost to respiratory infections in swimmers supplementing with bee pollen.

Allergic reactions including anaphylaxis have been reported in people taking bee pollen supplements (Mansfield and Goldstein, 1981). The limited empirical research suggests that bee pollen supplementation affords no additional benefit to athletic performance beyond that provided by a balanced diet.

Competing interests   None

β-ALANINE AND CARNOSINE

Craig Sale and Roger C. Harris

Carnosine (β-alanyl-L-histidine, a dipeptide of β-alanine and histidine) is abundant in human muscle, with normal levels being 20–25 mmol·kg-1dm (Mannion *et al.*, 1992) and with type II muscle fibres having 1.5–2.0 times higher concentrations than type I fibres (Hill *et al.*, 2007). The imidazole ring of the histidine located in the carnosine molecule has a pKa of 6.83, making it an effective intramuscular buffer across the exercise-induced pH transit range.

Carnosine is synthesised in muscle by carnosine synthase and degraded by the extracellular dipeptidase, carnosinase. Synthesis in muscle is limited by the availability of β-alanine, produced from uracil degradation in the liver, which can be augmented through the hydrolysis of ingested carnosine found in meat, and by direct dietary supplementation. Deprived of a dietary source, vegetarians have lower muscle carnosine concentrations than meat eaters (Everaert *et al.*, 2011; Harris *et al.*, 2007), with Harris *et al.* reporting ~10–14 mmol.kg-1 dm.

Four weeks of dietary supplementation with β-alanine increased carnosine content of skeletal muscle by 40–60% (Harris *et al.*, 2006); with Hill *et al.* (2007) showing an 80% increase after 10 weeks. In the latter study, muscle content exceeded 40 mmol·kg-1dm but it is unknown as to whether there is a ceiling for muscle carnosine content. The increase occurred equally in muscle fibre types, despite higher concentrations in type II. When β-alanine supplementation ceases, muscle carnosine concentration declines slowly back towards the baseline (Baguet *et al.*, 2009), with a half-life of approximately nine weeks (Harris *et al.*, 2009). Stegen *et al.* (2014) showed that a 30–50% elevation in muscle carnosine concentration, following six weeks β-alanine supplementation at 3.2g·d-1, can be maintained with a dose of 1.2g·d-1.

Trained athletes have higher muscle carnosine concentrations than their untrained counterparts (Bex *et al.*, 2014), although training alone has little effect on muscle carnosine concentrations and acute training has no additional effect on the increase in muscle carnosine with β-alanine supplementation (Kendrick *et al.*, 2008, 2009). β-alanine supplementation seems every bit as effective in improving high-intensity cycling performance in trained as in untrained subjects (de Salles Painelli *et al.*, 2014).

The capacity to undertake strenuous cycle exercise increases with the increase in muscle carnosine following supplementation (Hill *et al.*, 2007). Total work done in a cycle exercise test performed at 110% power max (expected duration of two to four min) increased by 13% after four weeks (mean increase in muscle carnosine, 58.8%) and 16.2% after ten weeks (mean increase in muscle carnosine, 80.1%), with Sale *et al.* (2011) showing a similar effect of β-alanine on the same test. Evidence from Baguet *et al.* (2010) suggests that this is likely mediated via an effect on intramuscular pH buffering, since they showed β-alanine attenuated the reduction in blood pH during high-intensity exercise, without affecting blood lactate or bicarbonate concentrations. In line with this hypothesis, the majority of the ergogenic effects of β-alanine have been reported on high-intensity exercise lasting between two and six minutes and rarely on single efforts shorter than this or on repeated sprint performance (Sale *et al.*, 2013). A meta-analysis of 15 studies (Hobson *et al.*, 2012) found that β-alanine supplementation enhances exercise of this nature with a moderate effect size of 0.37 (0.14–0.75).

Competing interests   None

BORON

Nigel Mitchell and Joseph Lockey

Boron, an element with the atomic number 5, is an essential nutrient for plants but the physiological role in humans is not fully understood. Boron can be considered as an ultra trace element, therefore requirements are low (Nielsen, 2008). Dietary daily human intake is estimated to range from 2.1–4.3mg boron/ kg body weight/day (Naghii, 1999).

Boron enters the food chain via its incorporation into plant structure and subsequent consumption by humans. There is little evidence of boron deficiency in humans, however oral boron supplementation is used in the general health and sports market.

Boron has been linked to increased endogenous testosterone levels but there are few reports on athletes to support this. Nielsen *et al.* (1987) investigated boron supplementation in postmenopausal women after a boron-restricted diet. Supplementation of 3mg/day was associated with an increase in testosterone levels. No proposed mechanism for increased testosterone was reported: however, the authors suggested that maintenance of adequate boron levels in postmenopausal women might prevent calcium loss and bone demineralisation. Indeed, Newnham (1994) found that 6mg/day significantly improved osteoarthritis symptoms in a small double-blind placebo-controlled study of 20 patients over just eight weeks.

Few studies have investigated the effects of boron supplementation on increasing testosterone levels in an athletic population. Ferrando and Green (1993) randomized participants who regularly weight trained for at least one year to either 2.5mg/day boron ($n=10$) or placebo ($n=9$) for seven weeks. The results suggested an increase in strength (based on one repetition maximum, squat and bench press), increases in lean tissue and testosterone in both groups. However, there was no evidence that boron supplementation had any additional effect. Therefore, the changes appeared to be due only to a training effect.

A 10-month boron supplementation study in young female athletes, vs. sedentary women, produced a modest effect on mineral status (Meacham *et al.*, 1995). This included a decrease in serum phosphorous and increased urinary calcium excretion which was greater in athletes than controls.

There is currently little evidence to support the use of boron supplementation in the athletic population.

Competing interests   None

BRANCHED CHAIN AMINO ACIDS

Eva Blomstrand

The three branched chain amino acids (BCAA; leucine, isoleucine and valine) are essential amino acids, that is, they cannot be synthesised by the human body and must therefore be provided in the diet. Food sources containing BCAA are dietary proteins such as meat, poultry, fish, eggs, milk and cheese, which contain 15–20g BCAA/100g protein. The BCAA are metabolised mainly in skeletal muscle, which means they largely escape uptake by the liver, and ingestion of BCAA causes a rapid increase in the plasma level.

The anabolic effect of BCAA on human skeletal muscle was first demonstrated under resting conditions, followed by studies showing similar effects in the recovery period after endurance exercise (Blomstrand and Saltin, 2001). More recent data indicate that the effect of BCAA is mediated through activation of regulatory enzymes in the protein synthesis machinery (Karlsson *et al.*, 2004). However, administration of BCAA may also reduce muscle proteolysis, which has been demonstrated both at rest and during eccentric exercise (Louard *et al.*, 1995; MacLean *et al.*, 1994). Moreover, recent data indicate that intake of BCAA can influence the gene expression of the muscle-specific ubiquitin ligases, MAFbx and MuRF-1, suggesting a possible inhibitory effect of BCAA on breakdown of proteins involved in the degradation processes (Borgenvik *et al.*, 2012).

The BCAA can also influence the metabolism in the brain, such as the synthesis of neurotransmitters. The rate-limiting step in the synthesis of 5-hydroxytryptamine (5-HT) is the transport of the precursor tryptophan across the blood-brain barrier (see section on tryptophan). The large neutral amino acids share a common transport mechanism into the brain and competition for entry may occur (Fernstrom and Wurtman, 1972). Increasing the plasma concentration of BCAA during exercise may therefore reduce the transport of tryptophan into the brain and the synthesis of 5-HT (Choi *et al.*, 2013). 5-HT has been suggested to be involved in central fatigue, that is, fatigue emanating from the brain rather than muscle (Newsholme *et al.*, 1992). BCAA supplementation to human subjects during sustained physical activity has exerted positive effects on cognitive performance and perceived exertion (Blomstrand *et al.*, 1997; Portier *et al.*, 2008). Under certain conditions, ingestion of BCAA can also improve physical performance, although the majority of studies have found no effect of BCAA on performance when supplied together with carbohydrates (Meeusen *et al.*, 2006).

The amount of BCAA recommended is 0.03–0.05g/kg bodyweight/hour or 2–4g/hour ingested repeatedly during exercise and recovery, preferably taken as a drink. Large doses of BCAA (~30g/day) are well tolerated; however, they may be detrimental to performance due to increased production of ammonia by the exercising muscle.

Competing interests None

CAFFEINE

Louise M. Burke and Lawrence L. Spriet

Caffeine has been used as an aid to sports performance for more than a century and studied by exercise scientists for half of this. From 1980–2003 it was included on the list of substances banned by the International Olympic Committee, with a urinary caffeine threshold above which it would be deemed to be a doping offence. This threshold was intended to discriminate against the intake of large caffeine doses – typically, above 6–9mg/kg body mass (BM). In 2004, however, caffeine was removed from the List of Prohibited Substances and Methods of the World Anti-Doping Agency allowing athletes who compete under this code to consume caffeine, either in their background diets or intentionally for performance enhancement, without fear of sanctions.

Several aspects about caffeine are intriguing and differ from other ergogenic aids. First, caffeine exerts positive effects over a diverse range of exercise protocols. It can increase *endurance* during sub-maximal exercise (> 90 min), sustain high-intensity work (20–60 minutes) and short duration (one to five min) supra-maximal exercise (Graham, 2001). More importantly to athletes, laboratory and field studies (Burke, 2008; Burke *et al.*, 2013) show that caffeine supplementation can enhance *performance* across a range of sports including endurance events, 'stop and go' events (e.g. team and racquet sports) and sustained high-intensity activities of one to 60 min (e.g. swimming, rowing, middle and distance running races). However, effects on a single effort involving strength and power such as lifts, throws and very brief sprints are unclear.

Second, the benefits of caffeine are achieved by a number of different protocols of use with variables including the timing and amount of caffeine intake. Although traditional regimens involved a single caffeine dose of ~6mg/kg BM, one hour pre-exercise (Graham, 2001), recent studies show that ergogenic effects of caffeine occur at very modest levels of intake (1–3mg/kg BM or 70–200mg caffeine)(Cox *et al.*, 2002; Kovacs *et al.*, 1998). In fact, it appears that benefits for endurance exercise plateau at ~3mg/kg or ~200mg doses (Cox *et al.*, 2002; Graham and Spriet, 1995; Kovacs *et al.*, 1998). The caffeine content of traditional sources (coffee, tea and cola drinks) is typically around 50–150mg/serving but some newer products can provide 300–500mg/serving. At least in endurance sports, caffeine can be consumed pre-event, as single or multiple doses spread throughout the event, or around the onset of fatigue (Cox *et al.*, 2002; Kovacs *et al.*, 1998). Caffeine has long-lasting effects; caffeine taken to enhance a morning exercise task was shown to also assist a session undertaken later in the day (Bell and McLellan, 2003).

Part of caffeine's intrigue is that, because of its numerous effects on body tissues, there has been some confusion about the exact mechanism by which it enhances performance. The principal effects are likely to occur via its chemical similarity to adenosine; by binding to adenosine receptors in many organs, as caffeine blocks the action of this ubiquitous chemical. Potentially beneficial effects include mobilisation of fat from adipose tissue and muscle, stimulation of the release and activity of adrenaline, effects on cardiac muscle, changes to muscle contractility, and central nervous system alterations which change perceptions of effort or fatigue (for review, see Burke *et al.*, 2013; Spriet, 1997). Most scientists believe this last factor is the most important and consistent factor in explaining performance enhancement. However, as with many drugs, individuals respond differently to caffeine, ranging from positive to negative outcomes, and some tissues become tolerant to repeated caffeine use while others do not. A range of polymorphisms in genes related to adenosine receptors or liver metabolism of caffeine have been identified, and account for some of the differences in habitual intake patterns (Cornelis *et al.*, 2007) as well as caffeine's performance benefits (Womack *et al.*, 2012). Further work in this area is needed.

Recent evidence has changed our perspective on two of the widely promoted effects of caffeine. Whereas caffeine was believed to enhance endurance exercise by increasing the utilisation of fat as a muscle substrate, thus reducing the reliance on limited muscle glycogen stores, studies now show that 'glycogen sparing' during sub-maximal exercise following caffeine intake is short-lived and inconsistent (Chesley *et al.*, 1998). Furthermore, despite warnings that caffeine-containing drinks have a diuretic effect leading to dehydration, moderate doses of caffeine actually have minor effects on urine losses or the overall hydration of habitual caffeine users (Armstrong, 2002). In addition, caffeine-containing drinks such as tea, coffee and cola provide a significant source of fluid in the everyday diets of many people (see Figure 13).

This table presents the caffeine content of the smallest commonly available serving size; caffeine in larger serving sizes can be multiplied up.

Traditionally, in caffeine research or in actual competition use, athletes withdraw from caffeine use for 24–48 hours prior to exercise to remove their habituation to repeated use. However, no consistent differences in the performance effects of caffeine between regular users and non-users of caffeine, or as a result of withdrawal from regular caffeine use are apparent (Graham, 2001). Indeed, a study which directly compared the effects of caffeine on a one-hour cycling time-trial, with or without a four-day withdrawal period, found that a 3mg/kg dose enhanced performance regardless of the preparation strategy (Irwin *et al.*, 2011). Avoiding or withdrawing caffeine prior to a performance trial may be associated with side-effects such as headaches and fatigue. In fact, there are suggestions that the benefits of caffeine seen in controlled studies may be overstated if they reflect the reversal of adverse withdrawal symptoms rather than an ergogenic effect of caffeine *per se* (James and Rogers, 2005). Withdrawal can also increase the risk that subsequent caffeine intake attracts the negative

Food or drink	Serving#	Caffeine content (mg)
Instant coffee	250 ml cup	60 (12–169)★
Brewed coffee	250 ml cup	80 (40–110)★
Brewed coffee (same outlet on different days)	250 ml cup	130–282★
Short black coffee/espresso from variety of outlets (AUS)	1 standard serving	107 (25–214)★
Starbucks Breakfast Blend brewed coffee (USA)	600 ml (Extra large size)	415 (256–564★)
Iced coffee – commercial brands (AUS)	500 ml bottle	30–200 depending on brand
Frappuccino	375 ml cup	90
Tea	250 ml cup	27 (9–51)★
Black tea	250 ml cup	25–110
Green tea	250 ml cup	30–50
Iced tea	600 ml bottle	20–40
Hot chocolate	250 ml cup	5–10
Coca Cola and Coke Zero	355 ml can (12 fl oz)	34
Pepsi Max	355 ml can	68
Pepsi	355 ml	38
Red Bull energy drink	250 ml can	80
V Energy drink (AUS/NZ)	500 ml can	155
Vitamin water – energy	500 ml bottle	82
Powerade Fuel+ sports drink	300 ml can	96
PowerBar caffeinated sports gel	40 g sachet	25–50
PowerBar caffeinated gel blasts	60 g pouch (~9 lollies)	75
Gu caffeinated sports gel	32 g sachet	20–40
Musashi Re-activate Hard core pre-workout supplement	15 g powder serving	120
Body Science (BSc) K-OS	13 g powder	150
Jack3D pre-workout	5 g powder	100
No-Xplode pre-workout	18 g	Not disclosed on label
BSc Hydroxyburn Hardcore fat burner	1 capsule	70
Shred Matrix fat burner	1 capsule	Not disclosed on label
Stay Alert chewing gum	1 stick	100
No Doz (USA)	1 tablet	200
No Doz (Australia)	1 tablet	100
Excedrin Extra Strength	1 tablet	65

FIGURE 13 Caffeine content of common foods, drinks and non-prescription preparations

★ Denotes range of values from studies in which standard servings of the same beverage were analysed.

Soda and energy drinks are available in a range of individual serving sizes ranging from 150ml–750ml.

effects often seen with large caffeine doses (irritability, tremor, heart rate increases).

In summary, there is clear evidence that caffeine is an ergogenic aid for a variety of sports, although studies involving elite athletes and field situations are lacking. Further research on individual trialling by athletes is needed to define the range of protocols or sports activities associated with benefits from caffeine supplementation, with particular interest in the concept that optimal outcomes are seen at small to moderate caffeine doses (2–3mg/kg). Such intake is well within the normal daily caffeine intakes of the general population justifying the decision to remove caffeine from the Prohibited List in sports as pragmatic. The views expressed here apply only to adult athletes who already consume caffeine within their normal dietary practices. It is inappropriate and unnecessary for children and adolescents to consume caffeine as an ergogenic aid, especially since younger populations have the potential for greater performance enhancement via their maturation in age and experience in their sport. In addition, there are worrying scenarios of excessive caffeine use and misuse in the general population as well as athletes. These include the use of exotic caffeine sources, e.g. fat-loss and pre-workout supplements with undisclosed doses of caffeine (often in combination with other stimulants), the vicious cycle of use of caffeine and sleeping tablets where one is used to counteract the effect of the other, and the use of caffeine to increase tolerance for excessive alcohol intake (Burke *et al.*, 2013). Although caffeine is generally regarded as a safe substance that provides benefits to everyday life when used appropriately, individuals should regularly examine their caffeine intake habits.

Conflict of interest   The authors declare their royalty rights to a book on the topic of *Caffeine and Sports Performance* (Human Kinetics Publishers, Champaign, Illinois, 2013).

CALCIUM

Linda K. Houtkooper and Melinda M. Manore

Adequate levels of calcium throughout life are critical to bone health although other nutrients are also important (USDHHS, 2004; IOM, 2011; Prentice, 1997). Much of the work on examining the effect of nutrition on bone health has focused on calcium and phosphorus, due to them being major constituents of bone tissue, and vitamin D due to its role in calcium absorption. Other trace elements, such as zinc, manganese and copper are necessary for growth, development and maintenance of healthy bones; whereas dietary components such as vitamin C, vitamin K, magnesium and fluoride have biological actions that are at the level of bone itself; with vitamins A and B_6 also being linked to bone (Prentice, 1997). See elsewhere in the book for key topics. Other nutrients are also important due to their influence on calcium absorption. While many nutrients play a role in bone health, this article will focus on calcium and the associated role of vitamin D.

Calcium is the fifth most abundant mineral in the human body, accounting for 1–2% of adult body weight, with over 99% of total body calcium being found in the inorganic phase of bones and teeth. The crystal structure of bone salt resembles hydroxyapatite $Ca_{10}(PO_4)_6(OH)_2$, which contains calcium and phosphorus in the proportion of 2.15:1g/g (Prentice and Bates, 1994). The remainder (~1%) of calcium is found in the blood, muscle and extracellular fluid. The plasma ionized calcium concentration is maintained within narrow limits by the complex and integrated hormonal regulation of intestinal calcium absorption, urinary calcium excretion, and bone formation and reabsorption.

Calcium enters the body via the diet and is absorbed depending on its interaction with other dietary constituents, and on physiological factors such as calcium-regulating hormones (in particular parathyroid hormone, calcitonin and 1,25-dihyroxyvitamin D) and age (see section on vitamin D). Calcium losses occur through urine, faeces and sweat. There are two routes of dietary calcium absorption in the intestine: one is an active, saturable, transcellular process that occurs mainly in the duodenum and proximal jejunum, and is regulated via the vitamin D endocrine system; the other is a passive, non-saturable, paracellular route that is independent of vitamin D regulation and occurs throughout the small and large intestines. Active calcium absorption is affected by the physiology of the individual, particularly their calcium and vitamin D status, and their age, being at its highest during infancy, puberty and pregnancy (Weaver, 1994). The amount of passive diffusion, however, depends primarily on its quantity and bioavailability, and therefore becomes more important at higher calcium levels. Overall, roughly 20% of dietary calcium is absorbed through various absorption and reabsorption routes. Although calcium losses through the skin are generally regarded as small (~15mg/day), they will increase substantially with severe sweating (see section on electrolytes).

The new 2011 U.S. and Canadian Dietary Reference Intakes (DRIs) and current UK Reference Nutrient Intakes (RNIs) for calcium listed in Figure 14 will meet the nutrient needs for most healthy adults, including athletes (IOM, 2011; Department of Health, 1991). Australia and New Zealand have similar DRI recommendations for these nutrients, with calcium recommendations for children and adults aged 9 to 70 years ranging from 1,000–1,300mg/day (Australian Government, 2006). The debate about calcium requirements has been going on for years, and is reflected in the differences in recommended intake levels for calcium, through the years and between national committees issuing the recommendations. There is no doubt that adequate intake of calcium is important for skeletal growth and bone mineralisation, especially during growth years if optimal peak bone mass is to be achieved. The concern is that many children and adolescents are not meeting the recommended calcium intakes (USDHHS, 2004; IOM, 2011). However, excessive nutrient intake does not have any additive benefit, and can have negative effects on health (USDHHS, 2004; IOM, 2011). Tolerable Upper Intake Levels (UL), which are the highest levels of daily nutrient intakes that are not likely to pose a risk of adverse health effects for almost all individuals in the general population, are listed in Figure 14. As intake increases above the UL, the potential risk of adverse effects increases (IOM, 2011). See section on vitamin D for further discussion regarding intake levels.

Nutrient	Life Stage Group	US/Canada RDA	United Kingdom RNI	Upper Limit
Calcium (mg/day)	1–3 y	700	350	2,500
	4–8 y	1,000	450 (4–6y)	2,500
	9–13y	1,300	550 (7–10y)	3,000
	14–18 y	1,300	800 (11–18y F)	3,000
			1,000 (11–18y M)	
	19–30 y	1,000	700 (≥19 y)	2,500
	31–50 y	1,000		2,500
	51–70 y M	1,000		2,000
	51–70y F	1,200		2,000
	>70y	1,200		2,000

FIGURE 14   Recommended dietary reference intakes for calcium

Key: mg = milligrams; RDA =Recommended Dietary Allowances; RNI = Recommended Nutrient Intakes; UL = Tolerable Upper Intake Levels; F = female; M = male.

Sources: IOM, 2011; Department of Health, 1991.

Calcium plays a major role in forming and maintaining healthy bone tissue (USDHHS, 2004; IOM, 2011; Palacios, 2006). The major food source for calcium is generally from dairy products (i.e. milk and milk products such as yoghurt and cheese, and foods prepared with milk), with other sources including green leafy vegetables, fruits, fish with bones, dried beans, calcium-rich mineral water and calcium-fortified foods. Low-fat or non-fat versions of milk and milk products have the same amount of calcium as whole milk, but lower fat content. In some countries, a few foods such as white flour (UK), cereal and orange juice are fortified with calcium. Fortification of white flour in the UK is historic due to it being added to bulk up flour during wartime, but has remained because of the additional health benefits.

The absorption of calcium from food depends on its bioavailability. The bioavailability from non-dairy sources is poor, which has led to the concern that individuals, including vegans, who avoid dairy products, may have low calcium intakes and therefore have compromised bone health. For example, active females and males who restrict energy intake to maintain a low body weight or eliminate food groups, especially dairy, are at risk for poor bone mass (Mountjoy et al., 2014; Nattiv et al., 2007). Higher intakes of calcium (1,500mg/day) and vitamin D (1,500–2,000mg/day) may be required, to restore bone loss in these individuals. One alternative source is calcium-rich mineral water, where the calcium has been shown to be as well absorbed and retained as that from milk (Heaney and Dowell, 1994; Couzy et al., 1995). Other food constituents affect the bioavailability of calcium, some increase it by either enhancing calcium absorption (e.g. calcium and vitamin D) or decreasing calcium excretion (e.g. boron and phosphate). In addition, some constituents can decrease its bioavailability by reducing calcium absorption (e.g. phytates, oxalates, phosphate and caffeine) or increasing calcium excretion (e.g. sulphur-rich proteins, sodium, caffeine) (see elsewhere in this book for some of these topics). However, it is a highly complex situation, with most evidence coming from balance studies that are fraught with methodological and interpretive issues, and hence the overall impact on calcium bioavailability is far from clear. In addition, some nutrients for example, phosphate, both increase and decrease calcium bioavailability, and so the overall effect is diminished. Furthermore, there seem to be differences between coffee and caffeine, with the detrimental effect of caffeine on calcium bioavailability being offset by increasing calcium intake through the addition of milk to coffee (Barger-Lux and Heaney, 1995). In contrast, high intakes of calcium may have adverse effects on the absorption of other nutrients, such as iron, zinc and magnesium (see elsewhere in the book for some of these topics). This needs to be taken into consideration when consuming any of these nutrients as dietary supplements. For this reason, it is important to consider consuming these dietary supplements outside meal times.

If necessary, calcium supplements can be taken to supplement dietary calcium. Several different kinds of calcium salts are used in calcium supplements, such as carbonate, citrate, gluconate and lactate, with calcium salt preparations being found to have at least as good calcium bioavailability as milk (Mortenson and Charles, 1996). The various calcium salts differ in amounts of mineral calcium, referred to as elemental calcium, with calcium carbonate being the highest (~40%) followed by calcium citrate (~20%). Although calcium citrate malate is considered slightly more soluble for some individuals (e.g. those with impaired HCl production), calcium carbonate supplements are inexpensive, commonly available and available in higher concentrations of elemental calcium. Absorption of calcium reaches a plateau at doses of about 500mg, therefore it is recommended that calcium tablets are better absorbed if provided in divided doses of not more than 400–500mg (Levenson and Brockman, 1994). It is also recommended that calcium supplements should be taken with meals in order to improve the reliability of absorption (Levenson and Brockman, 1994), but this does not take into account the adverse effects of extra calcium on the absorption of other minerals, especially iron, as discussed above. Potential side effects from calcium supplements include gastrointestinal bloating, constipation or gas, and are most commonly caused by calcium carbonate (NIH, 2014). However, rather confusingly, calcium carbonate is the active ingredient of indigestion medications.

In conclusion, since many nutrients in addition to calcium and vitamin D play a role in bone health, it is important to consume a nutritionally adequate diet containing a variety of food, rather than just focusing on one or two bone-related nutrients. A diet that contains vegetables, fruits, low-fat milk and milk products, whole grains and adequate levels of protein and calories to maintain a healthy body weight can provide the nutrients needed for the formation and maintenance of healthy bones. For otherwise healthy individuals, including athletes, if calcium or vitamin D needs are not met from foods and beverages, then supplements are recommended at levels that meet, but do not exceed, recommended intakes for these nutrients when added to intakes from foods. See section on vitamin D for further information on monitoring vitamin D levels if significant supplementation is required.

Competing interests None

CARBOHYDRATES

Ronald J. Maughan and Louise M. Burke

Carbohydrates are members of a large family of organic compounds composed of carbon, hydrogen and oxygen with the general formula $C_m(H_2O)_n$. Carbohydrates can exist as single molecules (monosaccharides) such as glucose (a six carbon sugar or hexose with the formula $C_6H_{12}O_6$), which can polymerise to form chains that vary in length from two (disaccharides) to tens of thousands of glucose units (polysaccharides). Sugars is the term used to refer to monosaccharides such as glucose (dextrose) and fructose (fruit sugar), and disaccharides such as sucrose (table sugar: one molecule of glucose and one of fructose) and lactose (milk sugar: glucose plus galactose). Five-carbon sugars (pentoses) include ribose, which forms an important part of several key molecules such as the adenine nucleotides (ATP, ATP and AMP) and ribonucleic acid (RNA). Glycogen, the storage form of carbohydrate in liver and in muscle, has a complex glucose polymer structure, and is in many ways similar to starch, which acts as a storage form of carbohydrate in plants. The polymerised form occupies much less space and, since it is almost insoluble, it can be stored without large amounts of extra water being retained by the cells.

The total amount of carbohydrate stored in the body is small, with a maximum of about 100g in the liver and 400–500g in the muscles: these amounts depend on the energy and carbohydrate content of the preceding diet, and will be reduced by fasting and by exercise. Liver glycogen can be broken down to glucose and released into the bloodstream where it is available to all tissues to act as a fuel. This is especially important for the brain, which relies heavily on blood glucose as a fuel, and for other tissues such as the red blood cells which, because of their lack of mitochondria, use blood glucose as their only substrate. The muscle store of glycogen is more immediately available when the muscles are called on to do work, but it is not so readily available to other tissues. Resting muscle can meet the majority of its energy demand by the oxidation of any available fuels, including fat as well as carbohydrate. During exercise, the rate of carbohydrate utilisation, and its contribution to the total fuel mix, varies according to a range of factors, including the intensity and duration of exercise, the training state of the athlete, the composition of the prior diet, and whether carbohydrate is ingested immediately prior to and during the exercise session (Maughan and Gleeson, 2010).

There are several ways in which body carbohydrate stores are critical for sports performance. In mammalian muscle fibres, the capacity for ATP resynthesis by oxidative metabolism using carbohydrate as a fuel is about twice as high as that when fat is used (see Figure 15). High power outputs can therefore be achieved

	Maximum rates of ATP resynthesis (μmol/min/gram muscle)
CP Hydrolysis	440
Lactate formation	180
CHO oxidation	40
Fat oxidation	20

FIGURE 15 Maximal rates of ATP resynthesis from different energy pathways

only when the carbohydrate availability is sufficient to meet the needs of the contracting muscle fibres. Carbohydrate is the primary fuel for high-intensity work when the metabolic demand requires the recruitment of high glycolytic muscle fibres; these fibres have a high glycolytic capacity relative to their capacity to oxidise the pyruvate generated by glycolysis: regeneration of NAD to allow glycolysis to continue is therefore achieved by conversion of a significant fraction of the pyruvate to lactate rather than via oxidation in the mitochondria. Inadequate muscle glycogen stores can therefore limit the performance of single or repeated high-intensity bouts of only a few minutes duration. At moderate exercise intensities of long duration, the depletion of muscle glycogen is associated with fatigue and reduction in work capacity as the muscle becomes more reliant on fat as an energy substrate. The oxidation of fat requires about 10% more oxygen for a given power output than the oxidation of carbohydrate: where oxygen delivery is limited, this difference becomes important.

Reductions in blood glucose concentration can also occur during prolonged exercise due to a mismatch between liver glucose release and muscle glucose uptake. In some athletes or events, this may progress to symptomatic hypoglycaemia and obvious signs of fatigue, disorientation and impaired work capacity. However, central fatigue (or sub-optimal performance) may occur with more subtle changes in blood glucose concentrations or carbohydrate availability to the central nervous system. The presence of glucose in the mouth is also known to stimulate oral receptors that can influence the central perception of fatigue (Carter et al., 2004). The effects of reduced carbohydrate availability can manifest themselves in terms of sub-optimal work capacity via reductions in pacing strategies or muscle fibre recruitment or as impairments of the skill and concentration which underpin the outcomes in many sports. Readers are referred to reviews on carbohydrate and metabolism during sports performance for a more in-depth discussion (Maughan and Gleeson, 2010).

Total body carbohydrate stores are limited and are often substantially less than the fuel requirements of intensive training and competition sessions, so when it is important to train well or compete optimally, athletes are guided to consume dietary sources of carbohydrates to avoid or delay the depletion of body carbohydrate stores during exercise (Burke et al., 2011). A summary of current recommendations for carbohydrate intake by athletes is provided in Figure 16.

Situation	Recommended carbohydrate intake
Acute situation	
Optimal daily muscle glycogen storage (e.g. for post-exercise recovery or to fuel up or carbohydrate load before an event)	7–12 g/kg body mass/day
Rapid post-exercise recovery of muscle glycogen, where recovery between sessions is <8 h	1–1.2 g/kg immediately after exercise; repeated each hour until meal schedule is resumed There may be some advantages to consuming carbohydrate as a series of small snacks every 15–60 min in the early recovery phase.
Pre-event meal to increase carbohydrate availability before prolonged exercise session	1–4 g/kg eaten 1–4 h before exercise
Carbohydrate intake during moderate-intensity or intermittent exercise of >1 h	Exercise of 1 h: small amounts of carbohydrate (including even mouth rinsing with a carbohydrate drink) Exercise of > 90 min: 0.5–1.0 g/kg/h (30–60 g/h) Exercise of >4 h: maximal rates of oxidation of ingested carbohydrate occur with intakes of ~ 1.5–1.8 g/min of multiple transportable carbohydrates
Chronic or everyday situation	
Daily recovery or fuel needs for athletes with very light training programme (low-intensity exercise or skill-based exercise). These targets may be particularly suited to athletes with large body mass or a need to reduce energy intake to lose weight	3–5 g/kg/day★
Daily recovery or fuel needs for athlete with moderate exercise programme (i.e. 60–90 min)	5–7 g/kg/day★
Daily recovery or fuel needs for endurance athlete (i.e. 1–3 h of moderate- to high-intensity exercise)	7–12 g/kg/day★
Daily recovery or fuel needs for athlete undertaking extreme exercise programme (i.e. >4–5 h of moderate- to high-intensity exercise such as Tour de France)	≥10–12 g/kg/day★

FIGURE 16 Summary of current guidelines for carbohydrate intake by athletes (adapted from Burke *et al.*, 2011)

★   Note that this carbohydrate intake should be spread over the day to promote fuel availability for key training sessions – i.e. consumed before, during or after these sessions.

It should be noted from this summary that sports nutrition guidelines no longer promote a 'high carbohydrate' diet for all athletes. Instead, carbohydrate intake should be judged relative to the varying fuel needs of an athlete's daily training or competition programme, with 'high carbohydrate availability' describing scenarios where the total amount of carbohydrate consumed over a day or around an exercise session keeps pace with muscle and brain fuel needs. Not only will carbohydrate intake targets differ between athletes, but they will also vary from day to day for the same athlete according to the changing substrate needs of a periodised training/event programme, and the importance of approaching a particular session or training block with high or low carbohydrate availability.

There is a sound body of evidence that carbohydrate intake strategies which maintain high carbohydrate availability during exercise and prevent carbohydrate depletion are associated with enhanced endurance and performance during many types of sporting activities. Such strategies include glycogen super-compensation prior to endurance and ultra-endurance events, the intake of a carbohydrate-rich meal in the hours before events of prolonged (> 90 min), sustained or intermittent exercise, the intake of carbohydrate during sustained high-intensity exercise lasting ~60 min or in prolonged sustained/intermittent exercise, and the intake of carbohydrate in the recovery period between two bouts of carbohydrate-demanding exercise (Coyle, 2004). Carbohydrate is an essential ingredient of effective sports drinks, and water and carbohydrate have independent and additive performance-enhancing effects when ingested during endurance exercise (Coyle, 2004). The evidence for the benefits of carbohydrate intake during many sport and exercise activities is robust (Cermak and van Loon, 2013; Stellingwerff and Cox, 2014), with a variety and combination of mechanisms in play depending on the protocol of intake and the type of exercise (Karelis *et al.*, 2010). Expert guidelines recognise differences in the amount and type of carbohydrate intake according to the duration/intensity of sport (Jeukendrup, 2011). In prolonged activities (~3 h duration and longer), there appears to be a dose effect (Smith *et al.*, 2013) on performance, and ingestion of large amounts of carbohydrate – up to 90g/h or even more – may be beneficial if these include varied carbohydrate types that can take advantage of the different intestinal transport mechanisms to maximise absorption and if the gut has been trained by repeated exposure to the high carbohydrate concentrations (Jeukendrup and McLaughlin, 2011).

Low-carbohydrate diets have been promoted for athletes in recent years (Brukner, 2013) without clear evidence of benefits to performance. Training with restricted carbohydrate availability may enhance the capacity for fat oxidation during exercise but it seems that a performance benefit does not necessarily result, at least under the protocols used in the currently available literature in which 50–100% of training sessions have been undertaken in this manner (Burke, 2010). It is more likely that benefits would be seen when it is integrated into the sophisticated and periodised training programmes undertaken by modern athletes with an artful blend where sessions are undertaken with different levels of carbohydrate availability during and after the session.

The primary source of carbohydrate comes from the diet, and sugar-rich and starch-rich foods can contribute to energy and fuel needs as well as providing other useful nutrients for health and performance. However, special sports products containing substantial amounts of carbohydrate provide a valuable nutrition aid in some situations (Figure 17). The advantages or value of these products include taste appeal, provision of a known amount of carbohydrate to meet a specific sports nutrition goal, simultaneous provision of other important nutrients for sports nutrition goals, and gastrointestinal characteristics promoting quick digestion and absorption. Other benefits relate to characteristics that make the products practical to consume around exercise sessions (low-bulk, conveniently packaged) or in the athlete's lifestyle (portable, non-perishable, minimal preparation). When these sports products are used by an athlete to meet the sports nutrition situations outlined above, they are likely to enhance performance. The performance benefits achieved by addressing a situation that would otherwise result in low carbohydrate availability are robust, ranking carbohydrate supplements among the performance enhancers with the strongest evidence base in sports nutrition.

In summary, carbohydrate is an essential part of the human diet and is the macronutrient that supplies the greatest fraction of total energy intake for most people. Because of its central role in energy metabolism during exercise, it plays a vital role in the athlete's diet. Well-chosen foods can meet carbohydrate needs in many situations, but carbohydrate supplements may be useful before, during and after exercise to help athletes achieve their nutrition goals. These supplements may be in solid, liquid or gel format (Pfeiffer *et al.*, 2010a, 2010b), and may or may not contain other nutrients. Judicious selection of carbohydrate-containing foods and supplements can help athletes to optimise training and competition performance.

Competing interests Louise M. Burke was a member of the Gatorade Sports Science Institute's Expert Panel from 2014–2015 for which her workplace (Australian Institute of Sport) received an honorarium.

Supplement	Form	Typical composition	Main sports-related use
Sports drink	Powder or ready-to-drink liquid	4–8% carbohydrate, as mixtures of glucose, fructose, sucrose and maltodextrins Electrolytes (sodium and potassium) May contain other compounds such as protein/amino acids or caffeine	Optimum delivery of fluid and carbohydrate during exercise for hydration and fuelling Post-exercise rehydration Post-exercise refuelling
Sports gel	Sachets (30–40 g) or larger tubes of thick carbohydrate liquid (gel)	60–70% carbohydrate solution (~25g carbohydrate per sachet) May contain other compounds such as electrolytes or caffeine	Fuelling during exercise
Sports confectionery	Jelly or jube confectionery	Typically contain ~ 5 g carbohydrate per piece May contain other compounds such as electrolytes or caffeine	Fuelling during exercise
Liquid meal supplement	Powder (to be mixed with water or milk) or ready-to-drink liquid	Drink made from powder with typical content per 100 g powder: 60–70 g carbohydrate, 20–30 g protein, low to moderate fat content Often fortified with vitamins/ minerals May contain (purported) ergogenic compounds	Low-bulk meal replacement (especially pre-event meal) Post-exercise recovery - promoting protein synthesis and refuelling Nutrient-rich supplement for high-energy/high carbohydrate diet (especially during heavy training/ competition or weight gain) Portable nutrition for travelling athlete
Sports bar	Bar (50–60 g)	40–50 g carbohydrate, 5–10 g protein (some bars may have higher protein content) Usually low in fat and fibre Often fortified with vitamins and minerals May contain (purported) ergogenic aids	Fuelling during exercise Post-exercise recovery – promoting refuelling and some protein towards protein synthesis goals Supplement for high-energy/high carbohydrate diet Portable nutrition for the travelling athlete

FIGURE 17 Sports supplements containing carbohydrate

L-CARNITINE

Francis B. Stephens and Paul L. Greenhaff

Ninety-five percent of the body's carnitine (3-hydroxy-4-N,N,N-trimethylaminobutyric acid; $C_7H_{15}NO_3$) store (~25g) exists within skeletal muscle where it plays a central role in fat and carbohydrate oxidation, particularly during exercise (for review see Stephens *et al.*, 2007a). The recommended upper limit of L-carnitine supplementation is 2g/day(Hathcock and Shao, 2006), but no adverse effects were reported following feeding up to 6g/day for one year (Hathcock and Shao, 2006; Wächter *et al.*, 2002). The main food source of carnitine is meat. Non-vegetarians ingest ~1mg/kg of dietary carnitine per day, whereas strict vegetarians ingest around 0.01mg/kg (Rebouche *et al.*, 1993). Research has been directed towards supplementing dietary L-carnitine to improve exercise performance. However, neither oral (2–6g/day for one day to four months) nor intravenous (up to 65mg/kg) L-carnitine administration *per se* has been found to alter fuel metabolism during exercise or, more importantly, increase muscle carnitine content in humans (Brass, 2000; Stephens *et al.*, 2007a; Wächter *et al.*, 2002).

Despite this, L-carnitine feeding as a tool to promote apparent fat loss remains the foundation of a multi-million dollar dietary supplement industry in the present day. Intravenous infusion of L-carnitine along with insulin (to stimulate Na+ dependent muscle carnitine transport) has been found to increase muscle total carnitine content by ~15% in healthy volunteers, and to have a measurable effect on muscle fuel metabolism at rest (Stephens *et al.*, 2007a). This stimulatory effect on muscle carnitine accumulation occurred in the physiological range for serum insulin concentration (50–90 mU/l). Furthermore, feeding L-carnitine (3g/day) together with carbohydrate (500ml solution containing 94g of simple sugars) for two weeks increased whole body carnitine retention compared to ingestion of L-carnitine alone (Stephens *et al.*, 2007b).

Orally administered L-carnitine has a poor bioavailability (<15% for a 2–6g dose), and therefore it is likely that any carnitine and carbohydrate supplementation regimen would take ~100 days to increase muscle carnitine content by ~10% alone (Stephens *et al.*, 2007b). In this respect, it has been shown that ingestion of 1.36g of L-carnitine in combination with 80g of carbohydrate twice daily for 168 days can increase muscle total carnitine content by 21% in healthy, young volunteers, whilst there was no impact on muscle total carnitine in a matched control group who ingested 80g of carbohydrate twice daily (Wall *et al.*, 2011). Moreover, during exercise at 50% VO_{2max}, muscle glycogen use in the carnitine loaded state was 55% less compared to control, and pyruvate dehydrogenase complex activation (PDCa) was blunted. Conversely, at 80% VO_{2max}, muscle PDCa was greater, whilst muscle lactate content was 44% less and the muscle PCr/ATP ratio was better maintained in comparison to control volunteers. Importantly, in the carnitine loaded state, work output during a validated cycling performance trial was increased by 11% from baseline, while the control group showed no change (Wall *et al.*, 2011). This was the first demonstration that human muscle total carnitine content can be increased by dietary means and results in muscle glycogen sparing during low-intensity exercise (consistent with an increase in lipid utilisation) and a better matching of glycolytic, PDC and mitochondrial flux during high-intensity exercise, thereby reducing muscle anaerobic ATP production and improving exercise performance.

More recently, it has been described that the increase in muscle total carnitine content achieved by daily combined L-carnitine and carbohydrate feeding can prevent the increase in body fat mass associated with daily ingestion of a high carbohydrate-containing beverage (Stephens *et al.*, 2013). Moreover, this maintenance of body mass was associated with greater whole-body energy expenditure during low-intensity exercise (accounted for by an increase in fat oxidation), and a marked adaptive increase in the expression of gene networks involved in insulin signalling, peroxisome proliferator-activated receptor (PPAR) signalling, and fatty acid metabolism over and above the decline observed when carbohydrate alone was ingested (Stephens *et al.*, 2013). Taken together these observations suggest that increasing skeletal muscle carnitine content can prevent the increase in adiposity associated with prolonged high carbohydrate feeding by maintaining the capacity to oxidise fat, which is entirely consistent with a carnitine-mediated increase in muscle long-chain acyl-group translocation via CPT1. Implications to health warrant further investigation, particularly in the elderly and obese individuals who have reduced reliance on muscle fat oxidation during low intensity exercise.

Competing interests None

CHINESE HERBS

David S. Senchina

'Chinese herbs' is a broad phrase encompassing species from eastern or central Asia purportedly possessing ergogenic, as well as other, properties. Supplements from these herbs are marketed globally. The main ones used by athletes are cordyceps (ophiocordyceps), ephedra. ginseng, rhodiola and tribulus (Bucci, 2000); and are discussed individually elsewhere in this book. Ginseng is probably the most widely reported Chinese herbal supplement used by athletes, with ginseng and rhodiola both frequently found in energy drinks.

Many sports professionals mistakenly perceive Chinese herbs the same way as prescription drugs. In contrast to drugs, herbs are commonly grown outdoors, where they may experience considerable variation in environmental, harvesting, storage and extraction methods, all of which impact upon potential ergogenic effects (Senchina, 2013). Considering that only a handful of studies exist for only a smattering of herbs, and that the studies themselves differ in experimental design and measures, on top of the variation discussed previously, it is not surprising that multiple groups studying the same species report different results (Senchina *et al.*, 2009b). Chinese herbs, in particular, are often used in proprietary formulations, sometimes with other species, each formulation harbouring different properties.

Consequently, the ergogenic effects of most popular Chinese herbs have not been substantiated. Athletes are also reminded that there is a risk that supplements can be contaminated with compounds prohibited by the World Anti-Doping Agency (WADA, 2014b). Indeed, among the reports of supplements that have been found to be contaminated, preparations of ginseng (Cui *et al.*, 1994) and *T terrestris* (Geyer *et al.*, 2000) have been noted.

Competing interests None

CHLOROGENIC ACIDS

Adrian B. Hodgson

Chlorogenic acids (CGA) are phenolic compounds that are quinic acid esters of hydroxycinnamic acid (Crozier *et al.*, 2012; Manach *et al.*, 2004). The major source of CGA in the human diet is from brewed coffee due to the high presence of CGA found in the green coffee bean prior to roasting (Crozier *et al.*, 2012). Recently, CGA have been cited to have beneficial effects on type 2 diabetes and weight loss which has led to the appearance of a variety of CGA and/or green coffee bean extract supplements on the sports nutrition market.

Currently there are no dietary recommendations for daily chlorogenic acid intake. It has been reported that CGA intake from a single serving of coffee can provide 20–675mg (Crozier *et al.*, 2012), with daily intake varying considerably. The large variation in CGA content is due to the source of the bean -oasting procedure (which reduces CGA content when compared to green coffee beans) and preparation method of coffee (Crozier *et al.*, 2012). Similar to many flavonoids, there are a number of different CGA found in green coffee beans. The major CGA is 5-caffeoylguinic acid (5-CQA) making up ~50% of green coffee bean CGA content (Hodgson *et al.*, 2013b). However, it is important to consider that the composition of CGA in coffee is vast and the subsequent metabolism of CGA is complex (Crozier *et al.*, 2012).

Chlorogenic acids are believed to give coffee its health-promoting effects, specifically for type 2 diabetes (Beaudoin and Graham, 2011). Data in animal models show that chlorogenic acids and quinides found in coffee have anti-diabetic effects (Andrade-Cetto and Wiedenfeld, 2001). Early pilot data in humans show improved glucose and insulin concentrations during an OGTT (Oral Glucose Tolerance Test) after acute CGA intake, but this data has not been replicated when consuming CGA as decaffeinated coffee (van Dijk *et al.*, 2009). Hence more human data is needed to substantiate further this potential metabolic effect of CGA.

Despite this, it is purported that chronic coffee intake and thus CGA intake helps reduce the absorption of glucose from the small intestine which, in turn, could also have benefits on weight loss (Greenberg *et al.*, 2006). Evidence in animals has shown early promise for green coffee extract supplementation on weight loss through: a reduction in glucose uptake; suppressing accumulation of hepatic triglycerides and lipogenesis; activation of fat oxidation via peroxisome proliferator-activated receptor alpha (PPARα); and activation of lipolysis *in vitro* (Shimoda *et al.*, 2006; Cho *et al.*, 2010; Flanagan *et al.*, 2014). A meta-analysis of three randomized clinical trials, of which one was unpublished, showed a significant reduction in body weight following chronic supplementation (four to 12 weeks) of CGA (180–200mg/day), but the effect size was small, which questions the clinical significance (Onakpoya *et al.*, 2011). More recently, Vinson *et al.* (2012) showed that six weeks supplementation of CGA as a low (350mg twice a day) or high dose (350mg three times a day) resulted in a significant reduction in body weight when compared with placebo. This study however suffered from a lack of strict dietary, exercise and supplementation control as well as a low (*n*=16) subject number (Vinson *et al.*, 2012). Therefore, to date, there is a paucity of evidence to support the recommendation of CGA as a successful weight-loss supplementation strategy.

In an exercise and sporting context, it has previously been shown *in vitro* that chlorogenic acids antagonize adenosine receptor binding of caffeine (de Paulis *et al.*, 2002). This causes blunting to heart rate, blood pressure and a dose-dependent relaxation of smooth muscle (Tse, 1992). Based on this early research it was thought that the ergogenic effects of caffeine when consumed as coffee were impaired due to the high presence of CGA (Graham *et al.*, 1998). More recently, Hodgson *et al.* (2013b) showed that both caffeine (5mg/kg/body weight) and instant coffee (5mg/kg/body weight) consumed one hour prior to exercise can improve endurance exercise performance, despite a high presence of CGA in the coffee trial (~393mg/serving). Taking this recent research, together with previous data to show improvements in exercise performance after coffee (Wiles *et al.*, 1992), it is unlikely the chlorogenic acids impair the beneficial effects of caffeine during endurance exercise performance.

At present, chlorogenic acids are frequently found in the human diet in individuals who habitually consume coffee. However, the evidence to support the isolated application and use of CGA as a supplement, at least in humans, on type 2 diabetes or on weight loss is largely unclear. In addition, there is also no reason to believe that CGA will alter the ergogenic effects of caffeine when consumed as coffee, thus, coffee is a practical and readily available ergogenic aid for athletes.

Competing interests   None

CHOLINE BITARTRATE AND ACETYLCHOLINE

Jeni Pearce

Choline, an essential micronutrient, is widely distributed in food fats (especially liver, egg yolk, peanuts, dairy products and human milk). The body synthesizes choline in the liver, and a deficiency due to dietary inadequacy is unlikely as choline (and lecithin, a common food additive and supplement containing low levels of choline) is ubiquitous in the food supply. Choline is consumed as phosphatidylcholine (constituent of cell membranes) and has both functional and structural roles in the body (found within cells and blood). As a precursor for the neurotransmitter acetylcholine (initiating muscle contractions), choline also has roles in cell membrane signalling phospholipids (phosphatidylcholine and spingomyelin), memory and mood, and is a donor of methyl groups. Choline assists in the recycling of homocysteine to methionine and creatine synthesis via the methyl group donation.

Available in a wide range of supplements as choline bitartrate and lecithin, choline is promoted to athletes to improve endurance performance and increase fat lipolysis. Acetylcholine production has increased muscle contractions, delayed fatigue and improved cognitive function memory in rats. A study in cyclists indicated improved mood state with 2.43g supplemental choline although no improvement in performance was seen (Warber *et al.*, 2000). Evidence does not support claims that choline has a role in reducing body adipose nor that high doses elevate fat metabolism in humans (Penry and Manore, 2008).

There are links between the decreased plasma concentration of choline (9–40%) in endurance exercise (>2hrs) in marathon runners, cyclists, triathletes and military personnel, and reduced performance or early fatigue (Conlay *et al.*, 1986, 1992; Buchman *et al.*, 1999). The exercise-related reductions are short term, returning to normal in 48 hours (Buchman *et al.*, 1999). Duration and intensity may be more relevant than mode of exercise for eliciting choline depletion. Neither prolonged low-intensity sessions, nor shorter, high-intensity sessions appear to deplete choline levels (Penry and Manore, 2008).

Insufficient availability of acetylcholine may contribute to fatigue, while increasing exogenous choline may enhance acetylcholine availability for neuromuscular transmission. Two well-designed studies involving exhaustive exercise protocols in cyclists and soldiers, used choline citrate/bitartrate intakes of 2.4–8.4g, consumed in beverages prior to exercise, which maintained the plasma choline concentration but failed to delay fatigue or show performance benefits (Spector *et al.*, 1995; Conlay *et al.*, 1986).

Free serum choline concentrations vary with dietary choline and lecithin intake. Supplementation is reported to raise blood levels within 45 minutes of choline ingestion (Spector *et al.*, 1995). Oral ingestion of some forms of choline supplements may cause gastrointestinal side effects leading to fishy body odours (a genetic disorder, trimethylaminuria). Small supplemental doses are not considered harmful at this time and the upper safe limit is set at 3–3.5g for adults (National Academy of Sciences, 2014). Athletes with gout are advised to avoid choline supplementation. Despite several studies showing choline supplementation elevating plasma choline concentrations there is no evidence this has translated into benefits in athletic performance or reductions in fatigue.

Competing interests   None

CHONDROITIN AND GLUCOSAMINE

James R. Borchers and Christopher C. Kaeding

Glucosamine, a primary building block for proteoglycans, is available as an oral supplement with approximately 90% gut absorption leading to uptake in several tissues including bone and articular cartilage. Oral administration results in absorption by several tissues including bone and articular cartilage (Setnikar *et al.*, 1993; Setnikar and Rovati, 2001). Chondroitin is a large molecule that is absorbed from the gastrointestinal tract but not as readily as glucosamine (Gorsline and Kaeding, 2005). Theoretically, it enhances proteoglycan synthesis and prevents cartilage degradation, whether due to damage or disease (Gorsline and Kaeding, 2005).

The overuse of non-steroidal anti inflammatories (NSAID) by athletes with degenerative joint disease is commonly seen and may lead to an increased risk of adverse events. The use of glucosamine and chondroitin as both treatment and disease-modifying agents for cartilage damage in athletes is therefore of interest. Much of the support for the disease- or damage-modifying aspects of glucosamine and chondroitin is derived from animal studies. Studies on rabbits suggest that there may be a role for glucosamine use in injury to articular cartilage (Oegema *et al.*, 2002; Shikhman *et al.*, 2005). Studies of joint stress in animal chondrocytes (Lippiello, 2003) suggest that treatment with glucosamine and chondroitin provides an enhanced protective metabolic response to various stresses (i.e. enzyme-induced matrix depletion, heat stress, mechanical compression and cytokine stress). These studies have led to the marketing of glucosamine sulphate and chondroitin to athletes for use in the modification of acute cartilage damage after an acute injury or cartilage damage due to repetitive loading. This is based on the hypothesis that glucosamine sulphate and chondroitin may stimulate chondrocytes to repair damaged cartilage more efficiently and completely. However, there are no current studies in athletes of any age for either supplement to suggest that these effects occur.

Pavelka and colleagues (2002) looked at the delay of knee osteoarthritis (OA) progression over a three-year period with 1,500mg/day of oral glucosamine sulphate. Many supplements contain lower amounts. Pavelka *et al.* (2002) observed no significant joint space narrowing after treatment, compared with significant narrowing in the placebo group. Similar results were observed by Reginster and colleagues (2001). In another study of chondroitin sulphate in knee OA, Uebelhart and colleagues (2004) found that similar joint space narrowing in the placebo group after one year was delayed by the treatment. Taken together, these studies demonstrate the potential of both glucosamine and chondroitin to delay radiographic findings of joint space narrowing in sedentary populations. This might be of interest to athletes with degenerative joint disease or damage regardless of age. Systematic studies of the use of these agents by athletic populations are needed before such treatment can be considered fully evidence-based.

There is conflicting evidence for the use of glucosamine and chondroitin as a symptomatic treatment of OA. There are studies that suggest both benefit and no benefit for the use of either glucosamine or chondroitin in the treatment of symptomatic knee OA. The large-scale Glucosamine/Chondroitin Arthritis Trial leaves doubt as to the effectiveness of glucosamine and chondroitin in the treatment of knee OA (Clegg *et al.*, 2006). There are data to support a combination of glucosamine and chondroitin as effective in those patients with moderate to severe knee pain. However, no benefit was observed with individual use of these agents in this population with respect to knee pain. Neither the combination nor individual-use showed benefit in those patients classified with mild knee pain compared to placebo. A more recent trial studying single and combination use of glucosamine and chondroitin for the treatment of osteoarthritis observed improvement in self-reported patient outcomes for single and combination use but this improvement was not statistically different from placebo (Fransen *et al.*, 2014). Multiple systematic reviews and consensus recommendations suggest uncertainty as to the effectiveness of glucosamine and chondroitin in the symptomatic treatment of osteoarthritis (McAlindon *et al.*, 2014; Nelson *et al.*, 2014a; Vangsness *et al.*, 2009). The reviews and guidelines report inconsistent results regarding improvement in pain and joint function in knee OA after the use of glucosamine and chondroitin. Current evidence from these reviews and guidelines suggests there is at best uncertainty regarding the effectiveness of glucosamine and chondroitin as a symptomatic treatment of osteoarthritis and any positive effect may not be more effective than placebo. Both supplements have an excellent safety profile. Therefore, if an athlete plans to use these products as an alternative to chronic NSAID or analgesic use, the authors suggest clinicians discuss whether or not there is potential for benefit in athletes with degenerative joint disease.

Competing interests   None

CHROMIUM PICOLINATE

Eric S. Rawson

Chromium (Cr3+) is a required trace mineral that potentiates the effect of insulin. A small number of patients on total parenteral nutrition have developed severe chromium deficiencies and subsequently presented with symptoms of diabetes. However, this was reversed with chromium supplementation (Jeejeebhoy *et al.*, 1977). Chromium levels in food are quite low, with highest levels found in egg yolk, brewer's yeast and beef. Although physical activity may increase chromium losses (Clancy *et al.*, 1994), and intestinal chromium absorption is low (0.5 to 2.0%), chromium deficiencies are uncommon and supplementation is generally not warranted. The Adequate Intake (AI) of chromium is 35 mg/day and 25 mg/day for adult (19 to 50 years) men and women, respectively.

Chromium picolinate, a complex of trivalent chromium and picolinic acid, is better absorbed (2–5%) than dietary chromium. As a dietary supplement, chromium picolinate has been heavily marketed for muscle building (Vincent, 2003), fat loss (Tian *et al.*, 2013) and, more recently, to manage insulin resistance/ type 2 diabetes risk in obese men and women with impaired glucose tolerance. Based on these claims, sales of chromium picolinate supplements soared, reaching $500 million dollars/year and representing 6% of mineral supplement sales (second behind calcium) in the United States. In terms of muscle building and fat loss, the overwhelming majority of the data do not support the purported benefits of chromium picolinate supplementation (Vincent, 2003; Tian *et al.*, 2013), and thus, supplementation is not recommended.

For management of diabetes, chromium picolinate supplementation may cause small improvements in glycaemic control (Suksomboon *et al.*, 2014), but the numerical versus clinical significance of these data are debatable, and are probably negligible in comparison to weight loss and exercise.

Adverse events related to chromium picolinate supplementation in humans are rare and based on case studies, but negative effects on iron status were noted in a double-blind placebo-controlled trial (Lukaski *et al.*, 1996). Data are unavailable regarding the safety of high-dose long-term chromium picolinate ingestion in both healthy and patient populations. More work needs to be done to understand fully any potential value of chromium picolinate in the management of diabetes. However, there is currently little evidence to support chromium picolinate supplementation by athletes.

Competing interests   None

CISSUS QUADRANGULARIS

Greg Shaw

Cissus quadrangularis (CQ) is an ancient medicinal plant found in warm regions of Asia and Africa. It has been used in traditional medicine for a variety of purposes from healing bones to treating asthma. Recently CQ has enjoyed popularity within the supplement industry due to its numerous reported actions and its range of constituents (Stohs and Ray, 2013). Various extracts of CQ have been reported to influence significantly the regulation of bone turnover. In rats CQ extracts have been shown to improve the healing time of bone fractures (Chopra *et al.*, 1976), as well as demonstrating significant anti-osteoporotic effects through the thickening of cortical and trabecular regions of bone (Potu *et al.*, 2009). Mechanisms suggested for these outcomes include: the increased proliferation and differentiation of mesenchymal stem cells to osteoblasts; a subsequent increase in bone mineralisation via enhanced alkaline phosphatase activity; or the enhanced regulation of the insulin-like growth factor system in osteoblast-like cells (Potu *et al.*, 2009; Muthusami *et al.*, 2011). The small number of human studies investigating the bone-influencing properties of CQ *in vitro* (Muthusami *et al.*, 2011) and *in vivo* (Singh *et al.*, 2011) seem positive.

Although commonly thought to contain 'anabolic steroidal substances' there is currently no evidence of these compounds being isolated in CQ extracts. The popularity of CQ in athletic circles is mainly focused on its purported anti-inflammatory action. Again, in animal models, CQ extracts have been reported to influence inflammation through the inhibition of COX1 and 2 related inflammatory pathways (Bhujade *et al.*, 2012) and via the attenuation of pro inflammatory cytokines (Banu *et al.*, 2012). More recently CQ has become a common ingredient in weight loss supplements with preliminary evidence suggesting that supplementation with CQ for a period of ten weeks in obese patients induced greater weight loss compared to a placebo (Oben *et al.*, 2007).

Recommended doses range from 100–500mg of CQ extract or 3–6g of the dried plant. Currently there is no evidence that CQ poses a safety issue in humans but data is limited (see section on hydoxycut in this book). Although animal and *in vitro* research is promising, well controlled research data in humans, particularly in the athletic population, are currently limited. With this in mind athletes should avoid this supplement until more evidence is available, particularly around safety.

Competing interests None

L-CITRULLINE

*Nikki A. Jeacocke, Stephen J. Bailey and
Andrew M. Jones*

L-citrulline is a non-essential α-amino acid ($C_6H_{13}N_3O_3$), found in a range
of protein-rich foods of both animal and plant origin. Endogenously,
L-citrulline is synthesised during the metabolism of L-ornithine by ornithine
carbamoyltransferase, a key reaction in the breakdown of L-glutamine, and is a
product of L-arginine oxidation via the nitric oxide synthase (NOS) enzymes
(Wu and Morris, 1998). L-citrulline can be recycled back into L-arginine through
the enzymatic activity of argininosuccinate synthase (yielding argininosuccinate)
and subsequently argininosuccinate lyase (yielding L-citrulline). Oral
supplementation of L-citrulline appears more effective at increasing circulating
and muscle [L-arginine] and nitric oxide (NO) biomarkers than L-arginine
supplementation (Schwedhelm *et al.*, 2008; Wijnands *et al.*, 2012). L-citrulline
is also an intermediate in the urea cycle; it attenuates the rise in circulating
ammonia during exercise (Takeda *et al.*, 2011). The potential for L-citrulline
to improve exercise performance may be linked to its ability to increase
L-arginine content, and hence NO and creatine synthesis substrates, and to
facilitate ammonia detoxification (Sureda and Pons, 2013). However, studies
investigating the potential benefits of L-citrulline supplementation on athletic
performance are limited.

Skeletal muscle power output and oxidative energy turnover are increased,
while the power output/pH ratio and ratings of perceived exertion are lowered
following short-term supplementation with L-citrulline malate (Bendahan *et
al.*, 2002). Another study found a 19% increase in the number of repetitions
performed until exhaustion during a bench-press test at 80% 1-RM, after a
single dose of 8g L-citrulline malate (Pérez-Guisado and Jakeman, 2010).
However, since malate can impact on muscle metabolic responses independent
of L-citrulline (Wagenmakers, 1998), it is not possible to discern the effect of
L-citrulline in these findings. Ingesting 6g of L-citrulline malate two hours
prior to a cycling event in well-trained endurance athletes increased plasma
[L-arginine] and NO metabolites post-race, but performance was not measured
in these studies (Sureda *et al.*, 2009, 2010). Surprisingly, acute ingestion of 3–9g
of pure L-citrulline compromises exercise tolerance during an incremental
running test together with a trend towards reduced NO bioavailability (Hickner
et al., 2006), as inferred from plasma [nitrate] + [nitrite].

The watermelon (*Citrullus lanatus*) is a rich source of L-citrulline, with
~2.33g L-citrulline/L of unpasteurized watermelon juice (Tarazona-Díaz *et al.*,
2013). Watermelon ingestion increases plasma L-arginine (Collins *et al.*, 2007),

but as yet, no published studies have investigated the effects of watermelon on exercise performance. Watermelon juice consumption (~1.17g/500ml L-citrulline) relieves muscle soreness after intense exercise (Tarazona-Díaz *et al.*, 2013), which together with the increased neutrophil oxidative burst observed with L-citrulline malate (Sureda *et al.*, 2009), suggests that L-citrulline might reduce immunodepression and aid recovery after intense exercise.

In summary, a dearth of studies has investigated the effects of L-citrulline on exercise performance. Based on these limited results, evidence to support the use of L-citrulline as an ergogenic aid is lacking. Moreover, the extent to which any positive effects of L-citrulline malate or watermelon consumption can be attributed to L-citrulline-mediated effects is complicated by the fact that malate can evoke positive metabolic responses, and watermelon contains a number of other potential 'active ingredients'. Irrespective of its form of administration, L-citrulline can increase L-arginine availability (Schwedhelm *et al.*, 2008; Wijnands *et al.*, 2012), and most studies observed increases in NO biomarkers (Wijnands *et al.*, 2012; Sureda *et al.*, 2009, 2010). Improvements in oxidative metabolism (Bendahan *et al.*, 2002), and metabolite clearance (Takeda *et al.*, 2011), have also been observed following L-citrulline administration. However, it is unclear whether this potential for increased NO synthesis and better maintenance of skeletal muscle homeostasis is related to improved exercise performance. Further research is required to establish potential ergogenic efficacy of citrulline.

Competing interests   None

CO-ENZYME Q10

Björn Ekblom

Co-enzyme Q10 (originally known as ubiquinone) is a co-enzyme in the electron shuttle system of the inner mitochondrial membrane and is part of the total antioxidant defence system. It protects different cell structures from free oxygen radicals produced during oxygen stress such as severe physical exercise. Therefore, athletes have used antioxidant supplements to strengthen their antioxidant defence during training and competition. However, more recently it was proposed that free radicals may provide useful functions in the body, particularly in the signalling pathways associated with the exercise stimulus. Thus, free radical production might be a prerequisite for the training effect in muscle (Gomez-Cabrera et al., 2008).

Effects of antioxidant (Q10) supplementation on exercise performance and metabolic adaptation to exercise are divergent. Some studies (Mizuno et al., 2008; Ylikoski et al., 1997) report enhanced exercise capacity and performance, while most others do not (Braun et al., 1991; Snider et al., 1992; Zhou et al., 2005). There is also evidence that Q10 supplementation may interfere with divergent adaptations to exercise, such as modulating inflammatory response signalling (Diaz-Castro et al., 2012), affecting lipid oxidation (Close et al., 2006) and enhancing mRNA responses (Hellsten et al., 2007). All these effects can interfere with the response to short periods of training. In addition, increased CK levels after Q10 supplementation denoted cell damage (Malm et al., 1996).

We carried out a double blind study: nine men received $2 \times 60mg$ Q10, and nine received placebo for 22 days with dietary control (Malm et al., 1997). Normal physical training was undertaken for ten days, followed by high-intensity anaerobic training (Days 11–14), and then recovery (Days 15–22). On Days 1, 11, 15 and 22, different high-intensity cycling tests were performed. On Day 15 the placebo group showed significantly greater improvements in the anaerobic test than the Q10 group. After recovery (Day 22) the improvement was maintained in the placebo group, while the Q10 group value was not different from Day 1. Total work performed during anaerobic training (Days 11–14) was significantly greater in the placebo group. There were no differences between groups in heart rate (HR) and rate of perceived exertion (RPE) during submaximal work rates in any test, nor with running VO_{2max}, which is in accordance with other studies. However, the Q10 group had significantly higher plasma creatine kinase activity, a crude marker of muscle damage, six hours after the Day 11 tests, and 24 hours after the Day 15 tests, which possibly was due to prooxidant free radical formation of Q10 supplementation in combination with anaerobic exercise/training. These values were normal on Day 22. The abolished training effect of Q10 supplementation is in line with corresponding abolished training effect on insulin sensitivity (Ristow *et al.*, 2009) and other cellular adaptations to exercise (McGinley *et al.*, 2009).

Based on available findings, and the recent general caution about antioxidant supplementation in combination with exercise (Gomez-Cabrera *et al.*, 2008), it is not recommended that athletes take coenzyme Q10 or other antioxidant supplements.

Competing interests   None

COLOSTRUM

Cecilia M. Shing

Colostrum is the milk produced by mammals in the first 24–72 hours after giving birth. It is rich in immune, growth and antimicrobial factors that support neonate development. While colostrum supplementation provides a concentrated source of protein, non-nutrient bioactive components of colostrum (i.e. lactoferrin, insulin-like growth factor-1 (IGF-1), immunoglobulin) may confer a physiological advantage. The primary source of colostrum for supplementation by athletes is bovine, which is very similar in composition to human colostrum, although the concentration of immune and growth factors is up to 100 times greater.

Colostrum contains growth factors that mediate protein synthesis, although increases in lean mass and growth factors are not consistently reported after supplementation. Increases in lean mass with colostrum supplementation combined with resistance training appear comparable to those seen when supplementing with whey protein (Brinkworth et al., 2004; Duff et al., 2014), although one study has reported a further increase in lean mass of 1.5kg (Antonio et al., 2001). While colostrum supplementation may increase lean body mass and circulating concentrations of essential amino acids, these changes have not translated into significant improvements in maximal strength. Longer-term supplementation (e.g. 10–60g per/day for eight weeks) resulted in improved vertical jump, peak sprint cycle power and repeat sprint and endurance performance in some studies but failed to enhance exercise performance in other studies with similar methodologies (Shing et al., 2009). Any increase in IGF-1 (Mero et al., 1997) that may mediate performance changes following supplementation is similar to the increase reported after a period of increased (10%) milk consumption (Heaney et al., 1999), and values remain within the normal reference range for adult males. Any increase in circulating IGF-1 is most likely to be attributable to enhanced endogenous production (Shing et al., 2009); high concentrations of IGF-1 in colostrum (120µg/day) did not produce a positive doping test after four weeks' supplementation (Kuipers et al., 2002).

Bovine colostrum is most likely to be beneficial during periods of intense training or competition (Shing et al., 2006, 2013), where athletes may experience increased susceptibility to illness or performance decrements. While short supplementation periods (<10 days) do not affect the acute immune response to exercise (Carol et al., 2011), a reduction in upper respiratory tract illness symptoms (URS) after 8 to 12 weeks' colostrum supplementation has been reported (Crooks et al., 2006; Jones et al., 2013). Reductions in URS appear to be independent of increases in salivary IgA and may be attributable to a dampening of the post-exercise decrease in salivary lysozyme, improved recovery of neutrophil function post-exercise (Davison and Diment, 2010) and/or reductions in mucosal bacterial load (Jones *et al.*, 2013). Colostrum has also been shown to dampen exercise-associated increases in gastrointestinal permeability (Marchbank *et al.*, 2011). Thus, alterations at the level of the gastrointestinal tract, our largest immune organ, may mediate some of the reported immune benefits of colostrum, preventing disturbances in autonomic function and the hypothalamic-pituitary-gonadal axis associated with intense periods of exercise (Shing *et al.*, 2013).

There is limited evidence to support consistent improvements in acute exercise performance after bovine colostrum supplementation. Supplementation does, however, appear to reduce URS, and may prove beneficial to improve recovery/ maintain exercise performance during periods of intensified exercise training or competition (Shing *et al.*, 2006, 2013). According to WADA, 'Colostrum is not prohibited per se, however it contains certain quantities of IGF-1 and other growth factors which are prohibited and can influence the outcome of anti-doping tests. Therefore WADA does not recommend the ingestion of this product.'

Competing interests   None

CONJUGATED LINOLEIC ACID

Philip C. Calder

Conjugated linoleic acid (CLA) is a term for a series of structural and geometric isomers of linoleic acid. The two double bonds in the acyl chain of linoleic acid are on carbons 9 and 12 (counting from the carboxyl terminal carbon), separated by two single carbon-to-carbon bonds, and both are in the *cis* conformation. In CLA the double bonds are separated by only a single bond (i.e. the double bonds are conjugated) and each may be in either the *cis* or *trans* conformation. Thus there are a large number of possible forms of CLA. The major naturally occurring form in the human diet is *cis*-9, *trans*-11 CLA. This is produced as a result of rumen biohydrogenation and is found in ruminant milks, milk products and meats. These foods also contain several other CLA isomers. CLA in dietary supplements is mainly produced by chemical treatment of sunflower oil and typically contains an equal mixture of *cis*-9, *trans*-11 and *trans*-10, *cis*-12 CLA and, frequently, smaller amounts of other CLA isomers.

Biological effects of CLA have been demonstrated in many animal models and, in some studies, in healthy human volunteers; effects are reported on body fatness, blood lipids, insulin resistance and markers of oxidative stress and inflammation, but these effects appear to be isomer specific and are not consistently observed in humans (Pariza *et al.*, 2001; Roche *et al.*, 2001; Tricon *et al.*, 2005; Tricon and Yaqoob, 2006; Bhattacharya *et al.*, 2006; McCrorie *et al.*, 2011). There has been substantial interest in reported effects of CLA on body fatness (Navarro *et al.*, 2006; Plourde *et al.*, 2008). A systematic review of human trials of CLA supplements or CLA-enriched products on body weight and body composition, as well as several other health-related outcomes, concluded that there is not enough evidence to show that CLA has an effect on weight and body composition in humans (Salas-Salvadó *et al.*, 2006). A more recent systematic review of seven human trials of CLA lasting at least six months identified small, but significant, weight and fat loss effects of CLA (mean −0.70 and −1.33 kg, respectively), but concluded that the evidence does not convincingly show that CLA intake generates any clinically relevant effects on body composition in the long term (Onakpoya *et al.*, 2012).

Findings of studies of CLA conducted among individuals who regularly exercise or in body builders have been inconsistent; some studies report decreased fat mass and increased fat-free (lean) mass with CLA supplementation (1.8 to 6g/day of mixed isomers but predominantly an equal mix of *cis*-9, *trans*-11 and *trans*-10, *cis*-12) for about three months (Thom *et al.*, 2001, Colakoglu *et al.*, 2006), although this is not seen in all studies (Kreider *et al.*, 2002; Lambert *et al.*, 2007). CLA has also been used in combination with creatine (Tarnopolsky *et al.*,

2007), and with creatine and whey protein (Cornish *et al.*, 2009) in other studies reporting reduced fat mass and increased fat-free mass. CLA may (Cornish *et al.*, 2009), or may not (Kreider *et al.*, 2002), increase muscle strength.

It is likely that the level and duration of intake of specific biologically active CLA isomers is important, and differences in these factors may explain the contradictory findings in the literature. It is currently not possible to make a firm statement about the role of specific CLA isomers in athletic training and performance or to recommend a specific CLA isomer or intake level.

Competing interests   None

COPPER

Nathan A. Lewis

The importance of the mineral copper for human health can be deduced from its role as a co-factor in numerous metalloenzymes involved in antioxidant defence, oxygen transport and utilisation, immune function, catecholamine and connective tissue synthesis (Uauy *et al.*, 1998). Copper deficiency in adults has been described as secondary to malabsorption (Kumar and Low, 2004), zinc supplementation (Willis *et al.*, 2005) and excessive soft drink consumption (Nuviala *et al.*, 1999). Severe copper deficiency is associated with wide-ranging clinical manifestations: iron-resistant anaemia, pancytopaenia, neuropathy, hypercholesterolaemia, and osteoporosis (Kumar and Low, 2004; Uauy *et al.*, 1998; Willis *et al.*, 2005). However, copper toxicity has been associated with water contamination over 1.6mg/L (Department of Health, 2001).

Dietary requirements for adults have been set at 1.2mg per day in the UK with a Tolerable Upper Intake at 10mg/day (Department of Health, 2001), with no specific recommendations for athletes. Copper status studies in male and female athletes across a variety of sports via blood/dietary analysis have yielded mixed results (Clark *et al.*, 2003; Gropper *et al.*, 2003; Koury *et al.*, 2004; Nuviala *et al.*, 1999), but confirm that self-reported dietary intakes cannot reliably predict actual micronutrient status. Copper deficiency affects immune function. Indeed, athletes who restrict total energy and nutrient intake for long periods to reduce their body mass may be at greater risk of copper deficiency and its associated immunological effects (Lewis *et al.*, 2010). Copper supplementation may help to reduce loss of bone mineral density (Eaton-Evans *et al.*, 1998). It is advised that copper status should be assessed in athletes with chronically restricted energy intakes, those who report persistent fatigue, frequent infections and stress fractures. Despite potential for poor copper status in some athletes, copper supplementation should not be undertaken without clinical justification, given the fact that it can be toxic.

Competing interests   None

CORDYCEPS (*OPHIOCORDYCEPS*)

David S. Senchina

Cordyceps is labelled an ergogenic herb by many; however, *Ophiocordyceps sinensis* is actually a fungus (not a plant) commonly called caterpillar fungus. Cordycepic acid and mannitol are the most frequently cited bioactive compounds. It may affect oxygen metabolism. Results from recent investigations have been equivocal, but differ in their experimental designs and used *O sinensis* in combination with other purportedly ergogenic substances, making it difficult to ascertain the ergogenic effects of *O sinensis* individually. One study using single-dose supplementation showed no effect of *O sinensis* on anaerobic test outcomes in young males (Herda *et al.*, 2008), whereas a separate study using three-month supplementation showed improved reduced oxidative following a ~100 km race in young or middle-aged male cyclists (Rossi *et al.*, 2014).

Competing interests   None

CREATINE

Jacques R. Poortmans and Eric S. Rawson

About 20 years ago, Harris and colleagues (Harris *et al.*, 1992) introduced creatine as a nutritional supplement for athletes or individuals involved in physical training. Its commercial development worldwide has drawn it to the attention of athletes, from beginners to elite, as an ergogenic aid to enhance exercise performance. Creatine is a compound produced naturally by the body and its supplemental form is allowed under the WADA code. While some individuals and scientific media argue that there are potentially detrimental side effects, the past two decades of research have produced new insights into this compound (Poortmans *et al.*, 2010).

Creatine, a derivative from three amino acids, is distributed at approximately 95% in skeletal muscle mass; the remainder is located in the brain, the testes and the kidneys. Its synthesis starts mainly in the kidneys from glycine and arginine, forming α-methylguanidoacetic acid, which is conducted through the blood to the liver where it reacts with S-adenosylmethionine to synthesise creatine. Approximately 1–2g of creatine is produced over 24 hours and released mainly to the skeletal muscle system. Some creatine is also added to the pool by adequate dietary intake, predominantly from meat and fish, with a typical diet supplying approximately 1–2g of creatine daily. It may be assumed that there is a total creatine pool of approximately 120g in a man of 70 kg body weight. In skeletal muscle, creatine is slowly degraded to creatinine (approximately 2g/day), a reaction without any enzyme intervention, and is released to the blood and the kidney to be expelled through the urine.

Creatine is involved in the regulation of cellular energy demand. Under resting conditions, ATP is mainly formed in mitochondria through oxidative phosphorylation with ADP. Transported in sarcoplasm, some ATP molecules react with creatine, via the enzyme phosphorylcreatine kinase, to form phosphocreatine and ADP until equilibrium is reached. When ATP is needed for cellular energy, such as for muscle contraction, the phosphorylcreatine kinase reverse reaction replenishes the ATP content. Creatine thus acts indirectly to maintain a phosphorylcreatine reservoir for energy needs, more specifically to supply the muscle system with ATP.

In 1992, Harris *et al.* (1992) demonstrated that oral creatine supplementation could increase muscle creatine levels by approximately 20%. Subsequently, many studies have demonstrated that oral creatine supplementation can maximise muscle creatine levels by either: a 'loading' dose of 20g/day for approximately five days followed by a 'maintenance' dose of 2–3g/day; or by the 'maintenance' dose of 2–3g/day for approximately 30 days. These regimens lead to improved performance of repeated high-intensity exercise, increased strength and lean body mass and enhanced fatigue resistance for exercise tasks lasting 30 seconds or less, particularly when combined with progressive resistance training (Branch, 2003). The mechanisms through which creatine supplementation improves exercise performance and body composition include metabolic enhancements (increased pre-exercise phosphorylcreatine, increased pre-exercise muscle glycogen), molecular adaptations (increased gene expression of growth factors) and reduced muscle damage (Rawson and Persky, 2007). However, creatine supplementation does not increase skeletal muscle protein synthesis (Louis *et al.*, 2003; Parise *et al.*, 2001). As a result of these benefits, many sports competitors use creatine monohydrate as an ergogenic aid to boost their training and performance outcomes.

Although the focus of this review series is the sports-related uses of supplements, it is worth commenting that creatine supplements have potentially greater and more mainstream value than as performance enhancers for athletes. Creatine supplementation can improve muscle mass and fatigue resistance in sarcopenic older adults in whom a better function means an enhanced ability to perform activities of daily living (Rawson and Venezia, 2011). The benefits of creatine ingestion have been extended to patient populations as well, and there are many reports of improved muscle function in patients with various muscle disorders, e.g. muscular dystrophy, and degenerative central nervous system disorders, e.g. Parkinson's and Huntington's disease (Gualano *et al.*, 2010; Tarnopolsky, 2007). Promising new data have emerged demonstrating that creatine supplementation can improve cognitive processing in older adults (McMorris *et al.*, 2007).

In spring 1998, two British nephrologists initiated concerns about the possible deleterious consequences of oral creatine supplementation, citing a kidney-diseased individual. They suggested there was 'strong circumstantial evidence that creatine was responsible for the deterioration in renal function'. The Agence Française de Sécurité Sanitaire et Alimentaire (AFSSA) claimed that 'one should not encourage publicity of creatine in order to protect sport participants to any potential pathological consequences' (AFSSA, 2004). Anecdotal reports from athletes have claimed that creatine supplementation may induce muscle cramps. However, over the past 20 years the effects of creatine monohydrate on renal, hepatic, cardiovascular and muscular outcomes have been assessed, and creatine has been shown to have a good safety profile (Persky and Rawson, 2007).

For instance, despite allegations of detrimental effects of oral creatine supplementation on liver metabolism, studies on humans have not shown any significant increase in plasma urea, nor liver enzyme activity, during five years of creatine supplementation (Poortmans and Francaux, 2008). No reports have observed a modification of the glomerular filtration rate, nor the presence of microalbuminuria (Portmans and Francaux, 2000, 2008). All values remained within the normal range adapted for the age range. Experimentally, an excess conversion of creatine to sarcosine may result in cytotoxic agents such as methylamine. However, in humans taking up to 20g creatine per day for two weeks (Poortmans *et al.*, 2005; Sale *et al.*, 2009), urine methylamine excretion remains largely under the upper limit for healthy individuals.

Even if there are no health risks induced by oral creatine supplementation, it is safer to remain cautious when this substance is administered chronically. We advise that creatine supplementation should not be used by individuals with preexisting renal disease or those with a potential risk of renal dysfunction (hypertension, reduced glomerular filtration rate). Regular check-ups should be undertaken to monitor potential dysfunction, which could appear with some individuals less prone to compensate any homeostatic imbalance. Great care should also be taken as far as the purity of exogenous creatine supplements is concerned. Analytical tests must prove their unique nutraceutical composition, as safety is not assured in some preparations.

Competing interests   None

CYSTEINE AND CYSTINE

Kevin Currell

Cysteine is a non-essential amino acid and, together with glycine and glutamic acid, is an important precursor of the tripeptide glutathione. Glycine and glutamic acid are readily available within the body and it is thought that the limiting step in the synthesis of glutathione is the availability of cysteine (Rimaniol *et al.*, 2001). Glutathione is one of the key antioxidants within the body (Powers and Jackson, 2008), and is an essential component of immune function (Droge *et al.*, 1994).

Reid *et al.* (1994) intravenously infused 150mg/kg body weight of N-Acetyl-Cysteine (NAC) prior to electrical stimulation of the tibialis anterior to fatigue at either 10 or 40 Hz. NAC infusion increased force output during electrical stimulation at 10 Hz by 15% but failed to affect performance at 40 Hz. Medved *et al.* (2003) showed an improvement in blood redox status with NAC infusion during intermittent sprint cycling, but performance in the final sprint effort was not affected. However, these subjects were untrained and it is possible that the effect of NAC on delaying fatigue is greater with improved training status (Medved *et al.*, 2003). Oral intakes of NAC to obtain similar plasma levels seen during infusion would be very difficult and might lead to side effects such as nausea, bloating and diarrhoea (Medved *et al.*, 2003).

More recent research has investigated the effect of cystine, a dipeptide of cysteine, supplemented in conjunction with theanine, on the immune response to intense exercise training. Initial results suggest that immune function improved with oral cystine/theanine supplementation during intense training periods (Murakami *et al.*, 2009).

In conclusion, more work needs to be done in this area, particularly looking at oral cysteine ingestion and exercise performance and the effect of cystine supplementation on the immune response to training.

Competing interests   None

CYTOCHROME C

Christine E. Dziedzic

Cytochrome C, a small haeme protein, is found in the mitochondria where it is involved in the electron transport chain (Malatesta *et al.*, 1995). Endurance training (Holloszy and Coyle, 1984), and antioxidant supplementation (Davis *et al.*, 2008), have been shown to increase muscle cytochrome C concentrations. It has been hypothesised that supplementation with cytochrome C may also increase muscle levels, enhancing exercise performance by increasing maximum oxygen-carrying capacity, reducing blood lactate accumulation and raising anaerobic threshold (Snider *et al.*, 1992; Faria *et al.*, 2002).

In one of the few studies of supplementation in trained subjects, triathletes consumed a supplement providing cytochrome C (6430mg/day) in addition to inosine, vitamin E and coenzyme Q10 for 28 days prior to undertaking submaximal running followed by cycling to exhaustion (Snider *et al.*, 1992). No difference in cycling endurance was detected compared to performance in a placebo trial. Similarly, a six-day supplementation protocol by endurance runners, with cytochrome C as the main component (800mg/day plus a further 800mg one hour prior to testing) saw no benefits on run time to exhaustion, anaerobic threshold or blood lactate levels compared to a placebo trial (Faria *et al.*, 2002). Muscle cytochrome C concentrations were not measured in either of these studies.

On this basis, the use of cytochrome C as an ergogenic aid to enhance aerobic exercise capacity cannot be supported.

Competing interests   None

DEHYDROEPIANDROSTERONE (DHEA)

Douglas S. King

Dehydroepiandrosterone (DHEA) is a 'prohormone' or precursor of testosterone that is available as an over-the-counter supplement in many countries. It is promoted as a wonder supplement capable of promoting youthfulness, virility and enhanced strength or body composition. In men aged 20–70 years, ingesting a single dose of 50–100mg DHEA increases serum DHEA concentrations up to sevenfold and increases serum androstenedione concentrations approximately fourfold, but serum testosterone and dihydrotestosterone (DHT) concentrations are not changed (Brown et al., 2006). In older men (50–70 years), ingesting a single dose of 50–100mg DHEA raises serum oestradiol concentrations by 24–39% to the upper normal range. Prolonged ingestion of DHEA in doses ranging from 50 to 1,600mg/day in men (20–65 years) produces dose-dependent increases in serum DHEA, DHEA sulphate, and androstenedione, but has no effect on serum testosterone or DHT (Brown et al., 2006).

Thus, ingestion of DHEA in men increases only weak precursor hormones, with little or no increase in more potent androgens or oestrogens. More chronic intake of DHEA in doses of 50–1,600mg/day in men does not alter energy or protein metabolism, body mass or lean body mass (Welle et al., 1990). Intake of DHEA during resistance training does not augment the gains in lean mass or muscle strength in male college students or middle-aged men (Brown et al., 1999). It appears that DHEA does not promote fat loss or muscle gain or augment adaptations to resistance training in healthy men.

In women of all ages DHEA intake increases serum DHEA, DHEA sulphate, androstenedione, testosterone and oestradiol concentrations in a dose-dependent manner (von Mühlen et al., 2007). DHEA intake in women may cause negative side effects similar to those seen with anabolic steroid abuse (such as increased facial hair, oily skin and unfavourable changes in the blood lipid profile). There is no evidence that DHEA supplementation enhances athletic performance in women.

In summary, there is reasonably strong evidence of a lack of anabolic or ergogenic effects in supplement form at supraphysiological doses. There is also strong evidence of dose and time-related widespread adverse effects resulting in several negative health consequences. Surprisingly, DHEA is classified as an androgenic/anabolic steroid and included on the WADA Prohibited List (WADA, 2014) and other anti-doping codes, and may cause an athlete to fail a urinary screening for anabolic steroids, but DHEA is not included as a controlled substance in the United States Anabolic-Steroid Control Act of 2004. DHEA is being evaluated for treatment of depression and as an aid for fertility treatment, but these data are too preliminary to draw a conclusion.

Competing interests   None

DIHYDROXYACETONE PHOSPHATE AND PYRUVATE

Lawrence L. Spriet

Dihydroxyacetone phosphate (DHAP) and pyruvate are three-carbon metabolites in the glycolytic pathway. In skeletal muscle, the glycolytic pathway metabolises glucose from the blood and stored glycogen. DHAP is formed at an intermediate step, and pyruvate is produced in the final step of glycolysis. During aerobic exercise, pyruvate enters the mitochondrion and is oxidised to produce ATP. It is not immediately clear how ingesting oral doses of DHAP/pyruvate could influence athletic performance, as it is unlikely that the ingested compounds could reach skeletal muscle and have a direct effect on metabolism. Pyruvate undergoes acid hydrolysis in the stomach and gut with the liberation of carbon dioxide gas, and ingestion of large amounts of pyruvate results in gastrointestinal distress (Morrison *et al.*, 2000). In addition, the pyruvate that is absorbed into the blood could be taken up and stored by the liver, as even the highest tolerable acute dose of pyruvate (~25g) represents a small amount of glucose (~12.5g). In support of this, no increases in whole blood and plasma pyruvate were reported during a four-hour period after the acute ingestion of 7, 15 and 25g doses of pyruvate (Morrison *et al.*, 2000). It is not clear what happens to the ingested DHAP. Typically, a more successful approach is the ingestion of the six-carbon molecule glucose which has been repeatedly shown to accumulate in the blood and be taken up and oxidised by skeletal muscle (Jeukendrup *et al.*, 1995).

Only three studies have examined the potential for DHAP/pyruvate to improve exercise capacity. Despite no plausible ergogenic mechanism, two studies reported an improvement in exercise time to exhaustion (~20%) after the consumption of ~75g DHAP/25g pyruvate for seven days (Stanko *et al.*, 1990a, 1990b). The authors attributed the improvement to increased skeletal muscle glucose utilisation and this work has been summarised in a review by Ivy (1998). However, these studies used untrained subjects who were not blinded to the treatments. A later study examined the effects of pyruvate only and had well-trained subjects ingest 7g/day pyruvate or placebo for one week followed by cycling to exhaustion at 75–80% VO_{2max} (Morrison *et al.*, 2000). There was no difference in cycling endurance (~90 min) between the trials, and the subjects were not able to identify the supplement they received.

Two studies have examined a combination of supplemental creatine and pyruvate on the anaerobic exercise performance and body composition of American football players (Stone *et al.*, 1999) and cycling performance in well-trained cyclists (Van Schuylenbergh *et al.*, 2003). In the first study, the presence of pyruvate in the supplement had no effects above those of creatine alone, and in the second study, the creatine-pyruvate supplement did not improve endurance capacity or intermittent sprint performance. It has been argued that the addition of pyruvate to the creatine supplement was to improve the water solubility and possibly increase the availability of the ingested creatine, and not because of any purported independent ergogenic effect of pyruvate.

On the basis of these few reports and no apparent mechanism to alter metabolism, several reviews have concluded that oral pyruvate is not ergogenic (Dyck, 2004; Juhn, 2003; Sukala, 1998). Not surprisingly, there has not been recent research in this area. In summary, there is currently no scientific basis for the use of DHAP/pyruvate as an ergogenic aid.

Competing interests   None

1,3-DIMETHYLETHYLAMINE (DMAA)

Ano Lobb

1,3-Dimethylethylamine (DMAA), also known as methylhexanamine, is an amphetamine derivative originally patented as a nasal decongestant, then subsequently withdrawn as an approved pharmaceutical (Cohen, 2012; Gee *et al.*, 2012). DMAA has recently reemerged as an ingredient in dietary supplements, especially products aimed at weight loss and exercise performance (e.g. pre-workout products and energy drinks). Its presence in supplements was considered legitimate because trace amounts were reported as naturally occurring in oil from the geranium plant (*Pelargonium graveolens*), suggesting DMAA was a natural product. There has been significant controversy about whether geranium oil does in fact contain DMAA, with some studies saying yes (Fleming *et al.*, 2012; Gauthier, 2013; Li *et al.*, 2012; Rodricks and Lumpkin, 2013), and some saying no (Austin *et al.*, 2014; Cohen, 2012; Zhang *et al.*, 2012).

At least four small, short duration studies in healthy subjects funded by the manufacturer suggest that DMAA does not significantly increase blood pressure or cause other significant side effects (Farney *et al.*, 2012; McCarthy *et al.*, 2012; Schilling *et al.*, 2013; Whitehead *et al.*, 2012b). However, DMAA-containing supplements are now banned in several countries, including the USA after being linked to 86 adverse events, including hypertension, stroke, heart attack, seizure, psychiatric disorders and death (USFDA, 2014a; Gee *et al.*, 2012; Young *et al.*, 2012). DMAA was also suspected of 56 cases of poisoning reported between 2010 and 2011 in the state of Texas alone (Forrester, 2013). Authorities in the EU, UK, Australia, New Zealand and Canada have also taken steps to remove DMAA-containing supplements from consumer reach (Cohen, 2012; Eliason *et al.*, 2012). No reliable evidence from controlled trials in humans has found meaningful athletic performance enhancement from DMAA. DMAA is included on the WADA Prohibited List as a stimulant (WADA, 2014b), and a sudden increase in the number of Anti-Doping Rule Violations for this compound has led some countries to issue specific warnings about it and supplements in which it has been found (ASADA, 2014a).

Competing interests None

DIMETHYLGLYCINE

James Collins and Joseph Lockey

Dimethylglycine (N,N-Dimethylglycine, DMG) is a dimethylated derivative of the amino acid glycine. Found naturally in animal and plant cells, it is an intermediate in glycine synthesis from the degradation of choline. Indirectly it is involved in a wide range of metabolic pathways through transmethylation. DMG is also an active ingredient in pangamic acid (see section on pangamic acid). It is proposed that DMG may enhance metabolic variables of aerobic performance in humans, and historically, supplementation has been used by Soviet athletes (Graber *et al.*, 1981) and American Football players (Bishop *et al.*, 1987).

Studies using trained subjects found no difference in running performance (time to exhaustion), or associated metabolic variables (heart rate, VO_{2max}) following 21 days of 200mg/day DMG (Harpaz *et al.*, 1985) or when 135mg DMG was administered acutely prior to a treadmill test to exhaustion (Bishop *et al.*, 1987). Potential immunomodulating capacities of DMG in humans (Reap and Lawson, 1990) may have been masked by the study design. Animal studies have failed to demonstrate an enhancement in specific or non-specific immunity (Weiss, 1992).

Although little is known about the effects of DMG and general health outcomes, a recent study has demonstrated a consistent relationship between plasma concentration and an adverse cardiovascular risk profile. Within two cohorts totalling over 7,000 patients with cardiovascular disease, elevated plasma DMG was associated with higher mortality. It also improved risk prediction beyond traditional cardiovascular disease risk factors (Svingen *et al.*, 2014). Whilst this does not imply causation, caution should be used when considering DMG as a supplement until its role in cardiovascular disease has been further studied.

There is currently insufficient evidence to support DMG supplementation in athletic populations.

Competing interests   None

ECHINACEA

David S. Senchina

Echinacea is believed to strengthen the immune system against upper respiratory infections. Taxonomically, *Echinacea* is an American angiosperm genus of nine species, but vernacularly, 'echinacea' commonly refers to three species (*Echinacea angustifolia*, *Echinacea pallida* and *Echinacea purpurea*). Purported bioactive molecules include alk(yl)amides, caffeic acid derivatives and polysaccharides. Clinical studies of echinacea supplements typically utilize commercial whole herb formulations from above-ground parts, and less commonly roots.

Research on athletes given echinacea supplements (doses varied or not given) reported upper respiratory tract infection prophylaxis, reviewed elsewhere (Senchina *et al.*, 2009b; Senchina, 2013), and good tolerability with few adverse effects (Schoop *et al.*, 2006). Research using blood leucocytes isolated from athletes pre- and post-exercise, then stimulated with echinacea extracts *in vitro*, suggested that echinacea alkamides and caffeic acid derivatives may stimulate cytokine production or cell proliferation (Senchina *et al.*, 2009a). Athletes treated with echinacea for four weeks demonstrated a shorter duration of infections and improved post-exercise salivary antibody levels compared with athletes given placebo, though both groups had a similar number of infections (Hall *et al.*, 2007). The effects of echinacea on VO_{2max} appear equivocal (Bellar *et al.*, 2014; Whitehead *et al.*, 2012a), though it may increase erythropoietin (Whitehead *et al.*, 2007, 2012a). Echinacea alkamides appear to be responsible for the bulk of echinacea bioactivity in clinical and *in vitro* athlete studies (Senchina *et al.*, 2013a), but few of the athlete clinical trials reported extract composition. More numerous studies of echinacea in non-athletes vary greatly, complicating direct comparisons between studies, but overall show none or minimal effects of echinacea supplements on prevention and treatment of the common cold (Karsch-Völk *et al.*, 2014).

It is presently unclear why clinical studies of echinacea in athletes show stronger effects than in non-athlete populations, though discrepancies may stem from unaccounted preclinical factors, such as agricultural, production, storage, or clinical population factors (Senchina *et al.*, 2009b; Senchina, 2013).

Competing interests None

ELECTROLYTES

Michael F. Bergeron

Electrolytes are negatively (*anions*) or positively (*cations*) charged substances that, when in solution, conduct an electric current. Major physiological electrolytes include Na^+, K^+, Cl^- and HCO_3^-, while other electrolytes such as Ca^{2+}, Mg^{2+} and trace elements are also found in the body in significant amounts. Na^+, K^+, Cl^- and HCO_3^- are primarily responsible for normal water distribution and homeostasis throughout the body via their effect on osmotic pressure. These major electrolytes also play an essential role in regulating heart and muscle function, maintaining pH and a number of other important biochemical reactions. Calcium, the most abundant mineral in the body, plays an important role in vascular and muscle function, nerve transmission and intracellular signalling. However, the bulk of the body's vast reserve of Ca^{2+} is stored in the bones and teeth as an integral component to structure and function, including bone remodelling. About half of total body Mg^{2+} is found in bone, providing support for bone strength; whereas the rest is mostly inside tissue and organ cells, with around 1% in the blood. Mg^{2+} plays a critical cofactor role in numerous biochemical reactions, including those supporting muscle, nerve and immune function, blood glucose control, energy metabolism and protein synthesis. (See relevant electrolyte sections elsewhere in this book.)

An athlete's demand for electrolytes increases with exercise and heat stress, as extensive sweating can mean both large water and electrolyte losses in addition to related changes in extra- and intracellular water distribution. During long duration (e.g. >1 hour), moderate-intensity exercise in the heat, hypotonic sweat secretion and renal sodium conservation tend to elevate serum Na^+ concentration and decrease urinary Na^+ excretion. Dehydration and an increase in plasma osmolality, which is primarily driven by Na^+, will concomitantly stimulate osmoreceptors prompting an athlete to drink to maintain further or defend plasma volume (Stachenfeld, 2008). The primary electrolytes in sweat are Na^+ (20–70 mmol/l) and Cl^-, with comparatively much lower levels of K^+ (~5 mmol/l) and even less Ca^{2+} (~1 mmol/l) and Mg^{2+} (~0.8 mmol/l) (Sawka and Montain, 2000). As the sweating rate increases, the concentration of Na^+ in sweat increases correspondingly, even with the lower sweat Na^+ concentrations observed after heat acclimation (Buono *et al.*, 2007). With Na^+ being the major cation of extracellular fluid, despite renal Na^+ conservation, copious sweating can lead to a sizable sweat-induced whole-body exchangeable Na^+ deficit. In sports such as tennis, substantial sweat losses and extensive related body water and electrolyte deficits are not uncommon, especially when players compete in extended and multiple same-day matches (Bergeron, 2014). It is worth noting that such a deficit is not usually indicated by lower plasma osmolality or circulating Na^+ levels. A significant Na^+ deficit (e.g. 20–30% of the exchangeable Na^+ pool), combined with a loss in plasma volume prompting water to shift to the intravascular space, can lead to a contracted interstitial fluid compartment and possible widespread skeletal muscle cramping. Athletes affected with exertional muscle cramping related to significant water and/or sodium deficit(s) can be effectively treated with an oral high-salt solution or intravenously (Bergeron, 2008).

Being a predominantly intracellular cation, losses of K^+ in sweat are generally low enough to be adequately met by a normal diet. Moreover, as with Na^+, plasma K^+ levels are acutely affected by exercise – notably, in proportion to exercise intensity as well as the muscle mass involved and the interplay of K^+ release and reuptake by muscle during and after exercise. Associated fluid shifts and related changes in plasma volume are also influencing factors (Atanasovska *et al.*, 2014). Undue exercise strain and/or hyperthermia can elicit excessive skeletal muscle fibre breakdown and rhabdomyolysis. An influx of Ca^{2+} in these circumstances would promote further muscle damage and fibre necrosis, and the release of muscle fibre intracellular contents (myoglobin, creatine kinase, phosphate *and* K^+) into the circulation could potentially lead to acute renal failure and death. This is often preceded by severe hyperkalaemia (very high levels of K^+ in the blood) prompting cardiac arrhythmia and arrest (Sauret *et al.*, 2002).

The major source of electrolytes comes from our diets; and the dietary guidelines for maintaining water and electrolyte balance for health and performance in active people are well-defined (American Dietetic Association *et al.*, 2009; Sawka *et al.*, 2007; Whiting and Barabash, 2006). Although certain electrolytes (especially sodium) are frequently consumed well in excess of requirements, athletes often look for supplementary forms of electrolytes to replace those lost in sweat. This is sometimes justified when the timing and amount of necessary electrolyte replacement during or after an exercise session cannot be provided easily by food sources. The body normally conserves enough extracellular Na^+ and Cl^- through reabsorption by the kidneys as is needed to maintain whole-body Na^+ and water balance. However, an accumulating sodium deficit often needs to be offset with supplemental dietary NaCl intake during and after exercise or other physical activity when sweat losses are great (Valentine, 2007). The presence of moderate amounts of sodium (and other electrolytes) in a sports drink, or the addition of electrolyte supplements to other beverages, can increase voluntary intake of fluid and enhance the retention of fluids consumed to restore hydration status more completely after exercise or other dehydrating activities (Shirreffs *et al.*, 2004). Accordingly, the value of simultaneous replacement of electrolytes with fluid intake in situations requiring restoration of moderate to large fluid deficits is well accepted.

Excessive intake of water or low-sodium fluids (such as most sports drinks) over a short period of time, in measurable excess of sweat and urinary water losses can readily lead to water overload, a condition known as hyponatraemia. Exercise-related hyponatraemia typically indicates an excess of total body water compared with total body exchangeable Na^+ and sometimes, in a much lesser contributing way, a measurable sweat-induced exchangeable Na^+ deficit. Severe hyponatraemia can lead to serious consequences. This is because a significant decrease in plasma Na^+ concentration and consequent osmotic gradient can cause brain swelling and altered mental status, seizure, respiratory distress, coma or even death. But less severe exercise-related hyponatraemia (when plasma Na^+ concentration is 125–130 mmol/l) resulting from moderate overconsumption of fluid during physical activity can still prompt nausea, vomiting and headache. Its prevalence is increasingly recognized at endurance events in slow and inexperienced athletes who have low sweat rates and generous opportunities to consume fluid. This clinical situation often needs to be corrected by intravenous saline administration after being verified by a plasma or serum Na^+ measurement (Hew-Butler et al., 2005).

Competing interests   None

EPHEDRA

David S. Senchina

Ephedra, Asiatic in origin and widely popular historically, often refers to a single Asian species (*Ephedra sinica*, Ma Huang) or sometimes a supplement containing one isolated alkaloid, though the genus *Ephedra* is a global gymnosperm genus of ~50 species. Ephedra is billed to promote alertness, endurance and strength. Ephedra sympathomimetic alkaloids (ephedrine, pseudoephedrine, phenylpropanolamine) are structurally similar to methamphetamine, releasing catechoalmines and acting on cellular α and β receptors and adrenoreceptors; these actions increase cardiovascular variables (Avois *et al.*, 2006). Ephedra alkaloids are components in cough syrups, decongestants and diet aids. Supplements are most often made from ephedra stems.

Studies investigating ergogenic effects of ephedra by dosing athletes with isolated alkaloids (usually pseudoephedrine, usually up to 120mg) have reported non-significant and often heterogeneous results, reviewed elsewhere (Magkos and Kavouras, 2004). One study that supplemented athletes with a whole herb supplement found no effect of 60mg of ephedra when used in conjunction with 300mg of caffeine on strength or power (Williams *et al.*, 2008). Some *in vitro* data suggest ephedra supplements or isolated alkaloids may modulate athlete immune function, possibly through anti-inflammatory mechanisms, though a recent review concluded the data was not consistent and that *in vivo* effects had yet to be demonstrated (Senchina *et al.*, 2014).

Despite widespread public belief, ephedra does not have ergogenic properties in applicable contexts. However, it does carry serious adverse effect risks (Jenkinson and Harbert, 2008). Ephedrine, methylephedrine and pseudoephedrine are specified on WADA's stimulants prohibited in competition list with urinary concentrations being prohibited at >10μg/ml for ephedrine and methylephedrine and >150μg/ml for pseudoephedrine (WADA, 2014b). Consequently, due to the occurrence of ephedra alkaloids in many every-day medications, both OTC (over the counter) and prescribed, athletes always need to check their medications with their sports physician and obtain a Therapeutic Use Exemption (TUE) certificate if the product contains a prohibited substance but is essential for medical purposes. Athletes are also cautioned about buying products, even seemingly the same brand, whilst travelling abroad as some products may contain different substances when purchased abroad. Sadly there are cases of athletes' athletic careers ending abruptly due to testing positive for a banned substance after taking a cold remedy.

Competing interests   None

FATTY ACIDS

Philip C. Calder

Fatty acids are a major component of most diets and can be synthesised endogenously in the human body (Calder and Burdge, 2004). They are found in all cells and tissues and are transported between tissues in the bloodstream. Fatty acids are usually linked to other structures, frequently but not exclusively by ester linkages, to form more complex lipids like triglycerides, phospholipids and sphingolipids. Non-esterified fatty acids (NEFAs), often called 'free fatty acids', circulate in the bloodstream and are an important source of energy for skeletal muscle and heart cells.

All fatty acids have a common general structure: a hydrocarbon chain (termed the acyl chain) with a methyl group at one end and carboxyl group at the other (Calder and Burdge, 2004). It is this reactive carboxyl group that readily forms ester links. Individual fatty acids are distinguished by the length of their hydrocarbon chain, and by the absence, presence, number and configuration (*cis* or *trans*) of double bonds within that chain. Fatty acids have systematic and trivial names and there are also several shorthand nomenclatures based upon structural features (Calder and Burdge, 2004).

Saturated and monounsaturated fatty acids can be synthesised *de novo* from precursors like glucose (Gurr *et al.*, 2002). This occurs mainly in the liver and is promoted by insulin. The simplest polyunsaturated fatty acids (PUFAs), linoleic acid (18:2n-6) and α-linolenic acid (18:3n-3), cannot be synthesised in animals including humans. However, they can be synthesised in plants, often abundantly. Because they have important roles in animals but cannot be synthesised *de novo*, linoleic and α-linolenic acids are essential in the diet. Essential fatty acid deficiency is manifested by typical nutrient deficiency symptoms. However, this condition is rare in humans, being avoided by relatively low intakes of the essential fatty acids. Animals can metabolise essential fatty acids further, inserting additional double bonds (desaturation) and extending the hydrocarbon chain (elongation). Through these processes linoleic acid can be converted to arachidonic acid (20:4n-6) and α-linolenic acid to eicosapentaenoic acid (EPA; 20:5n-3). Further metabolism to longer chain, more unsaturated derivatives is possible; for example, the conversion of EPA to docosahexaenoic acid (DHA; 22:6n-3), although the extent of this conversion is not clear in humans. There is competition between the n-6 and n-3 fatty acid families for metabolism and therefore the ratio or balance between these fatty acids appears important.

Fat makes an important contribution to dietary energy intake, typically providing 30 to 40% in most Western diets. Most dietary fat occurs as fatty acids esterified into triglycerides. All diets contain many different fatty acids, the relative abundance reflecting the fatty acid composition of the foods eaten. Triglycerides must be extensively hydrolysed before the body can assimilate their constituent fatty acids. This hydrolysis is catalysed by lipase enzymes, chiefly pancreatic lipase, operating in the small intestine. The process of triglyceride digestion is very efficient in most humans. After entering the absorptive cells (enterocytes), fatty acids with hydrocarbon chains of < 12 carbons are absorbed directly into the portal blood. However, transport of longer chain fatty acids is more complex. They are first re-esterified into triglycerides, then packaged with phospholipids and apolipoproteins to form chylomicrons which are secreted into the lymphatic circulation and then enter the bloodstream, having bypassed the liver. Fatty acids within chylomicrons are targeted for uptake and storage in adipose tissue, promoted by lipoprotein lipase action at the endothelial surface. Once taken up, fatty acids are re-esterified to triglycerides within the adipose tissue and stored in this form. These processes are promoted by insulin. Hydrolysis of stored triglyceride releases the fatty acids which enter the bloodstream in the non-esterified form: this is promoted by adrenaline, noradrenaline and other stress hormones. Some triglyceride stored within skeletal muscle serves as a local reservoir of fatty acids.

The principal roles of fatty acids are as energy sources and membrane constituents (Gurr et al., 2002; Calder and Burdge, 2004). Many types of fatty acid can fill these roles. Certain fatty acids have additional, specific roles, such as serving as precursors for the synthesis of bioactive lipid mediators (e.g. prostaglandins), and influencing membrane and intracellular signalling processes, the activation of transcription factors and gene expression (Calder and Burge, 2004). Through these different actions, fatty acids are able to influence cellular functions and thus physiological responses.

Fatty acids are oxidized by the process of β-oxidation which occurs within mitochondria. Oxidation of fatty acids generates more energy than the oxidation of glucose (~9 cal/g vs. ~4 cal/g, respectively). Two key points control the rate of fatty acid oxidation: 1) intracellular fatty acid concentration which, in turn, is determined by their concentration in the blood, so that a rise in circulating NEFA concentration increases fatty acid oxidation in the tissues using them; 2) transport of NEFAs (as their coenzyme A esters) from the cytosol into the mitochondria via the carnitine acyl transferase system (Gurr et al., 2002; Frayn, 2010). NEFAs become important energy sources during starvation, endurance exercise and other situations where carbohydrate supply is limiting (Frayn, 2010). Glucose and NEFA oxidation are inversely related, so that energy demands of different tissues in different physiological situations can be met by an appropriate, but changing, fuel supply. Importantly, the oxidation of fatty acids requires concurrent glucose oxidation because the movement of acetyl-coenzyme A from fatty acid β-oxidation into the Kreb's Cycle needs a supply of oxaloacetate provided from pyruvate, derived from glucose. Fatty acid oxidation cannot maintain the same power output as glucose oxidation and so performance is decreased as fatty acids contribute increasingly to meeting the demand for energy. It is well known that endurance training regimens can enhance the number of mitochondria and enzyme activities of the Kreb's Cycle and the β-oxidation pathway, thus improving NEFA utilisation as a fuel (Frayn, 2010).

Other training and supplement strategies that have been investigated with the intention of enhancing fatty acid oxidation either fail to increase fat utilisation or fail to result in performance enhancement (Hawley *et al.*, 1998). Among these are 'fat loading' (high fat consumption), which may bring about metabolic alterations to increase fatty acid use during exercise, but does not improve performance, perhaps even impairing the ability to undertake high-intensity exercise when required during an endurance event (Burke and Kiens, 2006). Oral L-carnitine has poor bioavailability and little impact on tissue carnitine content unless taken under specific conditions (see section on carnitine); this does not appear to be an easy strategy to increase fatty acid oxidation. Caffeine promotes NEFA release from stored triglycerides and is well-supported as an ergogenic aid across a variety of sports (see section on caffeine), although the effects vary across individuals (Ganio *et al.*, 2009) and are unlikely to be related to effects on fat oxidation (Graham *et al.*, 2008).

Increased dietary intake of fatty acids normally consumed in low amounts (e.g. long chain n-3 PUFAs like EPA and DHA) results in the incorporation of these fatty acids into cell membranes, and this might be one mechanism by which dietary fat affects cell function, physiological responses and health (Calder, 2012). One study suggested that differences in fatty acid profiles of skeletal muscle between trained and untrained individuals, despite similar dietary fatty acid composition (Andersson *et al.*, 2000), were a direct consequence of changes in fatty acid metabolism due to increased physical activity.

There is no role for supplements aimed at providing saturated or monounsaturated fatty acids or linoleic acid, since these are all consumed in significant amounts from a mixed healthy diet and the former two classes of fatty acid can be synthesized *de novo*. There may be a role for supplements aimed at providing those fatty acids which are consumed in lower amounts from the diet and which have general or specific physiological functions or roles in human health or athletic performance. Examples would be: 1) α-linolenic acid, found in significant amounts in certain plant oils (e.g. flaxseed), which acts to increase status of its derivative EPA: EPA status increase is linearly related to the amount of α-linolenic acid provided; 2) the long chain highly unsaturated n-3 PUFAs EPA and DHA found in fish oils and similar supplements (see section on fish oils); and 3) conjugated linoleic acids (see section on conjugated linoleic acid).

Competing interests   None

FERULIC ACID AND γ-ORYZANOL

Siobhan Crawshay

γ-oryzanol, a mixture of a plant sterol and ferulic acid ester first isolated from rice bran oil in the 1950s, is now known to be found in various vegetable oils and products. The phytosterol base, structurally similar to cholesterol, has been promoted as having cholesterol-lowering and testosterone-enhancing activities, but these have not been substantiated in humans. Like other plant sterols, γ-oryzanol is poorly absorbed from the gastrointestinal tract. However, it has been proposed that the well-absorbed ferulic acid is the active agent in γ-oryzanol, having antioxidant properties (Fry *et al.*, 1997; Wheeler and Garleb, 1991). As a result, ferulic acid has been isolated and marketed as a separate supplement.

Despite a lack of evidence or consistent explanation of mechanisms underpinning claimed benefits, γ-oryzanol and ferulic acid have been used by body builders and strength-training athletes in the hope of increasing muscle mass and strength, reducing body fat, speeding recovery and reducing post-exercise soreness. Endorphin release is also claimed. Only one study testing these claimed effects on athletic performance has been published in peer-reviewed literature. This involved 22 recreationally weight-trained male college students who undertook a nine-week resistance training protocol, combined with daily intake of 500mg of γ-oryzanol or placebo. Both groups improved their muscle strength and vertical jump power, while increasing body mass and decreasing skinfold fat (Fry *et al.*, 1997). Resting testosterone and cortisol concentrations were decreased at the end of the testing period in both groups, with no other alterations in hormone, lipid or blood parameters. These findings recognize the benefits of training, but do not support additional effects from γ-oryzanol ingestion. Other information in abstract form also fails to support benefits from ferulate supplements. Six highly trained male distance runners supplemented with either placebo or 50mg of ferulate daily for three weeks in a cross-over design. Although workouts increased blood concentrations of cortisol, testosterone and β-endorphins, there were no differences in the response between ferulate and placebo trials, with the exception of an increase in post-exercise β-endorphin concentrations during some sessions in the final week of intensified training (Bonner *et al.*, 1990). A further multi-centre trial involved supplementation of a placebo or ferulate treatment (15mg twice daily) for eight weeks by a small number of weightlifters. The authors reported a significant increase in body weight and shoulder press strength in the supplemented group ($n=6$) compared to the placebo group ($n=4$), but no differences in leg and chest strength (Bucci *et al.*, 1990).

In summary, the effects of supplementation with γ-oryzanol and ferulic acid on athletic performance have not been well studied, and there is no current evidence to support their use in sport.

Competing interests   None

FISH OILS

Philip C. Calder and Martin R. Lindley

Fish oils contain the long chain highly unsaturated omega-3 (n-3) fatty acids eicosapenteanoic acid (EPA) and docosahexaenoic acid (DHA), although EPA and DHA amounts and their ratio vary according to origin: type of fish; season; location where the fish is caught, etc. (Calder and Yaqoob, 2009). Many commonly available fish oils contain about 30% EPA plus DHA; more concentrated preparations are available. Most fish oils present fatty acids in triglyceride form although some supplements provide them as phospholipids, free fatty acids or ethyl esters. All forms have good bioavailability, although there may be small differences in this. Fish liver oils, e.g. cod liver oil, contain higher amounts of vitamins A and D than fish body oils. Typical daily intakes of EPA and DHA in people not consuming oily fish are likely to be < 200mg/day, perhaps even lower than this, which is below the recommendation of ~500mg/day. Thus, supplements can make a substantial contribution to the recommended n-3 fatty acid intake. When fish oil supplements are consumed, EPA and DHA become enriched within blood lipids, cells and tissues, and influence many aspects of metabolism and physiology; the changes induced are considered to lead to improved health or lowered risk of disease (Calder and Yaqoob, 2009). A daily intake of at least several hundred mg of EPA and DHA is apparently required to induce health benefits, but clear threshold doses and dose-response relationships are not established.

Exercise- or athlete-specific benefits of fish oils are not clear due to inconsistencies in the scientific literature. They may improve metabolic changes that occur with exercise (Peoples *et al.*, 2008), or reduce exercise-induced inflammation (Phillips *et al.*, 2003). Enhanced cardiac function during exercise, perhaps resulting in better oxygen delivery to tissues, has been described following fish oil supplementation in healthy non-athletes (Walser and Stebbins, 2008). Other studies report no effect of fish oil on maximum aerobic power, anaerobic threshold or exercise performance in athletes (Oostenbrug *et al.*, 1997; Raastad *et al.*, 1997; Huffman *et al.*, 2004; Nieman *et al.*, 2009b). One study reported that fish oil reduced exercise-induced delayed onset muscle soreness (Tartibian *et al.*, 2009), but another study found no effect (Lenn *et al.*, 2002). A recent study reported that fish oil could prevent some, though not all, of the exercise-induced impairments of immune function in untrained individuals (Gray *et al.*, 2012), but had no effect on exercise-induced muscle soreness in these individuals (Gray *et al.*, 2014). These studies typically used moderate (1.8g/day) to high (4g/day) doses of EPA plus DHA over several weeks or months but many studies have studied only a small number of subjects. One area yielding some positive results for fish oil supplementation is exercise-induced bronchoconstriction (EIB). A high dose (3.2g EPA plus 2.0g DHA daily) for three weeks markedly improved lung function post-exercise in non-atopic elite athletes with exercise-induced bronchoconstriction (Mickleborough *et al.*, 2003), and in asthmatic athletes (Mickleborough *et al.*, 2006). Cell culture work suggests that EPA rather than DHA may be responsible and the benefit may involve novel EPA-derived mediators.

Competing interests   None

FLAVONOIDS

David C. Nieman

Phytochemicals are chemicals produced by plants, and include tannins, lignins and flavonoids. The largest and best studied polyphenols are the flavonoids, with more than 6,000 identified and classified into at least six subgroups: flavonols, flavones, flavanones, flavanols (and their oligomers, proanthocyanidins), anthocyanidins, and isoflavonoids (Figure 18). Flavonoids are widely distributed in plants and function as plant pigments, signalling molecules, and defenders against infection and injury. Dietary intake of flavonoids ranges from 50 to 800mg/day depending on the consumption of fruits and vegetables, and the intake of tea (Chun *et al.*, 2010; Zamora *et al.*, 2010). In the USA, total flavonoid intake averages 210mg/day (Chun *et al.* 2010) and in Spain 313mg/day (Zamora-Ros *et al.,* 2010), with important sources including tea, citrus fruit and juice, beers and ales, wines, melon and berries, apples, onions and bananas.

A high intake of fruits and vegetables has been linked in numerous studies to reduced risk of cardiovascular disease and various types of cancer. The disease-reducing influence of fruits and vegetables may be due in part to high levels of flavonoids. Although cell culture and animal scientific evidence is promising in support of the role of flavonoid intake in disease prevention, human studies are mixed and inconclusive when taken as a whole (Hooper *et al.*, 2008; Wang *et al.*, 2009). Part of the problem is that flavonoid data are limited to a modest number of foods, hampering efforts to estimate total flavonoid intake in human subjects.

Flavonoid subgroup	Specific flavonoids	Food sources
1. Flavonols	Quercetin, Kaempferol, Myricetin, Isorhamnetin	Onions, apples, leafy vegetables, berries
2. Flavones	Luteolin, Apigenin	Parsley, hot peppers, celery, artichokes, spices
3. Flavanones	Hesperetin, Naringenin, Eriodictyol	Citrus fruits and citrus juices
4. Flavan-3-ols	Catechins, Epigallocatechins, Theaflavins	Tea, chocolate, tree fruits, grape seed
5. Anthocyanidins	Cyanidin, Delphinidin, Malvidin, Pelargonidin, Peonidin, Petunidin	Most berries, cowpeas
6. Isoflavones	Daidzein, Genistein, Glycitein	Soybeans, soyfoods

FIGURE 18 Flavonoid subgroups and food sources

Source: Adapted from USDA Nutrient Data Laboratory (2007).

Many flavonoids possess strong anti-inflammatory, anti-viral, antioxidant, anti-obesity and anti-carcinogenic properties when studied *in vitro* using large doses of the purified form. Inflammation and oxidative stress are key mechanisms in the pathogenesis of certain disease states, supporting the proposed strategy of increased flavonoid intake for prevention of cancer, diabetes mellitus and cardiovascular disease. However, results from randomized, double-blinded studies in humans with large doses of purified flavonoids such as quercetin have been disappointing (Shanely *et al.*, 2010). Flavonoids vary widely in bioavailability, and most are poorly absorbed, undergo active efflux, and are extensively conjugated and metabolically transformed, all of which can affect their bioactive capacities (Zhang *et al.*, 2007). Despite low bioavailability of the parent flavonoid, some of the *in vivo* metabolites may accumulate in tissues and produce bioactive influences, but conclusive human data are lacking. For example, animal data indicate that quercetin metabolites accumulate in the vascular tissue and act there as complementary antioxidants, with plasma albumin facilitating the translocation of quercetin metabolites to the vascular target (Terao *et al.*, 2008).

There is a growing realization that the bioactive influences of individual flavonoids are potentiated when mixed with other flavonoids (e.g. the flavonol quercetin with the flavanol epigallocatechin 3-gallate or EGCG) or included in a cocktail or extract of other polyphenols and nutrients (Lila, 2007). Two or more flavonoids ingested together may increase bioavailability and decrease elimination via competitive inhibition of glucuronide and sulphate conjugation in both the intestine and liver, and by inhibiting efflux transporters such as P-glycoprotein, breast cancer resistance protein (BCRP), and multidrug resistance protein 2, i.e. MRP2 (Kale *et al.*, 2010).

The health-protective effects of plant foods are not produced by a single component but rather complex mixtures of interacting molecules (Lila, 2007). The polyphenols and natural components provide a multifaceted defensive strategy for both plants and humans. Thus the 'pharma' approach of using large doses of a single bioactive molecule is seldom successful in the application of nutrition to human health and performance. Additionally, a metabolomics or nutrigenomics approach is needed to improve the capacity of investigators to capture the complex and subtle influences of flavonoid supplements or flavonoid-rich extracts, foods and beverages on whole-body metabolism and physiology (Bakker *et al.*, 2010).

Flavonoids and exercise

Various nutritional agents have been tested for their capacity to attenuate oxidative stress, inflammation and immune changes following intensive exercise, and thus lower the magnitude of physiologic stress and risk of upper respiratory tract infection (URTI; Nieman, 2008). Some question the value of using nutritional supplements as countermeasures to exercise-induced oxidative stress and inflammation because these may interfere with important signaling mechanisms for training adaptations (Ristow *et al.*, 2009). Another viewpoint is that nutritional supplements attenuate but do not totally block exercise-induced oxidative stress and inflammation, analogous to the beneficial use of ice packs to reduce swelling following mild injuries (Yfanti *et al.*, 2010).

Pure flavonoids such as quercetin, EGCG and isoflavones, or flavonoid-rich plant extracts, are being tested by an increasing number of investigative teams as performance aids and countermeasures to exercise-induced inflammation, delayed onset of muscle soreness (DOMS), oxidative stress, immune dysfunction and URTI (see Figure 19 for a summary including references of individual studies). Most studies have focused on the ability of flavonoid-rich tea, fruit and vegetable extracts to counter oxidative stress, and as summarized in Figure 19, the majority indicate an effective response. The second most common outcome measure is related to inflammation and DOMS, and again, most studies support protective effects when flavonoid mixtures or plant extracts are ingested prior to demanding bouts of exercise (see Figure 19 for indication of individual studies). Results are mixed for performance outcomes, and few studies have included immune and URTI measures (see Figure 19).

For any particular flavonoid or plant extract studied within an exercise context, few papers are available, and research designs vary widely in regards to the supplementation dose and regimen, the mode of exercise stress, and outcome measures. The flavonoid supplementation period in the studies listed in Figure 19 varies from 15 minutes to 60 days prior to an exercise challenge, with most studies clustered between 7 and 21 days. Nonetheless, the data in general support that flavonoid-rich plant extracts and unique flavonoid-nutrient mixtures (e.g. quercetin with green tea extract and fish oil, or isoflavones with lycopene) help counter exercise-induced oxidative stress and inflammation/ DOMS. A large proportion of ingested plant polyphenols reach the colon, and there is a growing realization that the metabolites created from colonic bacterial degradation can be reabsorbed and exert bioactive effects, especially following exercise when gut permeability is increased (Nieman *et al.*, 2013). Future research should focus on the gut-derived phenolic signature measured following polyphenolic supplementation and exercise, especially at the tissue level.

More exercise-related research has been conducted with quercetin than any other flavonoid (MacRae *et al.*, 2006; Cureton *et al.*, 2009; Nieman *et al.*, 2007a, 2007b, 2009a, 2010a; Nieman, 2010). In one of the earliest studies with exercise-stressed cyclists, supplementation with pure quercetin (1,000mg/ day) over a five-week period reduced illness rates but did not counter post-exercise inflammation, oxidative stress, or immune dysfunction (Nieman *et al.*, 2007a). In a follow-up study using a similar design, quercetin supplementation combined with green tea extract, isoquercetin and fish oil did cause a sizeable reduction in exercise-induced inflammation and oxidative stress, with chronic augmentation of innate immune function (Nieman *et al.*, 2009a). Quercetin's

Flavonoids and flavonoid-rich extracts	Performance (aerobic or muscular)	Exercise-induced Inflammation / DOMS	Oxidative stress	Immune dysfunction	URTI	References
Apple polyphenols	↑	→				Nakazato et al., 2007, 2010
Artichoke extract		→	↔			Skarpanska-Stejnborn et al., 2008
Beer polyphenols		→	→		→	Scherr et al., 2012
Black currant extract		→	→			Lyall et al., 2009
Black grape, raspberry, red currant beverage			→			Morillas-Ruiz et al., 2005, 2006
Blueberry polyphenols			→			McAnulty et al., 2004; Hurst et al., 2010
Cherry juice blend		→				Connolly et al., 2006
Chokeberry juice			→			Pilaczynska-Szczesniak et al., 2005
Cocoa drink			→			Wiswedel et al., 2004
Green tea extract (EGCG)	↔↑	→	→			Murase et al., 2006; Panza et al., 2008; Dean et al., 2009; Eichenberger et al., 2010; Richards et al., 2010
Isoflavones, lycopene			→			Di Giacomo et al., 2009
Mixed fruit, vegetable concentrate			→			Bloomer et al., 2006
Pomegranate extract		→				Trombold et al., 2010
Quercetin (pure)	↔↓	↔	↔	↔	↔↓	Cuerton et al., 2009; Nieman et al., 2007a, 2007b, 2010; Nieman, 2010
Quercetin, EGCG, fish oil	↔↑	→	→	↔		MacRae et al., 2006; Nieman et al., 2009a
Rhodiola rosea L. extract			↔			Skarpanska-Stejnborn et al., 2009
Soy protein isolate/isoflavones	↔	↔	↔			Lenn et al., 2002; Chen et al., 2005a; Kok et al., 2005; Beavers et al., 2010

FIGURE 19 Influence of flavonoids and flavonoid-rich extracts and products on exercise performance and as a countermeasure to exercise-induced inflammation, delayed onset of muscle soreness (DOMS), oxidative stress, immune dysfunction and upper respiratory tract infection (URTI) Key: Blank = no published data; ↔ = data indicate no influence; ↔↓ = mixed results; ↑ = data support increase or ↓ decrease in outcome measure Note: In terms of exercise-induced factors a, '↓' decrease in outcome measures may be beneficial.

role as a performance aid has been tested by several research teams with mixed results (Cureton *et al.*, 2009; Nieman *et al.*, 2007a, 2007b, 2009a, 2010a; Nieman, 2010). Animal studies support a role for quercetin as an exercise mimetic for mitochondrial biogenesis and enhanced endurance performance (Nieman, 2010). One study with untrained human subjects indicated a modest enhancement in skeletal muscle mitochondrial density and endurance performance, but far below what was reported in mice (Nieman *et al.*, 2010b).

Flavonoid-rich extracts when consumed as an acute dose, or chronically for days or weeks, before heavy exertion partially counter post-exercise inflammation and oxidative stress. Research is needed to define better optimal dosing regimens and whether unique flavonoid mixtures that include several of the most bioactive flavonoids across different subgroups amplify these influences, while also bolstering immunity and operating as exercise mimetics for mitochondrial biogenesis.

Competing interests   None

FOLATE

Melinda M. Manore

Adequate folate intake is important for athletes and active individuals because of its role in red blood cell (RBC) production and in tissue repair and maintenance. Folate plays a significant part in cell division, especially in tissues with rapid turnover such as RBCs. Folate deficiency leads to anaemia, caused by failure of the red cell precursors to develop into functional RBCs. The result is abnormally large RBCs that cannot effectively transport oxygen or remove carbon dioxide.

For many countries, the recommended dietary allowance (RDA) for folate is 400 μg/day for individuals >19 years (IOM, 1998). Folate is found in many foods but is especially high in leafy green vegetables, nuts, legumes and liver. The bioavailability of folate in food is ~50% (IOM, 1998), but reduced by prolonged cooking. Many foods, such as breakfast cereals, are fortified with synthetic folic acid (~50–100% of the RDA for folate), which is highly bioavailable (~85%). Some countries have also made fortification of folic acid in enriched breads, flours and other grain products compulsory. Thus, our diets contain a mixture of food folate and synthetic folic acid with differing levels of bioavailability.

Overall, the apparent intake of dietary folate is adequate in active males as long as energy intake is adequate (Joubert and Manore, 2008), but below recommendations for active females (Beals and Manore, 1998; Clark et al., 2003; Heaney et al., 2010; Joubert and Manore, 2008), which can be due either to energy restriction for weight loss and/or underreporting of food intake in food records. Blood levels of folate are normal, even when seven-day dietary intakes appear to be low (Joubert and Manore, 2008). However, in female marathon runners, although folate supplementation (5g/day for ten weeks in conjunction with iron) improved blood folate levels, there was no effect on performance (Matter et al., 1987). Finally, it has been well documented in the research literature that low blood levels of key blood nutrients, including folate, impair exercise performance (Vaz et al., 2011). When normal blood status of these micronutrients is improved, performance improves.

Elevated plasma homocysteine (Hcy), an intermediate metabolite in the methionine pathway, has been suggested as a potential risk factor for cardiovascular disease (Clarke et al., 2010, 2011). Folate is required for methionine metabolism, so low dietary folate could increase plasma Hcy levels, alongside other factors that increase methionine catabolism, such as high-intensity exercise. Research including active and sedentary individuals shows an inverse relationship between plasma folate and Hcy levels (Joubert and Manore, 2008; Di Santolo et al., 2009). Joubert and Manore (2008) found that highly active individuals (12–18h/week of exercise) had significantly higher Hcy levels compared to sedentary individuals. Conversely, Di Santolo *et al.* (2009) found that women with low blood folate levels (<3.0 μg/L) were 4.5-fold more likely to have elevated Hcy levels (≥15.0 μmol/L), regardless of activity level, but their athletes were only doing ~8h/week of exercise.

Competing interests   None

GARLIC

Stéphane Bermon

Garlic (*Allium sativum*) is a herb that is used as a food in many countries. From the early ages, it was believed to have different pharmaceutical and physiological properties. Raw garlic contains different compounds; the main one being alliin. It can be physically or chemically processed in order to obtain dry garlic powder, distilled oil, macerated oil or aged garlic extract. The latter is the most commonly used as a phytotherapeutic agent and has also been the most studied in human and animal models.

It is claimed that garlic and garlic extracts show pharmaceutical properties such as nutritional, immuno-modulatory, antioxidant, micro-vascular and rheologic properties. For these reasons, garlic has been promoted as an anti-fatigue agent and an ergogenic agent when consumed alone or mixed with other compounds. According to existing scientific literature, it appears that good evidence exists to conclude that regular and high intakes (6–10g of fresh garlic daily) may improve the peripheral circulation. This effect is achieved through a better vascular relaxation, a change in membrane lipids in red blood cells that could increase their flexibility and deformability and a negative effect on blood clotting and platelets adhesion (Bordia et al., 1998). Because of the vasoconstriction of the pulmonary vasculature leading to pulmonary hypertension associated with exposure to hypoxia, garlic extracts might show potential ergogenic effects for athletes undertaking hypoxic exercise. However, when measuring peripheral blood pressures, blood oxygen saturation, heart rate, oxygen consumption, and time to exhaustion during a progressive exercise test in humans under hypoxia, seven days of supplementation with garlic or placebo failed to show significant differences between treatments. These results do not support garlic consumption as a method for improving performance in hypoxia (Morris et al., 2013).

Regarding immuno-modulatory and anti-oxidative capacity, a meta-analysis (Fleischauer et al., 2000) showed anti-carcinogenic (colorectal and stomach tumours) effects of regular garlic intakes (approx 18g of fresh garlic or six cloves daily). However, although some *in vivo* or animal studies showed promising results in terms of physical performance or delayed fatigue, this has not been confirmed so far in human athletes. There are some human clinical studies on garlic supplementation and fatigue (Morihara et al., 2007) but the designs are dubious and, in some of them, garlic has been used in conjunction with other molecules, making the interpretation of the results complicated.

Competing interests None

GINGER

David S. Senchina

'Ginger' most often refers to the underground stem (rhizome, often incorrectly referred to as 'root') of *Zingiber officinale*. Alkaloids called gingerols are the purported bioactive molecules; they are structurally similar to capsaicin. Athletes may take ginger supplements for presumed pain management or anti-inflammatory effects. While one review concluded ginger does not reduce pain compared to placebo (Terry *et al.*, 2011), subsequent studies have shown that ginger supplementation significantly reduced pain after resistance exercise in young adults (Black *et al.*, 2010) and young female athletes (Mashhadi *et al.*, 2013). As reviewed elsewhere, ginger may reduce plasma levels of inflammatory molecules such as IL-6 in obese individuals, but those same results have not been shown in athletic individuals (Senchina *et al.*, 2014). Altogether, the evidence suggests ginger may exhibit analgesic or anti-inflammatory effects in specific contexts, but ergogenic properties are unproven.

Competing interests None

GINKGO

David S. Senchina

Maidenhair tree (*Ginkgo biloba*, spelled 'ginkgo' but often pronounced 'gingko') is native to eastern Asia. Traditionally, ginkgo leaves were extracted in teas to aid memory or improve circulation, but today supplements are more commonly tablets standardized for glycosides and lactones, the purported bioactive constituents. As an ergogenic aid, ginkgo has been considered for claudication (peripheral artery disease) therapy in older adults; however, studies have found that treatment with ginkgo+exercise therapy is equivocal to exercise therapy alone (Nicolaï *et al.*, 2013). Ginkgo extract has been considered for mountain sickness or to offset haemorrheological problems associated with exercise at altitude, with one study suggesting it may or may not mitigate altitude sickness contingent on product-specific differences, which may also explain heterogeneity in previous studies (Leadbetter *et al.*, 2009). Effects of ginkgo supplementation on blood pressure or salivary cortisol production differed by gender, nature of stress and time of day (Jezova *et al.*, 2002). The combined evidence suggests ginkgo may have some utility haemorrheologically, but effects are likely to be inconsistent due to the variation in manufacturing processes.

Competing interests   None

GINSENG

David S. Senchina

Ginseng is perhaps the most widely reported Chinese herbal supplement used by athletes. The common name encompasses both American and Asian species (genus *Panax*) as well as 'Siberian ginseng' (genus *Eleutherococcus*, formerly *Acanthopanax*), although *Panax ginseng* root material is most commonly used in ergogenic aids (tablets, extracts and 'energy drinks'). Ginseng is claimed to improve cardiorespiratory function, increase aerobic and anaerobic performance, and improve mental acuity via its ginsenosides (triterpenoid saponins, a subclass of glycosides). Ginsenosides are purported to be the primary bioactive compounds responsible for ginseng ergogenic properties, but other compounds such as caffeine and other methylxanthines are present in ginseng supplements.

However, reviews from ginseng supplementation in athletic contexts have reported heterogeneous findings (Bahrke *et al.*, 2009; Senchina *et al.*, 2013a). The most comprehensive review concluded that ginseng has not demonstrated efficacy as an ergogenic aid in athletes and, further, that the results of studies reporting benefits may be confounded by unsound methodologies such as inappropriate subject populations (e.g. non-athletes) or inappropriate/absent control groups (Bahrke *et al.*, 2009). Ginseng is an increasingly frequent ingredient of 'energy drinks' (along with caffeine, taurine and guarana). A recent review of performance-enhancing properties of energy drinks suggested glucose and caffeine, not ginseng, are most likely responsible for observed effects (Ballard *et al.*, 2010). However, it is difficult to pinpoint the effects of ginseng specifically, as it is often found in conjunction with numerous other ingredients. One study showed improvements in treadmill VO_{2max}, critical running velocity and lean body mass following a three-week ginseng-containing energy drink+training programme as compared with placebo (Smith *et al.*, 2010a), but with so many other ingredients in the supplement, it is difficult to ascertain ginseng-specific effects. Despite numerous testimonials, the ergogenic properties of ginseng have not been substantiated scientifically. The case of ginseng may be similar to that of ginkgo and other supplements where extraneous variability is confounding studies.

Competing interests None

GLANDULARS

Samantha J. Stear

Glandulars are extracts from animal glands, which are normally dried, ground-up and sold in powder or tablet form. The most common glandular supplements include: thyroid, adrenal, thymus, testis and ovary; followed by glandulars from the pituitary, kidney, liver, pancreas, spleen, lung, heart, brain, uterus and prostate. Glandulars are claimed to enhance the function of the equivalent gland in the human body. The theory is that glandular tissues contain intrinsic cell-specific, but not species-specific, factors that are distinct from vitamins and minerals.

Glandulars are popular with bodybuilders who believe that their ingestion will produce anabolic effects by boosting the body's production of hormones. However, glandular extracts are degraded during the digestive process and are inactive when absorbed. Therefore, it is not surprising that there is no scientific evidence that glandular tissue concentrates enhance organ and gland activities, nor work ergogenically, other than through their vitamin, mineral and protein content.

Competing interests None

GLUCURONOLACTONE

Stéphane Bermon

D-glucurono 3-6 lactone or glucuronolactone is a molecule with the following formula: $C_6H_8O_6$. The biochemical precursor of the glucuronolactone is the glucuronic acid which is involved in the liver metabolism and the glucuronidation process. This process is of utmost importance to eliminate xenobiotics and other natural compounds, making them more water-soluble and thus eliminated through the kidneys or faeces (bile salts). At physiological pH, the glucuronic acid and glucuronolactone remain in an equilibrium state. In animals, with the exception of primates and guinea pigs, glucuronic acid is a precursor of ascorbic acid.

Glucuronolactone is a lactone naturally produced by the liver during the glucose metabolism. It is thus involved in the glycogen metabolism at the liver level. As a lactone, it is also used in the food industry for its aromatic properties. Glucuronolactone can be found in cereal, and in wine with the highest source at 20mg/L. For more than 15 years, glucuronolactone has been a component of energy drinks and the concentration there can reach up to 2,000–2,400mg/L.

The only available data on glucuronolactone toxicity comes from rat and mouse studies where LD_{50} (oral) are reported at 10.7 and more than 20g/kg respectively. Renal toxicity was suspected with high intakes but was not proven. In 2003, the SCF (European Scientific Committee on Food) agreed with its earlier position in 1999 that there was a lack of scientific evidence to support the safety of glucuronolactone present in beverages at concentrations that may result in intakes several-fold higher than that usually obtained from the rest of the diet. For example, an estimated high chronic intake of glucuronolactone at 840mg/day and an acute intake of up to 1,800mg/day from consumption of 'energy' drinks, was compared with the estimated intake of glucuronolactone from naturally occurring sources in the diet of only 1–2mg/day. But, due to the lack of relevant data, it was not possible to set an upper safe level for daily intake of glucuronolactone.

Due to a lack of controlled studies, it is impossible to state a purported ergogenic effect of glucuronolactone. The only available studies linking physical and/or mental performance with glucuronolactone concern 'energy' drinks, which also contain other ingredients such as taurine, caffeine and vitamins, with caffeine likely to be the key bioactive ingredient influencing performance (see section on caffeine).

In athletes treated with drugs which are glucuronidated, a depletion of glucuronic acid and consequently glucose and glycogen is theoretically possible. In order to spare the glycogen stores necessary for physical performance, a supplementation with glucuronolactone would, in this particular case, appear appropriate but again controlled studies are lacking.

Competing interests None

GLUTAMINE

Linda M. Castell, Philip Newsholme and Eric A. Newsholme*

Glutamine, the most abundant amino acid in the body, has in recent years become regarded as conditionally essential rather than non-essential. Glutamine is synthesized, stored and released predominantly by skeletal muscle: it is taken up by organs including the intestine, liver, kidney, and by some key immune cells. From clinical studies, it is known that the plasma concentration of glutamine is decreased in trauma and starvation. There is considerable evidence that glutamine feeding has a beneficial effect on gut function (Castell, 2003); it has had a positive effect on morbidity, mortality and some aspects of the immune system; glutamine provision has also shortened the recovery time from surgery and maintained muscle protein mass. The main source of glutamine is meat, poultry and fish.

The normal resting, fasting plasma glutamine is 500–700μmol/L; 600–700μmol/L is often seen in athletes. Resting plasma glutamine is usually lower in athletes with unexplained underperformance syndrome (Parry-Billings *et al.*, 1992). The muscle concentration of glutamine can reach 20mM (60% of the intramuscular amino acid pool). During short-term strenuous exercise, plasma glutamine can be markedly increased, probably due to the release of glutamine into the circulation from skeletal muscle. However, plasma glutamine is usually substantially reduced by prolonged, exhaustive exercise: this decrease often occurs concomitantly with transient immunodepression (Castell, 2003). Immunodepression must be taken into account in terms of the ergogenic effect of supplementation in athletes, since its elimination will allow more effective training and thus better performance.

Glutamine is not a banned substance and has a good safety record. Supplementation with glutamine or a glutamine precursor reduced the self-reported incidence of illness in endurance athletes (Castell *et al.*, 1996; Bassit *et al.*, 2000). However, when glutamine given to athletes attenuated the exercise-induced reduction of circulating glutamine, few effects were observed on the immune parameters studied, apart from reduced neutrocytosis (Kryzwkowski *et al.*, 2001) which supports the notion that plasma glutamine influences neutrophil function (Castell *et al.*, 2004); and increased circulating IL-6 (Hiscock *et al.*, 2003), which might prove beneficial if the myokine IL-6 acts as an anti-inflammatory cytokine (Pedersen, 2006).

Glutamine is positively linked with heat shock proteins (HSP). Fehrenbach and Niess (1999) suggested a protective effect of HSPs in leucocytes in athletes after endurance exercise. Zuhl *et al.* (2014) demonstrated that glutamine supplementation decreased exercise-induced intestinal permeability and reduced NFκB activity in peripheral blood mononuclear cells. Both these anti-inflammatory actions of glutamine might be mediated through an increase in HSP70 levels and the heat shock response.

Muscle glycogen repletion is an important factor in recovery and subsequent performance after endurance exercise. Post-exercise intake of carbohydrate provides a substrate for glycogen synthesis and also stimulates insulin secretion which subsequently activates glucose transport and glycogen synthase in muscle. Varnier *et al.* (1995) suggested that glutamine supplementation might also promote glycogen synthesis – perhaps indirectly via promotion of insulin secretion. However, Marwood and Bowtell (2008) found no effect of glutamine supplementation on performance during high-intensity exercise when they gave athletes 0.125g/kg after glycogen depletion.

Acute glutamine administration (16–36mg/kg) increased both plasma bicarbonate and growth hormone (Welbourne, 1995). However, glutamine administration (0.03g/kg 90 min prior to exercise) did not improve maximum effort on a bicycle ergometer (Haub *et al.*, 1998). Glutamine, versus alanine, protected footballers against an exercise-induced increase in blood ammonia, which would have an impact on fatigue (Bassini-Cameron *et al.*, 2008).

Glutamine supplementation via the L-alanyl-L-glutamine dipeptide (at 0.05g/kg and 0.2g/kg) led to an ergogenic benefit by increasing time to exhaustion during a mild hydration stress (Hoffman *et al.*, 2010). This effect may have been mediated by enhanced fluid and electrolyte uptake.

A mixture containing 12 amino acids, including glutamine, was provided to improve training efficiency in athletes (Ohtani *et al.*, 2006). However, it is impossible to deduce whether any one amino acid had a more specific effect than another. The mixture also contained vitamins and minerals. When branched chain amino acids (BCAA; precursors for glutamine) were given, although plasma glutamine was increased and muscle recovery helped, supplementation did not enhance athletic performance (Negro *et al.*, 2008).

Overall, there is no consensus that exogenous provision of glutamine alone beneficially affects performance in athletes, although improvements have been reported when it is combined with COH, or other amino acids.

Although glutamine is effective in decreasing the self-reported incidence of URTI, little evidence has been obtained of an effect on specific aspects of the immune system. Glutamine does protect against an exercise-induced rise in blood ammonia. The effects of glutamine on performance *per se* are not convincing. More research is needed to back up the small amount of evidence already reported.

Competing interests   None

*Tribute to Professor Eric Arthur Newsholme

Eric Newsholme died on 17 March 2011. He was an innovative researcher, and an outstanding teacher (a lecturer in the Department of Biochemistry at the

University of Oxford since 1973). He published more than 300 research papers and some classic books: his book with Tony Leech *Keep on Running* in 1994 is typically practical with schedules and recipes for runners which could be applied to all athletes – but the biochemistry is there too, written in a way which makes it accessible to all. Exercise biochemistry was one of Eric's passions in life and his marathon running gave him considerable insight into energy metabolism. He was particularly interested in the role of amino acids in exercise, both in immunology and in central fatigue, and produced some novel hypotheses on which researchers all over the world have worked for many years. Thus, it is very appropriate to pay tribute to him, both in this article on glutamine and in this book stemming from the A–Z Series of Nutritional Supplements in *BJSM*, in which he was keenly interested. Eric is still greatly missed by those who were fortunate enough to have collaborated with him.

Linda M. Castell, 2014

GLUTATHIONE AND GLUTAMATE

Philip Newsholme and Mauricio Krause

Glutathione (g-glutamyl-cysteinyl-glycine; GSH) is the predominant low-molecular-weight thiol (0.5–10 mmol/L) in mammalian cells. Most GSH (85–90%) is cytosolic, with the remainder located in organelles, including the mitochondria, nuclear matrix and peroxisomes (Wu *et al.*, 2004). This tripeptide is a key antioxidant within cells, critical to the regulation of ROS (Reactive Oxygen Species) concentration (Krause *et al.*, 2007). Reduced glutathione (GSH) may be used to remove damaging ROS such as H_2O_2 and convert it to harmless H_2O, generating GSSG via glutathione peroxidase (Figure 20). Disulphide formation and glutathionylation are reversible forms of protein covalent modification dependent on glutathione and can provide mechanisms for regulation of metabolic, signalling and transcriptional processes (Ghezzi, 2005), including skeletal muscle adaptation to exercise and training (Ji, 2008). The cellular redox state is crucial for molecular signalling and glutathione is a key regulator/sensor for redox status, thus strategies aiming at increasing GSH synthesis should be beneficial to exercise performance.

Exercise, free radical production and dissipation

Exercise stimulates ROS and RNS (Reactive Nitrogen Species) production, dependent on exercise type, duration and intensity, culminating in changes in skeletal muscle redox state (Powers and Lennon, 1999). ROS/RNS production and various antioxidant roles are summarized in Figure 20. Excessive ROS and RNS production is associated with deleterious effects in many diseases including diabetes (Newsholme *et al.*, 2009; Krause and de Bittencourt, 2008). Antioxidant supplementation strategies have been assessed for their ability to decrease ROS levels and the deleterious effects of oxidative/nitrosative damage. While excessive ROS and RNS can exert harmful effects within skeletal muscle during exercise, lower levels are crucial for adaptation of metabolic and signalling pathways in response to exercise. For example, redox changes are essential for the production and release of myokines such as IL-6. IL-6 is a key signal molecule produced and secreted in exercise in part to optimise fuel provision for sustained activity (Pedersen, 2007). Although antioxidant supplementation may at first be considered as beneficial, the consequent reduction of ROS/RNS could actually have negative effects. Muscle redox state may be best improved by providing skeletal muscle cells with the key natural precursors for GSH synthesis and allowing the cells to synthesise what they actually require. Exercise-induced free radical production in

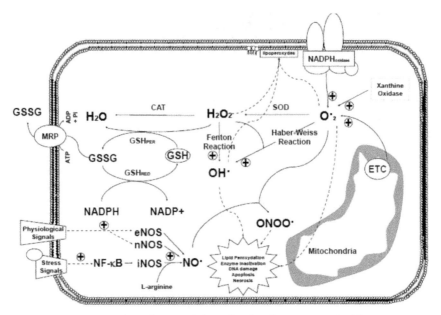

FIGURE 20 ROS/RNS synthesis and the role of endogenous antioxidants

Note: Cells require antioxidant systems to neutralize ROS and RNS. Superoxide ($O_2 \bullet$) is enzymatically converted into H_2O_2 by a Mn-SOD [manganese SOD (superoxide dismutase)] within mitochondria. H_2O_2 can then be rapidly removed by the mitochondrial enzyme GPX (glutathione peroxidase). Glutathione is a tripeptide (γ-glutamyl-cysteinyl-glycine) composed of glutamate, cysteine and glycine, with the amino group of cysteine joined in peptide linkage to the γ-carboxyl group of glutamate. A further antioxidant enzyme CAT (catalase) is the major H_2O_2-detoxifying enzyme found exclusively in peroxisomes. In addition to the classic antioxidant enzymes, MRP (multidrug-resistance proteins), such as the MRP pump (a transmembrane protein that acts by exporting intracellular glutathione disulfide, reducing accumulation and redox imbalance), are also important (Krause *et al.*, 2007).

skeletal muscle is not detrimental to human health, thus endogenous antioxidants may be sufficient to protect against exercise-induced oxidative damage.

Regulation of glutathione synthesis

The synthesis of GSH from glutamate, cysteine and glycine is catalyzed sequentially by two key cytosolic enzymes, g-glutamylcysteine synthetase (GCS) and GSH synthetase. The availability of these amino acids is essential for GSH synthesis (Figure 21). Supplementation with cysteine precursors, such as N-acetylcysteine (NAC), increases glutathione levels (Townsend *et al.*, 2003). However, *de novo* GSH synthesis depends on glutamate, because this amino acid is both a constituent of the GSH molecule and also acts as an amino acid donor in serine synthesis, which can subsequently be converted to glycine. GSH is a non-allosteric feedback inhibitor of GCS, but competes with glutamate, thus high intracellular glutamate concentrations will enhance GSH synthesis (Griffith, 1999).

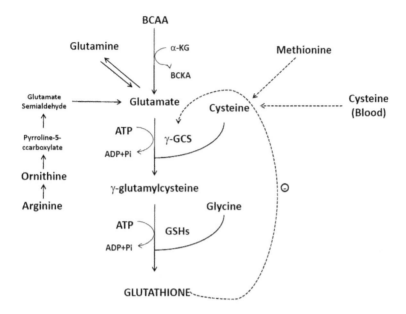

FIGURE 21   Glutathione synthesis and the possible amino acid candidates which may increase intracellular glutamate and glutathione

Note: (See main text for further explanations.) BCAA: Branched chain amino acids; BCKA: Branched chain keto acids; α-KG: α-ketoglutarate.

Supplementation with precursors of glutathione in exercise or disease treatment

A decreased availability of glutamine during disease progression or overtraining may depress the synthesis of several key molecules such as GSH, a key molecule in cellular resistance to lesions, oxidative stress, apoptotic processes and detoxification of xenobiotics (see section on glutamine). Supplementation with glutamine may serve as an alternative way to increase cellular levels of GSH and attenuate the oxidative stress that occurs in catabolic situations (Flaring *et al.*, 2003; Valencia *et al.*, 2002). Furthermore, supplementation with the dipeptide L-alanyl-L-glutamine (DIP) and free glutamine plus alanine before long-duration exercise resulted in an effective supply of glutamine and glutamate. This was associated with an increase in muscle and liver levels of GSH (↑~20%), and an improvement in the redox state of the cell (Cruzat and Tirapegui, 2009). N-acetylcysteine (NAC, a membrane permeable cysteine precursor, see section on NAC) supplementation, stimulated GSH synthesis and is widely used for increasing antioxidant status during exercise. Indeed, NAC attenuated the elevation of inflammatory markers of muscle damage and oxidative stress after intense eccentric exercise (Michailidis *et al.*, 2013). However, NAC also blunted the activation of key proteins for recovery and muscle growth (via reduction in phosphorylation of: PKB, mammalian target of rapamycin, p70 ribosomal S6 kinase, ribosomal protein S6, and mitogen activated protein kinase p38), thus delaying recovery. Although thiol-based antioxidant supplementation may enhance GSH availability in skeletal muscle, it may also disrupt the normal skeletal muscle inflammatory response and repair capability, potentially because of attenuation of activation of redox-sensitive signalling pathways (Michailidis *et al.*, 2013).

In addition to exercise, several other conditions are associated with reduced levels of GSH such as diabetes (Krause *et al.*, 2012, 2014a), HIV (Nguyen *et al.*, 2014), aging (Sekhar *et al.*, 2011b) and Gaucher and Parkinson diseases (Holmay *et al.*, 2013). For example, sustained hyperglycaemia is associated with low cellular levels of GSH (73% lower than control subjects), which leads to tissue damage (membrane lipid damage and protein oxidation in skeletal muscle, liver and kidney) attributed to oxidative stress. Indeed, it is known that patients with uncontrolled type 2 diabetes have severely deficient glutathione synthesis attributed to limited precursor (cysteine and glycine) availability (Sekhar *et al.*, 2011a). Dietary supplementation with both GSH precursor amino acids can restore GSH synthesis (↑ 85%), reducing oxidative stress and oxidant damage in the face of persistent hyperglycaemia (Sekhar *et al.*, 2011a). Similarly, in HIV-infected patients, diminished synthesis of GSH is attributed to decreased availability of cysteine and glycine. Interestingly, this glutathione deficiency was corrected (53% increase) after dietary supplementation with these amino acids (Sekhar *et al.*, 2011b).

Aging and diabetes share some markers of inflammation, metabolism and redox status (Krause *et al.*, 2014b). In both conditions, oxidative stress markers are elevated, and glutathione deficiency (46% lower in older subjects than young controls) is associated with a marked reduction in synthesis (Sekhar *et al.*, 2011b). Dietary supplementation with the glutathione precursor amino acids cysteine and glycine fully restored glutathione synthesis (94% increase) and concentrations and lowered levels of oxidative stress and oxidant damage (Sekhar *et al.*, 2011b). Finally, decreased nigral GSH in Parkinson disease (PD) and increased reactive oxygen species in blood and fibroblasts in Gaucher disease, are restored after NAC supplementation in human subjects (Holmay *et al.*, 2013).

Summary

In conclusion, amino acid supplementation that increases intracellular glutamate, glycine and cysteine could improve muscle GSH synthesis. Future studies need to determine which amino acids can increase intracellular glutamate and GSH synthesis in skeletal muscle without the risk of blunting essential redox changes required for exercise adaptation. Potential amino acid candidates are summarized in Figure 21 and include BCAA, arginine and glutamine.

Competing interests   None

GLYCEROL

Louise M. Burke

Glycerol is a 3-carbon sugar alcohol which provides the backbone of triglycerides and is naturally found in foods as a component of dietary fats. However, its various physical and chemical properties are valuable in food technology: glycerol is added to manufactured foods and drinks as an emulsifier, humectant, sweetener, filler and thickener. Its viscosity also makes it useful as a component of lotions and creams, explaining its common availability for purchase in purified form under the name of glycerine. Although it has been suggested as a gluconeogenic precursor that could provide a substrate for exercise, the ingestion of glycerol by athletes is best known for its role as an osmolyte. When ingested or released following lipolysis, glycerol contributes to the osmotic pressure of body fluids until it is slowly metabolised. When consumed simultaneously with a substantial volume of fluid, there is a temporary retention of this fluid and expansion of body fluid compartments. Effective protocols for glycerol hyperhydration are 1–1.5g/kg glycerol with an intake of 25–35ml/kg of fluid (van Rosendal *et al.*, 2010). Such a protocol typically achieves a fluid expansion or retention of ~600–1,000ml above a fluid bolus alone via a reduction in urinary volume.

Several challenging situations commonly arise in sport in which athletes have made use of these strategies to promote better hydration status. These include hyperhydration prior to exercise in hot environments where a large fluid deficit will otherwise accumulate, and the reduction of the diuresis associated with aggressive rehydration such as in post-exercise recovery or following weight-making practices in weight-category sports (van Rosendal *et al.*, 2010). Position stands on fluid intake in exercise typically discount the value of hyperhydration or fluid overloading strategies (ACSM *et al.*, 2007). Indeed, there are occasional side-effects of glycerol use including nausea, gut discomfort and headaches from increased intracranial pressure (Goulet *et al.*, 2007; van Rosendal *et al.*, 2010). However, more focused reviews of glycerol hyperhydration in specific situations in sport, including a meta-analysis of glycerol hyperhydration prior to exercise in hot environments, have reported evidence of enhanced fluid balance and endurance performance compared with intake of large volumes of water alone or no hyperhydration (Goulet *et al.*, 2007; van Rosendal *et al.*, 2010; van Rosendal and Coombes, 2012). There has been less focus, but some support, for the addition of glycerol to rehydration beverages to promote rapid reversal of dehydration and to assist the performance of subsequent exercise (Goulet *et al.*, 2007; van Rosendal *et al.*, 2010). Indeed, there are anecdotal reports that some athletes add glycerol to rehydration beverages for practical reasons; for example, to reduce the interruption to sleep patterns due to overnight diuresis when fluid is consumed after exercise sessions undertaken late in the day. The apparent contradictions in the literature may be due to the specificity of the situations in which glycerol hyper/re-hydration is beneficial.

The major problem related to the use of glycerol by athletes, however, arises because of recent changes to anti-doping codes. Since 2010, S5 (Diuretics and other masking agents) of the WADA Prohibited List has included glycerol within its examples of banned plasma expanders (WADA, 2014). This ban exists despite: 1) the conclusion of a meta-analysis of glycerol hyper-hydration studies which observed that, in comparison to the use of other plasma-volume expanding agents, glycerol has very limited potential in increasing plasma volume and altering doping-relevant blood parameters (Koehler *et al.*, 2013); and 2) the findings of an intervention study that chronic (one week) use of a glycerol hyperhydration protocol did not significantly alter doping-relevant blood parameters (Polyviou *et al.*, 2012b). Nevertheless, to distinguish normal dietary intake of glycerol and glycerol release from triglyceride breakdown from specific intake of glycerol to aid fluid balance, WADA has set a threshold for urinary glycerol at 1.3mg/ml and advises that the small quantities of glycerol consumed in everyday foodstuffs and toiletries will not cause an athlete to test positive (WADA, 2014b).

Competing interests   None

GLYCINE

Kevin Currell

Glycine is the smallest amino acid; it is non-essential and can be synthesised from serine. Glycine is present in most proteins and is particularly highly concentrated in collagen. Consequently, one of the highest food sources of glycine is gelatin. Glycine is also one of the three amino acid components of glutathione which is a key component of the body's defences against oxidative stress, however it is thought that glycine availability is not the limiting step in glutathione synthesis. Glycine ingestion increases plasma concentrations of insulin similarly to other amino acids (Gannon *et al.*, 2002). Glycine is also an inhibitory neurotransmitter.

There is little research on supplementation with glycine. Research which has been conducted has looked at its potential role in decreasing inflammation (Zhong *et al.*, 2003). Sport-specific research has focused on combining glycine with other nutrients. Glycine-Propionyl-L-Carnitine (GPLC) has been shown to influence exercise performance (Smith *et al.*, 2008b), decrease oxidative stress and potentially increase vasodilation through increases in plasma nitrate (Bloomer and Smith, 2009). Jacobs and Goldstein (2010) suggested that GPLC might enhance aerobic work capacity but that doses must be specific for exercise intensity and duration.

At present there is insufficient evidence to suggest the use of glycine as a supplement to enhance sporting performance. However, further research on the effectiveness of GPLC is warranted.

Competing interests None

GREEN TEA

David S. Senchina

Green tea comes from the leaves of *Camellia sinensis* of eastern Asia; this species is the same source for white tea, black tea, etc. A subclass of flavonoids called catechins, and specifically epigallocatechin-3-gallate (EGCG), are believed to confer many biological activities unique to green tea, but caffeine and other compounds are also present and may explain some observed effects (Senchina *et al.*, 2014). Though doses, extract and exercise protocol characteristics varied, in athletic contexts of young- to middle-aged individuals studied, green tea extracts generally do not show any effect on metabolism (Martin *et al.*, 2014; Randell *et al.*, 2014) or inflammation/oxidative stress (Jówko *et al.*, 2012; Nieman *et al.*, 2013). In single studies a green tea extract was shown to augment post-exercise salivary defense variables (Lin *et al.*, 2014), and an EGCG extract improved cycling VO_{2max} (Richards *et al.*, 2010). Studies in hypertensive, obese or older adults have often reported an effect of green tea or EGCG extract, suggesting that anthropometric and epidemiological characteristics are important variables in green tea clinical studies. Current research indicates green tea supplements are of little utility to healthy, athletic individuals.

Competing interests   None

GUARANA

Samantha J. Stear

Guarana (*Paullinia cupana*), a climbing plant in the maple family, native to the Amazon basin and especially common in Brazil, contains a high amount of guaranine, a chemical substance with the same characteristics as caffeine (Schimpl *et al.*, 2013; Smith and Atroch, 2007). Guaranine, a synonym for caffeine, is defined only as the caffeine chemical in guarana and is identical to the caffeine chemical derived from other sources (e.g. coffee, tea, yerba maté). Guarana features large leaves, clusters of flowers and a fruit similar in size to the coffee bean. As a dietary supplement, guarana is a useful caffeine source with the guarana seeds containing more caffeine than the seeds of any other plant in the world (2–7.5%), and greater than the 1–2% of caffeine found in coffee beans (Smith and Atroch, 2007). Figure 22 contains a partial listing of some of the main chemicals found in guarana seeds.

The table illustrates that guarana, alongside other natural sources of caffeine, also contains varying mixtures of other xanthine alkaloids such as theobromine and theophylline. Guarana is generally recognized as an acceptable ingredient and can be found in drinks, 'energy' shots/drinks, herbal teas or capsules.

Due to the popularity of this concentrated source of caffeine in supplements, particularly energy drinks, there have been a few recent reviews on its impact as an ergogenic aid in athletic performance and weight loss (Ballard *et al.*, 2010; Higgins *et al.*, 2010; McLellan and Lieberman, 2012). Guarana is best known for its stimulatory properties, providing similar benefits to caffeine such as reducing fatigue, increasing alertness, and as an ergogenic aid in the athletic arena (see section on caffeine). Also, as reviewed in the section on herbal weight

Chemical component	Parts per million
Ash	<14.200
Guaranine (caffeine)	9,100–76,000
Fat	<30,000
Protein	<98,600
Resin	<70,000
Starch	50,000–60,000
Tannin	50,000–120,000
Theobromine	200–400
Theophylline	0–2,500

FIGURE 22   The main chemicals found in guarana seeds

loss supplements, guarana either on its own or in combination with other ingredients such as caffeine, green tea and yerba maté, may be efficacious in weight loss (Senchina et al., 2013b), primarily due to its caffeine content and its proposed effect on increasing energy expenditure and fat utilization as a fuel source (Bérubé-Parent et al., 2005; Spriet et al., 2010; Outlaw et al., 2013).

However, isolated supplements of caffeine and guarana may also carry serious adverse risks (Senchina et al., 2013b). The maximal ergogenic benefits of caffeine and guarana can be seen at small to moderate caffeine doses (2–3mg/kg). Theoretically, it is possible to overdose on caffeine or guarana, with the fatal dose being estimated at a single dose of 10g pure caffeine or guaranine. Although the amounts of guarana found in popular supplements including energy drinks, are generally below the amounts expected to deliver therapeutic benefits or cause adverse events (Higgins et al., 2010), there have been some cases of young adults being admitted to emergency departments with overdoses of caffeine after overindulging in guarana-based energy drinks (Smith and Atroch, 2007).

Competing interests   None

HISTIDINE-CONTAINING DIPEPTIDES

Inge Everaert and Wim Derave

Carnosine (β-alanyl-L-histidine) and its methylated analogues anserine (β-alanyl-N-π-methylhistidine) and balenine/ophidine (β-alanyl-N-τ-methylhistidine) are histidine-containing dipeptides (HCD) abundantly present in mammalian skeletal muscles (Boldyrev *et al.*, 2013). Carnosine is the only HCD found in human skeletal muscles, while all three HCD are present in the human omnivorous diet (see section on β-alanine and carnosine).

Hill and co-workers (2007) showed that increased muscle carnosine content leads to better performance during high-intensity exercise; an outcome first shown by Harris *et al.* (2006) to be achieved by supplementation with β-alanine (4–6g/day for four to ten weeks). Carnosine loading is higher in trained than untrained muscles (Bex *et al.*, 2014), but seems to be independent of gender, baseline levels, age or the use of β-alanine supplements with different absorption characteristics (Del Favero *et al.*, 2012; Hill *et al.*, 2007; Stegen *et al.*, 2013, 2014). However, this β-alanine-induced muscle carnosine loading can be further optimized by taking β-alanine together with a meal (Stegen *et al.*, 2013). Based on a meta-analysis of 2012 (Hobson *et al.*, 2012) and subsequently published papers, it seems that β-alanine supplementation is most ergogenic for exercises lasting between one and ten minutes. The ergogenic mechanism of β-alanine supplementation may be the result of the attenuation of acidosis through the proton-buffering capacity of carnosine, whereas other physiological properties of carnosine cannot be excluded at present. Indeed, both *in vitro* and *in vivo* experiments on rodents revealed for example an improvement in calcium handling during muscle contractions (Dutka *et al.*, 2012; Everaert *et al.*, 2013). Further information on β-alanine supplementation can be found elsewhere in this book, leaving the remainder of this piece to discuss the acute or chronic dietary intake of the intact dipeptides, rather than only the rate-limiting precursor β-alanine.

HCD-rich meat or fish extracts, such as the chicken breast extract (CBEX), are popular supplements in Asia. CBEX, obtained via hot water extraction of chicken breast, is rich in anserine (1.4g/100ml) and carnosine (0.6g/100ml), and its chronic intake is likely to increase muscle carnosine content. Long-term CBEX supplementation enhanced the time to exhaustion during the last spurt of a relatively high-intensity endurance performance (Maemura *et al.*, 2006). Suzuki *et al.* (2006) showed further that the acute supplementation with CBEX, 30 minutes before 10x5s repeated sprints, decreased the bicarbonate buffering in blood but did not affect performance. Finally, acute supplementation with carnosine (20mg/kg BW) has been shown to enhance baseline blood bicarbonate levels without improving high-intensity cycling performance (CCT110%; Baguet *et al.*, 2014).

Concerning health, supplementation studies in rodents are very promising and reveal protective effects of carnosine-increasing supplements on aging, the development of diabetes (complications), atherosclerosis and tumor growth (Boldyrev *et al.*, 2013). The direct extrapolation of these results to humans is hampered by the fact that rodents lack the carnosine-degrading enzyme in the circulation. In conclusion, an increase in muscle carnosine levels, by chronic β-alanine and possibly by CBEX supplementation, seems to be ergogenic mainly in high-intensity exercises lasting several minutes.

Competing interests   None

α-HYDROXYISOCAPROIC ACID (HICA)

Antti A. Mero, Tuomo Ojala and Juha J. Hulmi

DL-α-hydroxyisocaproic acid (HICA), also known as leucic acid or DL-2-hydroxy-4-methylvaleric, is an α-hydroxyl acid metabolite of leucine. It is an end product of leucine metabolism in human tissues such as muscle and connective tissue with a molecular weight of 132.16g/mol (Sakko *et al.*, 2012). Although leucine (see section on leucine) has a unique role as a promoter of protein synthesis, early studies suggested that metabolites of leucine may be more effective in preventing breakdown of proteins, particularly muscle proteins (Tischler *et al.*, 1982). In a double-blind placebo-controlled study, Mero *et al.* (2010) investigated the effects of HICA on body composition, exercise-induced delayed onset of muscle soreness (DOMS) and athletic performance in soccer players. The four-week supplementation with HICA (1.5g/day) increased DEXA-derived measurements of lean body mass of soccer players, with the increase (~0.5 kg) being emphasized in lower extremities (i.e. the main trained muscles). Interestingly, the athletes in this study already had an average daily protein intake of 1.6–1.7g/kg BM: therefore, the HICA appeared effective even in the face of sufficient protein and leucine intake. Other outcomes of the study included a reduction in symptoms of DOMS, a sensation of muscular discomfort and pain during palpitation or active contractions that occur some time after strenuous exercise (Lieber and Friden, 2002), and an increase in training alertness. Despite these enhancements, there was no improvement in sports performance; a finding that was attributed to the short training period (Mero *et al.*, 2010). Similar results have been reported using KIC, another leucine metabolite (Yarrow *et al.*, 2007). Meanwhile, in another recent study in rats, HICA did not prevent immobilization-induced atrophy, but enhanced the recovery of muscle atrophy after cessation of immobilization (Lang *et al.*, 2013). The enhanced recovery was accompanied by a sustained increase in protein synthesis and mechanistic target of rapamycin (mTOR) signalling. Further studies are needed to compare HICA to other leucine metabolites, such as β-hydroxyβ-methylbutyrate (HMB; see section on HMB).

Competing interests   None

β-HYDROXY β-METHYLBUTYRATE (HMB)

Gary Slater

HMB is a metabolite of the essential branched chain amino acid leucine (LEU), the amino acid with the greatest ability to stimulate protein synthesis. Approximately 2–10% of LEU oxidation proceeds to HMB. Initial research on HMB focused on animals, assessing effects on immune function, morbidity/mortality, colostral milk fat content, growth rates, safety and toxicity. Despite unconvincing results in animal research, HMB supplementation was promoted to humans in the mid 1990s presuming that it might enhance gains in muscle size and strength while reducing muscle damage and soreness associated with resistance training (Nissen *et al.*, 1996), and possibly enhance aerobic capacity.

Supplementation with ~3.0g.day^{-1} of HMB was found to have a favourable impact on indirect indices of muscle protein breakdown and muscle damage, with concomitant trends for enhanced strength and skeletal muscle hypertrophy (Nissen *et al.*, 1996). Consequently, the popularity of HMB supplementation increased dramatically, becoming one of the most popular supplements in the late 1990s. More recently, interest in HMB supplementation amongst athletes has declined. Despite this, HMB research reports within the exercise environment continue to emerge, with recent research confirming HMB favourably impacts both protein synthesis and degradation, albeit to a lesser extent than LEU (Wilkinson *et al.*, 2013). Several recent HMB reviews have been published (Portal *et al.*, 2010; Zanchi *et al.*, 2011), with results of resistance training research from 2001 to 2007 consolidated into two meta-analyses (Nissen and Sharp, 2003; Rowlands and Thomson, 2009). Nissen and Sharp (2003) concluded that HMB supplementation augmented lean mass and strength gains associated with resistance training, although the magnitude of effect was trivial (0.28% increase in lean mass gain per week). Rowlands and Thomson (2009) identified similar small benefits from HMB supplementation in untrained males, but effects were trivial for strength and non-existent for body composition in trained lifters.

This disparity in responsiveness to HMB supplementation relative to resistance training status might be expected given the suppression in skeletal muscle protein breakdown as a consequence of resistance training adaptations (Phillips *et al.*, 1999). Furthermore, if HMB does enhance net protein balance following resistance training as a consequence of reducing protein degradation, any effect on adaptations is likely to be blunted compared to interventions that enhance protein synthesis as the protein synthetic response is many times more sensitive to nutrition interventions than degradation (Tang and Phillips, 2009).

An exception may be in clinical conditions in which skeletal muscle atrophy results from an elevation in skeletal muscle protein breakdown (Fitschen *et al.*, 2013).

Short-term HMB supplementation appears to be safe, with daily doses equivalent to ~6g.day^{-1} (76mg·kg^{-1}) having no impact on indices of hepatic, renal or immune function (Portal *et al.*, 2010). The free acid form of HMB appears to have more favourable bioavailability kinetics than the original HMB calcium salt (Fuller *et al.*, 2011).

Based on the literature currently available, the potential for HMB supplementation to enhance strength training adaptations appears to be small in previously untrained individuals and negligible in resistance-trained athletes. Given that the protein synthetic response is much more sensitive to nutrition interventions than protein breakdown, the resistance-trained athlete may prefer to focus on strategies with stronger evidential support such as post-exercise ingestion of high biological value proteins rich in leucine to maximize adaptation to the resistance training stimulus.

Competing interests None

γ-HYDROXYBUTYRATE (GHB) AND γ-BUTYROLACTONE (GBL)

Alex D. Popple and Michael J. Naylor

γ-hydroxybutyrate (GHB) is a short chain 4-carbon fatty acid found in the brain, mainly in the hypothalamus and basal ganglia, in the form of γ-hydroxybutyric acid. GHB has several precursors including γ-butyrolactone (GBL), that are metabolised into GHB upon ingestion through various pathways. Concurrently, GHB is transformed into the inhibitory neurotransmitter γ-aminobutyric acid (GABA), with preference for the $GABA_b$ receptor.

The precise mechanism of action of GHB remains unclear. GHB properties indicate a role in the brain as a neurotransmitter or neuromodulator (Vayer *et al.*, 1987). Additional research has shown it could influence serotonergic and dopaminergic activity, both directly and indirectly through interaction with other systems, e.g. $GABA_b$ receptors (Greiner *et al.*, 2003). Primary effects include lowered inhibition, induced feelings of euphoria and increased libido. GHB was identified and synthesised more than 40 years ago as a central nervous system depressant; it has been used as an anaesthetic adjuvant and to improve sleep patterns.

Links to athletic performance came from a study proposing that GHB administration increased growth hormone release (Takahara *et al.*, 1977). The drug was then marketed as a nutritional supplement alleging enhanced muscle growth, better sleep quality and improved sexual performance.

Simultaneously, GHB became popular during the 1980s with body builders due to the potential anabolic and performance-enhancing properties. These benefits have never been proven in athletic populations but, interestingly, a recent study that examined the effects of GHB on sleep and sleep-related growth hormone (GH) release found that low-dose supplementation (2.5–3.5 g day^{-1}) caused a two-fold increase in GH secretion during sleep (van Cauter *et al.*, 1997). An exact mechanism was not identified, but it was suggested that GHB augments GH release by inducing deeper phases of sleep.

GHB and its precursors are not typically present in the diet, but can be found in flavouring agents. It is typically taken as a liquid or powder and dosages range hugely from 12.5–100 mg kg^{-1} day^{-1}. It is rapidly absorbed and metabolised and effects occur almost instantaneously. After a single dose (12.5–50 mg kg^{-1}) maximal plasma concentrations are reached after approximately 30–40 minutes, and its elimination half-life ranges from 30–50 minutes (Brenneisen *et al.*, 2004).

Side effects include drowsiness, alcohol-like inebriation, dizziness and induction of sleep. In overdose it can cause coma, respiratory depression and death. Frequent and prolonged use has resulted in increased tolerance and dependence (Shneir, 2001). Currently, there is no available evidence to support the use of GHB in the athletic population.

Competing interests   None

HYDROXYCUT

Ano Lobb and Mark Ellison

Hydroxycut is a combination weight loss supplement whose active ingredients include *Cissus quadrangularis* (CQ) and caffeine (see respective sections in book). There are several subformulations containing various combinations of other botanical ingredients, including extracts of goji (*Lycium barbarum*), acerola (*Malpighia glabra*), wild mint (*Mentha longifolia*) and pomegranate (*Punica granatum*). Some of these botanical agents may have significant polyphenol/antioxidant component, which may be beneficial during hard training, but there is a lack of efficacy when used for weight loss (see section on herbal weight loss supplements).

A previous formulation of Hydroxycut was withdrawn from the market after being associated with 23 cases of hepatotoxicity and one death (Lobb, 2010; USFDA, 2011). The suspected hepatotoxic ingredients included hydroxycitric acid (HCA) extracted from the garcinia cambogia fruit, *Camellia sinensis* (green tea), and chromium (Dara *et al.*, 2008). These ingredients have been removed from the current formulation, although HCA continues to be available in other products, both alone and in combination with chromium and *Camellia sinensis*. Case reports of adverse events from HCA-containing Hydroxycut also continue to surface (Kaswala *et al.*, 2014; Narasimh *et al.*, 2013). Small, short-duration pilot studies have reported that eight weeks of HCA supplementation resulted in statistically significant weight loss compared with placebo (Preuss *et al.*, 2004).

With regard to the current formula, we could not find any reliable published studies assessing the product's safety and efficacy for weight loss in any population. In Hydroxycut's current formulation, HCA has been replaced with CQ, and chromium and *Camellia sinensis* have also been removed. Small, short-duration pilot studies of CQ have reported that ten weeks of supplementation resulted in statistically significant weight loss in obese patients compared with placebo (Oben *et al.*, 2007; Hasani-Ranjbar *et al.*, 2009). When taken as directed, the supplement provides 200mg of caffeine per dose, with two doses suggested per day. In athletes, modest caffeine supplementation has been found to be an ergogenic aid that positively affects exercise capacity and performance; potential side-effects include irritability, tremor and an increase in heart rate (see section on caffeine). As is the case with many weight loss supplements, Hydroxycut contains potentially powerful pharmacoactive ingredients, but has never undergone high quality study to assess its safety and efficacy. In addition to serious adverse effects linked to the earlier formulation containing HCA, at least one case report suggests the newer formulation may be associated with ischemic colitis (Sherid *et al.*, 2013). To date, the few published trials of the effectiveness of CQ (and HCA) in non-athletes have methodological weaknesses including short duration and small sample size, alongside potential conflicts of interest due to funding source (Lobb, 2010). Furthermore, as a product that receives minimal regulatory oversight or post-market surveillance (Lobb, 2009, 2010) there is an increased risk of issues with purity or potency, i.e. the supplement contains what it claims, and that there are no unlisted ingredients. Therefore, the true scale of any safety risk is not clear. Because of the lack of good evidence of safety and efficacy, herbal weight loss products are avoided by most performance nutrition practitioners in elite sport. Athletes seeking to lose weight should instead aim for a modest energy deficit via manipulations of diet and/or training.

Competing interests   None

INOSINE

Lars R. McNaughton and David Bentley

Inosine is a nucleoside that is formed when hypoxanthine is attached to a ribose ring (also known as a ribofuranose) via a β-N9-glycosidic bond. Inosine plays a role in a number of metabolic functions including increasing red blood cell concentrations of 2-3-diphosphoglycerate (2,3-DPG) which is involved in oxygen transport (Valeri, 1976). It may also potentiate the action of endogenously formed adenosine and inhibit its uptake and clearance. It has been proposed that inosine enhances exercise performance via the effects on 2,3-DPG, or by increasing ATP concentrations (Harmsen et al., 1984). An accumulation of inosine monophosphate, together with other factors, has been observed during prolonged exercise, suggesting a link with fatigue (Bowtell et al., 2007).

Little scientific investigation has been conducted on inosine as an ergogenic aid and there are few peer-reviewed papers. The available studies on trained individuals have investigated chronic intakes of large doses of inosine (e.g. 5–10,000mg d^{-1}), but these protocols have not been found to provide an ergogenic effect for endurance (Starling et al., 1996; Williams et al., 1990) or sprint activities (McNaughton et al., 1999a). Recent work (Avery et al., 2003) has also suggested that four weeks of inosine supplementation, taken in combination with vitamin E and a mixture of enzymes, had no effect on cycling performance time at 75% VO_{2max}. McNaughton et al. (1999a) suggested that high dose inosine, a uric acid pre-cursor, combined with elevated urinary excretion, could be detrimental and result in kidney stones or acute renal failure.

In summary there appears to be little support for the use of inosine as an ergogenic aid, though it is still used in some over-the-counter fitness products. Current clinical trials may indicate a future therapeutic effect as an antioxidant for exercise.

Competing interests None

INOSITOL

Shelly Meltzer

Inositol is sometimes referred to as vitamin B8, yet is not a true vitamin since it is ubiquitous in nature, and can be synthesized by the human body from D-glucose (Croze and Soulage, 2013; Higgins *et al.*, 2010). Of the nine different stereoisomer molecules of inositol, myo-inositol is the most commonly found in supplements. It is readily available in our food supply and a mixed diet supplies on average 1g/day. The highest levels are found in citrus fruits (except lemons), grains, beans and nuts (Croze and Soulage, 2013), plus it is an ingredient in some 'energy' drinks (Higgins *et al.*, 2010).

There is some evidence from human studies supporting a clinical role of myo-inositol, specifically with regard to its neurological and antidepressant effects using dosages from 12–20g/day (Croze and Soulage, 2013; Qureshi and Al-Bedah, 2013), and for treatment of polycystic ovarian syndrome, fertility, as well as for metabolic syndrome in postmenopausal women with dosages at 200mg–4g/day (Croze and Soulage, 2013). This is plausible considering its wide-ranging functions in the health of cell membranes, insulin signalling, nerve transmission, serotonin modulation and fat oxidation (Croze and Soulage, 2013; Higgins *et al.*, 2010). It is relatively non-toxic in healthy individuals and the mild gastrointestinal disturbances associated with higher doses can be overcome by using newer gel formulations (Carlomagno *et al.*, 2011; Croze and Soulage, 2013).

Since a major function of inositol is the mobilization of intracellular calcium, which is essential for muscle contraction (Maresh *et al.*, 1994), it is not surprising that it is sometimes also called 'muscle' sugar. However, sport-specific research is limited and until there are published human studies validating the benefits of a 'stand-alone' inositol supplement on performance, the claims remain speculative. When 2.2g inositol were combined with other ingredients including amino acids in an ATP-supplement administered to physically active men, their mean power output increased; however anaerobic blood levels of inositol were not examined, subjects were consuming a very modest intake of protein (1.5g/day) and the study was funded by the supplement company (Maresh *et al.*, 1994).

Competing interests None

IRON

Peter Peeling and Carmel Goodman

Iron deficiency is the most prevalent nutritional disorder in the world, and is particularly pertinent in athletic cohorts. An altered iron status may range in severity from iron depletion (ID; serum ferritin (SF) <35 μg/L, haemoglobin (Hb) >115g/L, transferrin saturation >16%) to iron deficiency anaemia (IDA; SF <12 μg/L, Hb <115g/L, transferrin saturation <16%) (Peeling et al., 2007).

It is well recognized that optimal physical performance is dependent on the efficient delivery and utilization of oxygen by the exercising muscle. Iron is a fundamental element to both of these processes due to its role as the functional component of Hb and myoglobin, as well as being a critical constituent of mitochondrial enzymes and cytochromes that promote oxidative phosphorylation. Insufficient iron stores may thus lead to feelings of lethargy and decrements in athletic performance.

There are several reasons why athletes may present with low iron stores. These may include: low dietary iron intake, low iron bioavailability and excessive iron excretion/loss. Furthermore, female athletes appear to be at a greater risk of iron deficiency due to menstrual blood loss and sub-optimal dietary iron intake. During exercise, iron losses can occur from several avenues such as red blood cell destruction (haemolysis), haematuria (blood in urine, possibly due to foot-strike haemolysis in athletes), gastrointestinal bleeding and sweating (for review see Peeling et al., 2008). Additionally, more recent research has demonstrated that the liver-produced hormone known as hepcidin is elevated in the 3–6 hour post-exercise period, which may negatively impact on the body's acute ability to absorb dietary iron, and to recycle iron from the macrophage subsequent to any exercise-induced haemolysis (for review see Peeling, 2010). Accordingly, both McClung et al. (2013) and Sim et al. (2014) have recently reported that the basal hepcidin levels of military personnel and athletes were increased after seven consecutive days of exercise. However, it appears that such hepcidin elevations are attenuated over a prolonged (i.e. eight weeks) training period (Auersperger et al., 2012). This is likely to be a result of a decline in iron status, stimulating the need for homeostatic iron regulation (Peeling et al., 2014). Regardless, it has been suggested that athletes presenting with sub-optimal iron stores (defined as a SF of 30–50 μg/L) will produce a post-exercise hepcidin response to the same magnitude as those considered to have healthy iron stores (SF >50 μg/L), which may contribute to the likelihood of developing an iron deficiency over time (Peeling et al., 2014). It is therefore suggested that practitioners consider the recommended timing for the consumption of high iron containing foods and supplements relative to the start or completion of exercise: this would provide iron sources at a more appropriate time than within the 3–6-hour post-exercise window, when hepcidin levels are likely to be elevated (Peeling et al., 2014).

To maintain sufficient iron stores, it is recommended that a dietary iron intake of 8mg/day for adult males and 18mg/day for adult females is consumed. The food choices used to attain this daily iron requirement may vary, and will include the ingestion of the more efficiently absorbed haem iron (derived from meat sources; accounting for ~20% of the daily dietary iron intake), and the less efficiently absorbed non-haem iron. The latter is derived from plant foods such as spinach, leafy greens, lentils and beans, which accounts for ~80% of the daily dietary iron intake (Beard and Tobin, 2000; Craig, 1994). However, with regard to iron supplementation, previous research has demonstrated that an oral iron supplement provided at a dose of 100mg of ferrous sulphate per day, may increase SF levels by 30–50% over a six to eight week period (Hinton et al., 2000; Klingshirn et al., 1992). The absorption of this iron supplement is considered to be more efficient when taken in conjunction with ascorbic acid (i.e. orange juice); and less efficient when taken with caffeinated products (i.e. teas and coffee). As a result, practitioners may wish to consider the prescription of an oral iron supplement that also contains vitamin C (e.g. ferrous sulphate with sodium ascorbate). Although it is recommended (and commonly practiced) to prescribe an oral iron supplement at 100mg/day of ferrous sulphate, an ill-tolerance of this supplement may result in side effects such as gastrointestinal distress, constipation and/or black coloured stools. In the event of such a response, the supplementation protocol may be reduced in consultation with the sports physician, to represent a dosage more tolerable to the individual athlete.

Although it is accepted that the consumption of an oral iron supplement might be effective in improving the physical performance of IDA athletes, there is still debate on the efficacy of such a regime in enhancing the physical performance of ID athletes. Some studies have demonstrated significant improvements in running energy efficiency, 15 km running time-trial performance, and maximal oxygen uptake as a result of oral iron supplementation in ID athletes (Hinton et al., 2000; Friedmann et al., 2001). However, other studies have demonstrated no improvement in athletic performance, despite a regime of oral iron supplementation significantly increasing SF levels (Klingshirn et al., 1992). The likely contrast in such outcomes may result from the different performance parameters and athlete characteristics measured within these studies; thus suggesting more research is warranted in this area. However, despite the equivocal research to suggest the influence of an oral iron supplement given to ID athletes, it is still encouraged that iron supplementation continues to be prescribed to such populations on the basis of preventing iron depletion from potentially progressing into IDA.

As established above, the use of an oral iron supplement may take at least six to eight weeks to improve the iron status of an athlete. However, should a faster increase in iron status be required (due to impending competition, extreme fatigue, etc.), the use of an intramuscular iron injection may be considered by the sports physician. When comparing such a strategy to the ingestion of oral iron tablets, it has been shown that 5×2ml intramuscular injections of aqueous Fe polymaltose (equivalent to 100mg of elemental iron), provided over a ten-day period, resulted in a significantly faster and greater increase in SF levels when compared to the ingestion of an oral iron tablet (105mg of elemental iron) consumed over a 30-day period (Dawson *et al.*, 2006). In support of such findings, a case-study by Garvican *et al.* (2011) treated an iron-deficient anaemic athlete with an intramuscular iron injection (aqueous Fe polymaltose: equivalent to 100mg of elemental Fe), followed by oral iron supplementation (325mg ferrous sulphate: equivalent to 105mg of elemental Fe) for a total of 15 weeks. Here, the SF levels of the athlete increased from 9.9 to 23.4 μg/L by two weeks post-injection, reaching a maximum level of 35.7 μg/L after seven weeks. Additional measures of Hb_{mass} showed a significant improvement of 49% within two weeks of the iron injection, thus highlighting the significance of iron to the adaptive ability of the erythropoietic pathway. Despite the positive outcomes on improving iron status, it should also be mentioned that the evidence to date for an improvement in athletic performance from such a supplementation regimen is not well documented, and as a result, more research is required into this area to assess its efficacy on performance.

Finally, it might also be mentioned that a more recent iron supplementation strategy trialled in athletic populations has involved the use of intravenous (IV) iron injections, as a fast and efficient method of increasing iron status. In fact, Garvican *et al.* (2014) assessed the efficacy of IV iron injections in comparison to a six-week oral iron supplementation protocol. The results of this study showed that the SF levels of both groups improved during the six-week intervention (IV: 31.7–167.5 μg/L; ORAL: 37.4–70.3 μg/L); however, the magnitude of this increase was substantially greater in the IV trial from week one onward. Such an outcome shows that improvements to iron status might be made in as few as seven days when using such a protocol, which may be promising for athletes presenting with compromised iron stores in relatively close proximity to competitive periods. However, such methods should only be carried out under the advice and guidance of a trained sports physician. Of course, such decisions to pursue these more recent methods of iron supplementation must always be checked against the ever-evolving substance and administration processes approved by the World Anti-Doping Agency.

Although in most instances the appropriate supplementation of iron in athletes presenting with compromised iron stores is positive, as mentioned earlier, the following should be noted: oral iron supplementation may result in GI distress, constipation and/or black coloured stools. Parenteral (intravenous) iron administration may carry a minor risk of infection at the site of injection, and may cause a degree of discomfort during administration. In severe cases, parenteral administration may result in anaphylactic shock, and thus must only be administered by trained medical personnel. Finally, indiscriminate iron supplementation carries a low risk of iron overload, whereby excessive iron stores accumulate and cause organ dysfunction through the production of reactive oxygen species. However, the risk of creating an iron overload issue in athletes is likely to be minimal given the numerous pathways of iron loss and limited iron intake reported in athletic populations. Regardless of this, since the iron overload disorder haemochromatosis is the world's most common genetic disorder, medical staff, dietitians and physiologists working with athletic populations are encouraged to know their athletes' baseline iron status prior to making recommendations on iron intake.

In conclusion, ID athletes should, in the first instance, increase their dietary intake of iron (preferably in the form of haem iron) on the advice of a sports dietitian. In addition, depending on the SF levels, clinical symptoms of fatigue, poor performance and the response to an increase in dietary iron intake, oral iron supplementation, intramuscular or IV iron injections should be considered in consultation with a sports physician.

Competing interests   None

JACK3D

Ano Lobb

Jack3D is a dietary supplement that claims to promote performance enhancement as a pre-workout product. It is widely available both in retail stores and on the internet, distributed by the manufacturer and large pharmacy and nutritional supplement chains. The current product may be found in different formulations, with the labelled ingredients including caffeine, creatine and β-alanine. While each of these compounds may enhance exercise in some way (see respective sections in this book), the exact dosages of these products in the supplement may not be readily apparent because it is described as a 'proprietary blend' and it may not therefore be clear whether they meet the accepted protocols for effective use. Jack3D also contains several botanical ingredients such as *pinus pinaster* whose effects on athletic performance are theoretical, not well documented, and also lack reliable recommended dosages. Any performance effects from this product would likely to be attributable to the effects of caffeine for fatigue resistance.

A previous formulation of Jack3D was linked to haemorrhagic stroke (Young *et al.*, 2012), acute myocardial infarction (Smith *et al.*, 2014) and two deaths (Singer and Lattman, 2013). The suspected cause of those adverse events was DMAA (see section on DMAA, which is included on the WADA Prohibited List: WADA, 2014a), possibly in combination with caffeine. Both substances are known to increase blood pressure and have previously been linked to stroke by independent researchers (Young *et al.*, 2012). Jack3D no longer contains DMAA, and we could find no published reports on the safety or efficacy of the current, DMAA-free formulation.

Competing interests   None

α-KETOGLUTARATE (AKG)

Mayur K. Ranchordas

α-ketoglutarate (AKG) is a five-carbon dicarboxylic acid produced in the citric acid cycle from the oxidative decarboxylation of isocitrate. AKG plays a central role in the oxidation of glutamine and glutamate in the small intestine, and the rate of AKG formation is important in determining the overall rate of the citric acid cycle (Wu *et al.*, 2009). AKG functions as an energy donor and ammonium scavenger, provides a source of glutamine that stimulates protein synthesis, inhibits protein catabolism in muscle, and constitutes an important metabolic fuel for cells of the gastrointestinal tract (Hixt and Müller, 1996).

The majority of studies investigating the effects of AKG supplementation have been conducted in animals. However, in humans, AKG has been shown to significantly increase plasma levels of several hormones such as insulin, growth hormone and insulin-like growth factor-1, although the mechanisms responsible are poorly understood (Moukarzel *et al.*, 1994). Research investigating the effects of AKG supplementation on athletic performance is scant and the limited studies that have been conducted have examined the effects of the co-ingestion of AKG L-arginine and/or with creatine. In one investigation involving an eight-week intervention (Campbell *et al.*, 2006), 12g/day of L-arginine α-ketoglutarate (AAKG) in three doses of 4g (2g L-arginine and 2g AKG) was found to be safe, well tolerated and to influence positively 1RM (One Maximum Repetition) bench press and Wingate peak power performance, but did not affect body composition or aerobic capacity. In another study, supplementation with creatine (0.1g.kg-1.d-1) and AAKG (0.075g.kg-1.d-1) for ten days was found to improve upper body muscle endurance and peak power output on repeated Wingate tests compared to a placebo (Little *et al.*, 2008). These findings, however, should be interpreted with caution because the individual effects of AKG cannot be isolated from these studies, and other investigations have found positive outcomes from creatine and L-arginine supplementation on exercise performance.

The effects of supplementation with either AKG or branched chain keto acids (BCKA) were recently examined in 33 untrained young men (Liu *et al.*, 2012). Participants received either AKG in doses of 0.2g/kg/d, BCKA in doses of 0.2g/kg/d, or a placebo for four weeks while undertaking a four-week resistance training programme. During the fourth week, training volume, maximum power output and muscle torque were higher in the AKG group (175 ± 42 min, 412 ± 49 Watts and 293 ± 58 Newton metres, respectively, P<0.05) and the BCKA group (158 ± 35, 390 ± 29 and 273 ± 47, P<0.05) than in the placebo group (92 ± 70, 381 ± 67 and 233 ± 43). After week three of the training programme both the general and emotional stress, assessed using the rest-stress-questionnaire-sport, increased in the placebo group while no changes were observed in the AKG and BCKA groups. These data suggest that AKG may be beneficial for resistance training and could have favourable effects on mental exhaustion over time as training intensity and volume increase.

Currently, there is insufficient evidence to support the use of AKG supplements to inhibit protein degradation in the muscle, increase muscle mass, promote positive training adaptations or enhance athletic performance. Further research is necessary to investigate the effects of AKG supplementation alone, or in combination with other nutrients.

Competing interests   None

α-KETOISOCAPROATE (KIC)

Mayur K. Ranchordas

α-ketoisocaproate (KIC) is a metabolite of the amino acid leucine. β-hydroxy-methylbutyrate (HMB) is produced from KIC by the enzyme KIC dehydrogenase ,and this route of HMB formation is dependent on liver KIC dioxygenase (Zanchi *et al.*, 2011). KIC has been found to have protein sparing and anti-catabolic properties through inhibition of muscle proteolysis and enhancement of protein synthesis. α-ketoisocaproic acid (α-KIC) supplementation has been suggested to enhance exercise performance by attenuating exercise-induced muscle soreness, promoting energy supply to the muscle, and potentially sparing muscle glucose utilisation (Ichihara *et al.*, 1973). More specifically, it has been purported that the liver can convert KIC to ketone bodies thereby increasing the energy supply during exercise.

Very few studies have examined the effects of α-KIC supplementation alone on athletic performance. Acute α-KIC supplementation at doses of 1.5g and 9.0g ingested immediately prior to exercise failed to improve moderate and high-intensity exercise performance in resistance-trained men (Yarrow *et al.*, 2007). α-KIC supplementation has been investigated in combination with HMB. Nunan *et al.* (2010) gave 14 men 3g HMB and 0.3g α-KIC vs. placebo, 11 days before and three days after a 40-minute downhill run, but failed to show differences in creatine kinase, delayed onset muscle soreness, mid-thigh girth, range of motion, and isometric and concentric torque. In contrast, van Someren and colleagues (2005) found that co-ingestion of α-KIC and HMB attenuated exercise-induced muscle damage and preserved fat-free mass.

Others have investigated the co-ingestion of α-KIC with glycine and L-arginine (GAKIC), and shown enhanced high-intensity exercise performance. Beis and colleagues (2011) investigated the effects of 11.2g GAKIC taken acutely 45 min before high-intensity repeated cycling, but failed to show differences on repeated cycling sprints, heart rate, fatigue index and rate of perceived exertion (RPE). Using 10.2g of GAKIC vs. placebo, Wax and colleagues have shown GAKIC supplementation to increase leg extension strength in nine resistance-trained females (2013a), and total load lifted when performing five sets of 75% 1RPM in seven resistance-trained men (2013b). Neither repeated-measures study was able to demonstrate changes in heart rate, blood lactate and blood glucose (Wax *et al.*, 2013a, 2013b).

However, it is unclear whether the benefits seen can be attributed to α-KIC supplementation or the other compounds. Acute doses of α-KIC, up to 9g/day, have been administered without any known side effects. At present there is insufficient evidence to support the use of α-KIC supplementation in enhancing exercise performance or reducing muscle damage.

Competing interests None

KETONE BODIES

Pete J. Cox and Kieran Clarke

Ketone bodies are water-soluble 4-carbon fuel substrates produced endogenously from fatty acids in the liver in response to low insulin and blood glucose concentrations. Ketone bodies D-β-hydroxybutyrate (βHB) and acetoacetate (AcAc) are always present in small amounts in our bloodstream (Robinson and Williamson, 1980), only increasing in response to energy deficit or some pathological conditions (Veech, 2004). Originally characterised in the odour of uncontrolled diabetes (Dreschfeld, 1886), the revelation of ketone metabolism as a vital evolutionary response to enhance survival duration in caloric deprivation took many decades to be recognised (Cahill and Owen, 1968). However, despite advances in clinical medicine, ketosis remains unfairly maligned as the 'grim reaper' of fuel substrates due to its association with poor clinical outcome in diabetic crisis (van Itallie and Nufert, 2003). This negativism, and the lack of practical utility to study ketone body metabolism outside starvation, high-fat diets, or ketone-salt intravenous infusion has meant that this fuel has, until recently, been largely ignored for its physiological potential.

Nutritional ketosis

Novel forms of edible ketone body are currently undergoing human trials (Clarke *et al.*, 2012; Cox, 2012) with promising results in exercise performance (Cox, 2012; Cox and Clarke, 2014). These dietary forms of ketone provide gut-absorbable βHB or AcAc as a novel dietary macronutrient. Delivered as a ketone body esterified to either fat (Hashim and van Itallie, 2014), or more usefully a ketone body precursor, such as the ketone monoester *R*-1,3,-Butanediol (Clarke *et al.*, 2012), blood ketone concentrations equivalent to that seen after weeks of total starvation are safely achievable in a matter of minutes (Clarke *et al.*, 2012).

Pleiotropic effects of ketone bodies on substrate metabolism

The conservation of carbohydrate reserves in the form of glycogen and gluconeogenic skeletal muscle protein is a hallmark of starvation-induced ketosis (Cahill, 1970), dramatically increasing survival duration in starving humans (Cahill and Owen, 1968; Felig *et al.*, 1969). Ketosis may also provide thermodynamic advantages over other carbon substrates by increasing the free energy conserved in ATP (ΔG_{ATP}) by the oxidation of ketones during mitochondrial oxidative phosphorylation (Veech, 2004; Sato *et al.*, 1995).

The combination of improved energetic efficiency and fuel sparing is vitally important not only during famine, but may also provide a new method of sustaining physical performance.

Athletes are ideally placed to use alternative energy sources

Athletic training increases the oxidative and enzymatic capacity of skeletal muscle for substrate combustion; in particular, blood borne nutrients (Holloszy and Coyle, 1984). While the athletic adaptations to harness greater energy requirement from fatty acids in endurance exercise are well known, ketolytic capacity also increases, with several-fold increases in ketolytic enzymes (Winder et al., 1974) and reduced ketone levels in athletes vs. controls during and after exercise, suggesting greater utilisation (Johnson et al., 1969). Furthermore the monocarboxylate transporters (SLC16 family) responsible for the transport of ketones through sarcolemmal and mitochondrial membranes (Halestrap and Meredith, 2004) are significantly upregulated by exercise.

Implications of ketosis for exercise performance

By their very nature as a substrate and signal in starvation, ketone bodies are oxidised by most body tissues to ease the use of carbohydrates and gluconeogenesis via proteolysis of muscle mass (Robinson and Williamson, 1980). The demands of endurance exercise place a premium on carbohydrate reserves, as skeletal muscle fuel selection during heavy exercise, such as during competitive sport, relies almost exclusively on glycogen and blood glucose for its energy requirements (Romijn et al., 1993; van Loon et al., 2001). In many ways, the metabolic demands of exercise parallel (albeit on a much more rapid scale) the metabolic conditions pertinent to survival in starvation.

Fuelling the engine: limitations to endurance performance

Intramuscular glycogen content is well known as a powerful determinant of endurance capacity (Bergström et al., 1967), with glucose oxidation during heavy exercise often exceeding 5–8g/min; depletion of this fuel store coincides with volitional fatigue. For decades, nutritional strategies for high-performance sport have focused on finding methods to spare glucose reserves, either by providing alternative energy sources to compete with glucose for respiration, or to enhance the contribution of exogenous fuels to total energy requirements (Jeukendrup, 2004). However, under conventional metabolic conditions, muscle fuel preference during high-intensity exercise remains stubbornly fixed to carbohydrates (Romijn et al., 1995; van Loon et al., 2001).

Ketosis alters muscular carbohydrate metabolism

Ketone bodies not only provide an alternative substrate for oxidative respiration, but also compete with pyruvate as a preferred substrate for mitochondrial oxidation (Robinson and Williamson, 1980). Strong evidence for the importance of ketosis in altering working muscle metabolism dates back in excess of 60 years; most notably the work of Randle and co-workers (1963), which demonstrated that ketone bodies inhibit glycolytic flux and increase glycogen in rat cardiac muscle and diaphragm. Maizels and colleagues (1977) subsequently demonstrated an increased glycogen concentration following exercise in rat soleus muscle when metabolising acetoacetate. This finding was repeated in an isolated perfused rat heart by Kashiwaya and colleagues (1997), who demonstrated that ketones in the perfusate have the ability to replicate the action of insulin in promoting glycogen synthesis. Perhaps most striking of all is the finding by Laughlin and colleagues (1994) that the addition of 1 mM D-β-hydroxybutyrate to a coronary artery perfusate of glucose and insulin in an *in vivo* anaesthetised dog heart raised glycogen synthesis rate six-fold. In humans, infusion of radiolabelled acetoacetate or βHB to ~5 mM during moderate exercise demonstrated a five- to eight-fold increase in $^{14}CO_2$ production from ketones, with an increased metabolic clearance (Fery and Balasse 1983). Such evidence suggests a sound rationale for the use of ketone bodies as a dietary supplement for exercise, as well as muscle recovery, and may challenge the accepted doctrine of fuel selection during exercise.

Duration vs. intensity

Effective oxidative respiration is clearly central to endurance exercise performance, of which the control of fuel homeostasis is an integral part. However, ketosis may not be advantageous to performance applications that rely almost solely on anaerobic glycolysis, or extremely high glycolytic flux for ATP production, such as sprint or middle distance events. Glucose is the only fuel which can be metabolised under anaerobic conditions to produce ATP, so ketone bodies would not be expected to contribute to energy transduction under these circumstances. Furthermore, highly glycolytic exercise may even be impaired if ketone body oxidation restricts glycolysis by negative feedback, either by an increase in NADH/NAD$^+$ or acetyl-CoA/CoA ratio (Randle *et al.*, 1963). Therefore the potential performance applications for ketosis appear more suited to sustained endurance, where incremental improvements in energy transduction/efficiency, or carbohydrate preservation, may translate to significant increases in performance.

Conclusion

While it is too soon to make conclusive statements regarding the role of supplemental forms of ketone bodies as a fuel in exercise, or their impact on performance, there is significant potential in exercise science for the considered application of this novel substrate. Preliminary studies on the safety of ketone body products, such as the ketone monoester R-1,3-butanediol, show it is generally well tolerated when consumed in the quantities needed to create significant increases in blood ketone concentrations. Both tests of efficacy and commercial production of such ketone bodies are required before they can be considered as useful for athletic performance. Multiple studies are underway to elucidate the potential of nutritional ketones in exercise, as well as their therapeutic utility in conditions of high energetic demand, or dysregulated substrate selection.

Competing interests   Professor Kieran Clarke is a non-executive director of TdeltaST, a spin out company of the University of Oxford who own the intellectual property rights to a D-3-β-hydroxybutyrate-1,3-butanediol ketone monoester.

LECITHIN

Mayur K. Ranchordas

Lecithin is a phospholipid that occurs naturally in foods of animal and plant origin such as egg yolk, soybeans and wheat germ. Lecithin is naturally high in phosphatidylcholine, which is required for normal cellular structure and function (Jäger *et al.*, 2007).

It has been suggested that strenuous exercise results in decreased plasma choline concentrations which is associated with decreased acetylcholine and delayed muscle contraction (Conlay *et al.*, 1992). Lecithin supplementation has been purported to possess ergogenic properties due to either its phosphate or choline content.

Very few studies have investigated the effects of lecithin supplementation on athletic performance. Trained triathletes were given a placebo and acute lecithin supplementation at a dose of $0.2\,g\,kg^{-1}$ one hour before exercise (von Allwörden *et al.*, 1993). The placebo condition decreased plasma choline concentrations by 17%; however, when lecithin supplementation was given, average plasma choline levels remained unchanged. In a similar study, 12 accomplished marathon runners were given either 2.2g of lecithin or a placebo one day before running a marathon (Buchman *et al.*, 2000). Runners given the lecithin supplementation maintained normal plasma-free choline levels compared to the placebo condition, however, there was no effect on performance. Another study found that 14 days of soya lecithin supplementation had no ergogenic effect on grip strength (Staton, 1951).

Acute lecithin supplementation at doses of 2.2g prior to exercise has been administered without any known side effects. Although lecithin supplementation appears to prevent the decrease in choline levels after exercise, there is no clear evidence to indicate any performance benefits.

Competing interests   None

LEPTIN

José A.L. Calbet

Leptin is a hormone secreted primarily by adipocytes from white adipose tissue in direct proportion to the amount of body fat. Leptin plays a crucial role in the regulation of appetite, body fat mass, basal metabolic rate and gonadal function (Friedman and Halaas, 1998). A rare congenital deficiency of leptin caused morbid obesity that normalized with subcutaneous leptin treatment.

Circulating leptin levels change acutely with energy balance: leptin increases with food ingestion and is reduced with prolonged exercise and fasting. With severe acute negative energy balance serum, leptin levels are dramatically reduced by 60–80%, despite small changes in total fat mass. Preventing this reduction in leptin levels could attenuate hunger in dieting athletes, facilitating the adjustment of body mass to specific targets. Nevertheless, there is no account of leptin use by athletes for this purpose.

Leptin receptors are more densely expressed in the cerebellum, than the hypothalamus, where it is supposed to exert its main action. Leptin-related changes in physical activity levels may promote structural changes in the cerebellum, which is strongly implicated in motor control and learning. Leptin receptors are also expressed in human skeletal muscle, more abundantly in women than men (Guerra *et al.*, 2007, 2008).

The main action of leptin in skeletal muscle is supposed to be the stimulation of fatty acid oxidation via activation of AMPK/acetyl-coenzyme A carboxylase β (ACCβ) signalling through the long isoform of the receptor. In cell culture, leptin can also elicit lipid oxidation via JAK2/p38 MAPK/STAT3 activation through a short isoform of the leptin receptor (Akasaka *et al.*, 2010). Interestingly, these pathways are also activated 30 minutes after sprint exercise (Guerra *et al.*, 2011); similarly, leptin induces PGC1α expression and mitochondrial biogenesis.

Exercise reduces leptin resistance in obese rodents or in rodents fed with high-fat diets (which cause skeletal muscle insulin and leptin resistance). Little is known about the influence of exercise on the regulation of leptin receptors and signalling in human skeletal muscles. In obese humans, leptin receptors are reduced in the m. vastus lateralis (Fuentes *et al.*, 2010), possibly by a mechanism related to reduced physical activity in obesity. However, 12 weeks of weightlifting combined with endurance training did not seem to induce changes in leptin receptors in the m. vastus lateralis of healthy men (Olmedillas *et al.*, 2011). Professional tennis players have increased expression of leptin receptors in the triceps brachi of the dominant compared to the non-dominant arm, suggesting that chronic loading may regulate the expression of leptin receptors in human skeletal muscle (Olmedillas *et al.*, 2010). An increased expression of leptin receptors in overloaded skeletal muscle may facilitate muscle growth by a mechanism involving leptin signalling through JAK2/PIK3/Akt elicited either by leptin itself or by IGF-1. Leptin increases the expression of IGF binding protein-2 (IGFBP-2) in human skeletal muscle, by a direct mechanism and also through the activation of the sympathetic nervous system (Yau *et al.*, 2014). Increased IGFBP-2 results in phosphatase and tensin homologue (PTEN) inhibition and increased Akt-mediated muscle hypertrophy (Sharples *et al.*, 2013). IGF-1 is able to induce leptin receptor phosphorylation by IGR-IR kinase, which is activated upon IGF binding to IGF-IR. Moreover, leptin could potentiate the anabolic response to leucine in skeletal muscles (Mao *et al.*, 2013).

Leptin has pleiotropic effects on the central nervous system far beyond the control of appetite, including the modulation of dopamine/serotonin pathways, which are implicated in sleep, fatigue and reward circuits. Leptin is reduced during exercise and this could contribute to the sense of effort. It remains unknown if leptin supplementation during exercise could have ergogenic effects.

Hypothetically, athletes could think of using leptin or leptin agonists to facilitate a reduction of fat mass, control hunger, promote muscle signalling similar to that induced by sprint training, stimulate mitochondrial biogenesis, and as an anabolic agent when combined with strength training and amino acid supplementation. Therefore, concerned authorities should keep track of potential misuse of leptin or leptin agonists.

Competing interests   None

LEUCINE

Eva Blomstrand

Leucine is one of the three branched-chain amino acids (BCAA; see section on BCAA) and is an essential amino acid that has to be provided in the diet. Besides serving as building blocks for protein synthesis, leucine can also regulate the rate of protein synthesis via a stimulatory effect on enzymes involved in the translation of specific mRNAs (Kimball and Jefferson, 2010). Direct stimulation by leucine of the rate of protein synthesis in muscle tissue was first demonstrated in various preparations from experimental animals and, later, in the intact animal after oral administration (Crozier et al., 2005). Infusion of leucine in human subjects was found to stimulate protein synthesis and activate the regulatory enzyme 70-kD ribosomal protein S6 kinase 1 (p70S6K1), but it was only recently shown that oral intake increased the rate of protein synthesis in resting human muscle (Greiwe et al., 2001; Smith et al., 1998; Wilkinson et al., 2013).

When leucine is ingested together with the other essential amino acids (EAA) following resistance exercise, the rate of protein synthesis increases to a larger extent than without nutritional supply, and a positive net protein balance is achieved during the period after exercise (Tipton et al., 1999). However, adding extra leucine to a complete protein or EAA mixture has no effect, or only minor additional effect, on the rate of protein synthesis in young subjects (Glynn et al., 2010; Koopman et al., 2006; Tipton et al., 2009). On the other hand, when leucine is excluded from an EAA mixture ingested in combination with resistance exercise, the stimulatory effect on mTORC1 signalling is reduced, as judged from a smaller increase in p70S6K1 phosphorylation following resistance exercise (Moberg et al., 2014). These results further emphasize that leucine has an especially important stimulatory effect on anabolic processes in human skeletal muscle. In elderly subjects, in whom the required amount of leucine to reach optimal stimulation on protein synthesis appears to be enhanced, leucine-enriched diet improves muscle protein synthesis acutely, whereas no effect on muscle mass is observed during long-term supplementation (Balage and Dardevet, 2010).

There is some evidence from animal studies that leucine can also inhibit muscle protein breakdown. In humans, leucine infusion reduces the rate of release of amino acids from the muscle, improving the net protein balance, which suggests a diminished protein breakdown (Nair et al., 1992). However, evidence for a direct effect of leucine on the degradation processes in human muscle has so far not yet been presented.

Intake of leucine together with the other EAA is recommended in connection with exercise. Available data indicate that the amount of leucine required to reach an optimal effect is 1.5–2.5g in young individuals, which is the normal content in ~20g of high quality protein. In elderly individuals the amount can preferably be increased.

Competing interests   None

LINOLEIC ACID

Philip C. Calder

Linoleic acid, the simplest member of the omega-6 polyunsaturated fatty acid family, is an essential fatty acid. It has a particular role in maintaining the integrity of the skin, so preventing water loss, as a result of its presence within the structure of skin-specific lipids. Linoleic acid is different in structure from conjugated linoleic acid (CLA; see section on CLA). Linoleic acid is the substrate for biosynthesis of arachidonic acid, the principal precursor of eicosanoids involved in a variety of physiological and pathophysiological responses. Linoleic acid is synthesised in plants. Consequently plant tissues, seeds and nuts; their oils (e.g. corn oil, sunflower oil, soybean oil); and foodstuffs produced from these oils (e.g. margarines) have a high content of linoleic acid (often > 50% of the fatty acids present). Inclusion of seeds, nuts, grains, vegetable oils and margarines in a variety of foods and the presence of linoleic acid in animal-derived foods as a result of animal foraging and modern farming practices (e.g. feeding on grains) means that linoleic acid is widespread in foods and in the diet.

The human requirement for linoleic acid is estimated to be 0.5% of energy, which in a typical Western adult equates to an intake of about 1g/day. The UK National Diet and Nutrition Survey indicated that the average intake of omega-6 fatty acids, most of which would be linoleic acid, among adults aged 19 to 64 years is about 5.4% of energy and that 97.5% of the population in this age range consume more than 2.7% of energy as omega-6 fatty acids, mainly linoleic acid (Henderson *et al.*, 2003). Average intakes in g/day were 12 in men and 9 in women, with 97.5% of men consuming more than 4.9g/day and 97.5% of women consuming more than 4g/day. Thus intake of linoleic acid among adults in the UK is greatly in excess of the estimated requirement. Intake in the USA is likely to be even higher than in the UK (Blasbalg *et al.*, 2011). A high intake of linoleic acid can competitively inhibit the biosynthesis of the omega-3 fatty acid eicosapentaenoic acid from its precursor α-linolenic acid (ALA). Given the widespread presence of linoleic acid in foods there does not seem to be a case for supplementation of linoleic acid amongst athletes.

Competing interests None

γ-LINOLENIC ACID

Philip C. Calder

Gamma (γ)-linolenic acid (GLA) is the desaturated derivative of linoleic acid. It is an omega-6 fatty acid. GLA is found in certain unusual plant oils like evening primrose oil and borage oil (sometimes called starflower oil) and is typically rare in the diet.

Experimental studies suggest an anti-inflammatory action mediated via prostaglandin E1 and analgesic effects. Low dose GLA supplementation during exercise had a therapeutic benefit in claudicants (individuals with pain primarily in the legs, which can impair walking and cause limping) undertaking standing leg exercises (Christie *et al.*, 1968). In a large rehabilitation study in patients with compressive radiculopathy syndrome (compression or irritation of a nerve as it exits the spinal column, causing pain, numbness, tingling, or weakness in the arms or legs) from disc-nerve root conflict, a daily supplement of 360mg GLA + 600mg alpha-lipoic acid improved neuropathic symptoms (Rainieri *et al.*, 2009).

Although GLA has been advocated by some as suitable for athletes with the aims of increasing performance and reducing inflammation, there is no scientific evidence to support this. High doses are thought to impair performance and have an adverse effect on mood, perhaps because GLA is the precursor of arachidonic acid. There are claims that GLA supplementation will help bodybuilders to lose fat, but there does not appear to be strong evidence to support this.

Competing interests   None

α-LIPOIC ACID

Karlien Smit and Shelly Meltzer

Alpha (α)-lipoic acid (ALA), not to be confused with alpha-linoleic acid, is a mitochondrial fatty acid that acts as an antioxidant and is also involved in a range of cellular actions as a metal chelator and mediator of cell signalling pathways. It is produced endogenously in small amounts and is also supplied via the diet by foods including red meat (specifically organ meat) and some fruits and vegetables (Shay et al., 2009). Supplementation of ALA has been shown to reduce symptoms in patients with diabetic neuropathy, but more human trials are needed to determine potential benefits for neurological disorders, weight loss and other chronic inflammatory conditions (Golbidi et al., 2011).

In terms of its application to sports performance, a study on recreational male weightlifters showed that five days of supplementation with 1,000mg ALA combined with creatine and sucrose significantly increased total creatine and phosphocreatine uptake in the muscle (Burke et al., 2003). However, subsequent studies on endurance-trained cyclists have shown this does not necessarily translate into thermoregulatory, cardiovascular or performance benefits (Polyviou et al., 2012a).

In double-blind placebo-controlled studies, 600–1,000mg alpha-lipoic acid/ day for eight to 14 days had a tendency to reduce markers of oxidative stress and selectively protect DNA and lipids after high-intensity muscle contractions in the quadriceps of untrained men (Zembron-Lacny et al., 2009; Fogarty et al., 2013). Antioxidant supplementation has been proposed to attenuate the physiological stresses of high altitude exposure (see section on antioxidants). However, evidence that alpha-lipoic acid reduces acute mountain sickness, when combined with vitamins C and E, is equivocal, with one study reporting favourable effects (Bailey and Davies, 2001) while another failed to find benefits (Baillie et al., 2009). The divergent results of these studies are not surprising given differences in the methodological design such as the duration of ascent, period of supplementation, physical effort and hypoxic exposure.

Finally, little is known about the long-term effects of taking high dosages of alpha-lipoic acid. In some situations, chronic antioxidant supplementation can dampen training adaptations (Fogarty et al., 2013). Thus, prudent advice would be to rather ingest an antioxidant-rich diet and, if going to high altitude, to use well proven therapies such as acetazolamide, rather than alpha-lipoic acid, until more rigorous studies have been performed (Baillie et al., 2009).

Competing interests None

MAGNESIUM

Frank C. Mooren

Magnesium (Mg) is an essential biological element which is predominantly located in bones (approx. 52%), in muscle cells (28%), soft tissue (19%), serum (0.3%; concentration range 0.75–1.1 mmol/l) and red blood cells (0.5%). Serum acts as a transit pathway between bone stores and actively metabolising tissues and is not representative of the body's Mg status. Intracellular Mg is under hormonal control in some cell types and regulated by a secondary active transport system, the Na^+-Mg^{2+}-exchanger. In both extra- and intracellular compartments, an equilibrium between ionized Mg^{2+} and bound Mg is established. Only Mg^{2+} is available to react in physiological and biochemical processes during cellular homeostasis by binding to organic substances, such as proteins, nucleic acids and nucleotides. In general, Mg^{2+} is an important regulator of three main complexes: 1) enzyme activation, e.g. during energy metabolism, 2) stabilizing membrane function and integrity, and 3) cell signalling, e.g. as a natural antagonist of intracellular calcium signals (Mooren et al., 2011). Regarding energy metabolism, Mg has been shown to be involved at several steps. At the insulin receptor level Mg enhances the cell's sensitivity towards an insulin stimulus thereby facilitating cellular glucose entry. Furthermore, Mg is an important cofactor of ATP generation at the inner mitochondrial membrane while Mg depletion seems to induce mitochondrial dysfunction.

Acute exercise induces a hypomagnesaemia (ten out of 18 studies) while total intracellular Mg ($[Mg]_i$) content of blood cells seems to be unchanged (seven out of 12 studies). Interestingly, ionized $[Mg^{2+}]_e$ decreased after high-intensity exercise while ionized $[Mg^{2+}]_i$ increased (Mooren et al., 2005). Results from animal studies suggest that Mg^{2+} is shifted from plasma into muscle and adipose tissue (Nielsen and Lukaski, 2006). Exercise-induced hypomagnesemia has been shown to coincide with alterations in ECG recordings, which may indicate an increased vulnerability for arrhythmias, as well as clinical signs of exhaustion such as muscle fatigue and collapse (Scherr et al., 2012; Siegel et al., 2008).

Longitudinal and cross-sectional studies suggest that chronic exercise training may be followed by Mg^{2+} depletion and that athletes are prone to Mg^{2+} deficiency, most likely due to Mg losses in sweat and urine. Dietary restrictions especially in athletes participating in sports requiring weight control may aggravate the situation. Using a Mg^{2+} loading test, an enhanced retention of the intravenously applicated Mg^{2+} for the athletes group compared to the control group was described indicating a depleted Mg^{2+} status (Saur et al., 2002).

Previously published reviews indicate no significant effect of Mg supplementation on endurance or strength performance, at least in athletes with balanced Mg status (Newhouse and Finstad, 2000; Nielsen and Lukaski, 2006). However, single studies indicate that Mg supplementation may improve exercise economy during submaximal aerobic exercise: lower VO_{2max} values at given intensity; better lactate clearance, etc. (Lukaski and Nielsen, 2002; Cheng et al., 2010). Moreover, recently published observational studies indicate an association between Mg intake and strength performance both in athletes and older adults (Santos et al., 2011; Dominguez et al., 2006). Therefore, Mg supplementation should be considered in athletes with Mg deficiency based on findings from animal experiments and in humans which suggest that magnesium deficiency can compromise exercise capacity. Mg^{2+} deficiency is characterized by an enhanced neuromuscular excitability including symptoms such as cardiac arrhythmias, headache, nervousness, and cramps of both smooth and skeletal muscle. The latter, however, have to be differentiated from exercise-induced muscle cramps for which Mg supplementation has not so far proved to be effective.

Important food sources of Mg include vegetables, fish, nuts and whole grains. Magnesium formulations include both inorganic and organic compounds of which the latter seemed to have a better bioavailability. A range between 350 and 400mg Mg/day is recommended as the upper limit. In case of a renal insufficiency the daily dosage has to be reduced adequately. Most common side effects include gastrointestinal side effects such as nausea and diarrhoea. Intravenous application may cause hypotension and cardiac arrhythmias (Guerrera et al., 2009). In contrast, Mg is recommended in the treatment of Torsades de Pointes, a type of malignant ventricular tachycardia. Finally, oral Mg supplementation is suggested as an effective co-medication for both prevention and therapy of diabetes mellitus by improving insulin sensitivity (Mooren et al., 2011).

Conflict of interest The author received grants from Verla-Pharm Arzneimittel GmbH & Co. KG, 82327 Tutzing and Hermes Arzneimittel GmbH, 82049 Großhesselohe, Germany.

MEDIUM-CHAIN TRIGLYCERIDES (MCT)

Louise M. Burke

Medium-chain triglycerides (MCT) are fats in which the fatty acids joined to the glycerol backbone are six to 14 carbon molecules in length. These fats are digested and metabolized differently from the long-chain fatty acids that make up most of our dietary fat intake. Specifically, MCT can be digested within the intestinal lumen with less need for bile and pancreatic juices than long-chain triglycerides, with the liberated medium-chain fatty acids (MCFA) being absorbed via the portal circulation. MCFA are then taken up into the mitochondria without the need for carnitine-assisted transport. MCT supplements derived from palm kernel and coconut oil are used in clinical nutrition situations as an energy source for patients who have various digestive or lipid metabolism disorders.

Sports-related applications of MCT include their marketing to body builders as an easily absorbed and oxidized fuel source that is less likely to deposit as body fat. More recently, MCT have been marketed as a 'superfood' suitable for intake in the high-fat low-carbohydrate and 'Clean Living' style diets which have crossed over to some athletic populations. Despite this resurgence in interest, there is no scientific evidence of any benefits to athletic performance from chronic use of MCT. In fact, there is little investigation of such chronic use by athletes apart from some evidence that a two-week protocol of intake of ~60g of MCT per day may be associated with deterioration in blood lipid profiles (Kern et al., 2000), without any benefit to exercise capacity (Misell et al., 2001).

The best studied use of MCT by athletes is as a source of rapidly accessible fat that could be consumed during exercise to increase fat availability during endurance and ultra-endurance events. In such events, there is both time to consume a fat source, and potential benefits if this leads to a sparing of muscle glycogen use. The maximum rate of oxidation of MCT occurs after about 120–180 min of exercise, and co-ingestion with carbohydrate can increase this rate, possibly by increasing the rate of MCT (Jeukendrup et al., 1995). The literature on supplementation with MCT and carbohydrate during ultra-endurance exercise is inconsistent, with the results appearing to depend on the amount of MCT that can be ingested and the prevailing hormonal conditions. Studies in which the intake of large amounts of MCT raised plasma-free fatty acid (FFA) concentrations and allowed glycogen sparing, reported enhancement of a performance trial undertaken at the end of prolonged exercise (van Zyl et al., 1996). However, these metabolic (and performance) benefits may be compromised when exercise is commenced with higher insulin levels, as is the case following a carbohydrate (CHO)-rich pre-exercise meal (Goedecke *et al.*, 1999; Angus *et al.*, 2000). The effectiveness of MCT is mostly limited by the inability of subjects to tolerate the substantial amount of MCT oils required to have a metabolic impact. A total intake of ~30g appears to be the limit of gastrointestinal tolerance of MCT, which would limit its fuel contribution to 3–7% of the total energy expenditure during typical ultra-endurance events (Jeukendrup *et al.*, 1995). Gastrointestinal reactions to larger intakes range from insignificant (van Zyl *et al.*, 1996) to performance-limiting (Goedecke *et al.*, 1999). Differences in gastrointestinal tolerance between or within studies may reflect differences in the type and intensity of exercise, the mean chain length of MCT found in the supplements or increased tolerance in some athletes due to chronic exposure to MCT. Despite some support for use during prolonged exercise, MCT appear to have limited application to most sporting situations.

Competing interests   None

MELAMINE

David S. Senchina

Melamine (2,4,6-triamino-1,3,5-triazine; tripolycyanimide) is used in the production of plastics and adhesives. It has no documented ergogenic capacity. Given its high nitrogen content, melamine has been illegally used to elevate food protein quantity (as in protein supplements). Melamine and derivatives (e.g. cyanuric acid) are toxic to humans even at low quantities, with strong effects on the kidneys (Hau *et al.*, 2009; Sharma and Paradakar, 2010). Tolerable daily intake amounts vary by country and consumer age, but a typical adult level is 0.5mg/kg/day (Hau *et al.*, 2009; Tyan *et al.*, 2009). Shortly after the 2008 Beijing Olympics, it was discovered that protein products from multiple Chinese manufacturers contained melamine and derivatives, and that those products were distributed internationally (Sharma and Paradakar, 2010). Although screening indicated that Olympic athletes were not exposed (Wu *et al.*, 2010), other populations (particularly Chinese infants) were clinically affected. Athletes should be aware of possible melamine contamination in protein-rich foodstuffs.

Competing interests None

MELATONIN

James C. Miller

Melatonin (N-acetyl-5-methoxytryptamine) is a pineal gland hormone with effects upon circadian rhythms, sleep onset and reproductive systems (Arendt, 1998; Chowdhury *et al.*, 2008). Blood levels of melatonin are generally undetectable during daytime, but rise sharply during darkness. Light–dark sensations at the retina are relayed to the suprachiasmatic nucleus of the hypothalamus. Fibres from the hypothalamus descend to the spinal cord and ultimately project to the superior cervical ganglia, from which sympathetic post-ganglionic neurons ascend back to the pineal gland. Melatonin peak amplitudes decrease with age (van Coevorden *et al.*, 1991) which may explain the flattening of the circadian rhythm also associated with aging. Melatonin is well-known as an antioxidant, immunomodulator and anti-cancer agent (Chowdhury *et al.*, 2008), and is hepato-protective (Mathes, 2010). Melatonin is available on prescription in the United Kingdom, Australia, New Zealand, Japan, Singapore, Canada and the European Union but is available for purchase over the counter in the USA, Hong Kong and Mexico.

Some effects of exercise on human biology may be mediated by melatonin (Escames *et al.*, 2012). Exercise causes a marked increase in the activity of the sympathetic nervous system and catecholamine secretion, potentially modulating melatonin secretion. Plasma melatonin increases after competition and after exercise not attenuated by regular training: this depends on the degree of utilization of melatonin in resisting oxidative damage. Melatonin's anti-oxidative properties may offer protective actions against free radical-mediated damage from exercise. Melatonin restores or preserves mitochondrial function after ischemia/reperfusion injury in skeletal muscle. Also, melatonin increases glucose uptake into skeletal muscle. In animal studies, melatonin administration protects against heart damage caused by acute exercise, as well as against age-related oxidative stress and inflammation. The levels of melatonin detected after exercise do not correspond to the melatonin produced by exercise itself, but perhaps to ambient lighting and time of day.

Mild heat loss initiation by peripheral vasodilation, modulated by melatonin secretion, may be the mechanism that initiates sleep (Kräuchi *et al.*, 2006). Supplemental melatonin could allow planned induction of this heat loss and potentially be advantageous to exercise performance. Provision of melatonin prior to exercise in the heat led to no reductions in core body temperature or improved performance. However, only low intensity exercise was performed in clothing that did not allow environmental heat loss (McLellan *et al.*, 1999, 2000). A further study looked at aspects of both physical and mental performance following daytime supplementation with melatonin and found decreased intra-aural temperature but without any change to short duration athletic performance. Notably, decrements in mental performance were identified (Atkinson *et al.*, 2005).

With increasing levels of international travel, optimizing recovery from jet lag may offer a significant performance advantage. Jet lag occurs in response to a minimum of a 3-zone change at a rate faster than one zone per day and has been suggested to cause decreased performance and increased injury risk, though direct evidence is limited (Paul *et al.*, 2010). Supplemental melatonin appears to reduce both subjective and objective symptoms of jetlag (Atkinson *et al.*, 2003). It is unclear at this point whether the main action is hypnotic, i.e. inducing sleepiness, or chronobiotic, i.e. helping to 'reset' the body clock to the new time zone. Rest–activity schedules and physical exercise potentiate entrainment of the circadian system (Escames *et al.*, 2012). However, they are weak *Zeitgebers* compared to the light–dark cycle. Night-time exercise of moderate or high intensity may cause a phase delay in dim light melatonin onset. A melatonin phase response curve for exercise needs to be clarified. There does not appear to be a performance 'hangover' from supplementation taken the night before exercise (Atkinson *et al.*, 2001). However, the use of daytime exogenous melatonin may be more likely to diminish cognitive performance variables than to enhance physical performance (Atkinson *et al.*, 2003, 2005).

Melatonin inhibits the secretion of luteinizing hormone and follicle-stimulating hormone from the anterior pituitary (Chowdhury *et al.*, 2008). Disturbances in melatonin production through continuous changes in time zone may also be linked to the frequency of amenorrhoea found in flight attendants (Harma *et al.*, 1994). There also appears to be a relationship between melatonin levels, exercise and amenorrhoea in female athletes that requires further investigation (Arena *et al.*, 1995).

Competing interests   None

METHIONINE

Nicholas A. Burd

Methionine is an indispensible amino acid that acts as a substrate, much like the other indispensible amino acids, for building functional muscle proteins. It is clear, however, that methionine also holds a unique role when compared against the other indispensible amino acids, as it serves as a methyl group donor for DNA/RNA intermediates and for the synthesis of cysteine (Stipanuk, 1986). Daily methionine requirement, reported as a constituent of the requirement for total sulphur amino acids, is 13–15mg·kg^{-1}·day^{-1} with the risk for toxicity manifesting only at levels exceeding >10-fold excess in humans (Garlick, 2006; Young et al., 2000). Daily requirements of methionine are easily obtained in the diet due to its widespread abundance in meats, eggs, cheeses, fruits and vegetables. However, vegan athletes may need increased self-awareness of daily methionine intake (Rodriguez et al., 2009b). In fact, the lower methionine by total amino acid content of plant-derived protein sources may lead to greater retention of dietary protein amino acids by the gut and ultimately contribute to the lower anabolic properties of vegetable versus animal derived proteins (Bos et al., 2003).

What purpose does supplemental methionine have in an athlete's diet for enhancing performance/recovery? Very little, provided the athlete is healthy and consuming a mixed diet containing an adequate amount of energy to meet training needs. Indeed, methionine is fundamental, together with arginine and glycine, for the endogenous synthesis of creatine (see relevant sections in book). However, there is no evidence to suggest that additional crystalline methionine to normal dietary intake would be more beneficial, or even helpful, than oral intake of creatine monohydrate; a supplement that has been shown to increase muscle strength and hypertrophy after a programme of resistance exercise training (Tarnopolsky et al., 2001).

Competing interests None

METHYLSULPHONYLMETHANE (MSM)

Kate Jackson

MSM (methylsulphonylmethane) is an organic sulphur compound. It is a metabolite of dimethyl sulphoxide (DMSO). MSM occurs naturally in certain foods including green vegetables, grains and milk (Cronin, 1999).

For over 30 years, MSM has been used as an oral daily nutritional supplement for various conditions including osteoarthritis, seasonal allergic rhinitis and autoimmune diseases. It has been used topically for the treatment of haemorrhoids (Joksimovic et al., 2012) and snoring. High quality randomized controlled trials (RCT) are lacking, but some evidence exists for an effect in osteoarthritic symptom relief.

Two small RCT (MSM groups $n=25$ and $n=26$) observed a statistically significant improvement in osteoarthritic pain scores with MSM compared to placebo. However, the clinical significance of the improved scores is unclear (Usha and Naidu, 2004; Kim et al., 2006). Participants received 3–6g daily in divided doses for 12 weeks. No studies on dose ranges have been conducted.

Brien et al. (2011) performed a meta-analysis of RCT using MSM or DMSO for symptomatic pain relief in osteoarthritis. However, no definitive conclusions could be drawn. Only 15% of DMSO is converted to MSM in the body, and other metabolites are also produced (Cronin, 1999). Thus, combining the studies may not be appropriate.

In 2011 a small RCT (MSM group $n=32$) compared extra-corporeal shock wave therapy (ESWT) plus a mixed dietary supplement (arginine, collagen, MSM, vitamin C and bromelain) with ESWT plus placebo in the treatment of insertional Achilles tendinopathy (Notarnicola et al., 2012). Both groups also did eccentric exercises. There was a small but significant improvement in pain scores and Ankle Hindfoot Scale at six months in the supplement versus the placebo group. The role of individual constituents of the supplement was not clear.

There is no long-term safety data from studies in humans. One RCT found that adverse events with MSM were equal to placebo in the short term (12 weeks) (Usha and Naidu, 2004). Most reported adverse events were minor and mainly gastrointestinal (Kim et al., 2006). In one case study a 35-year-old woman had acute angle glaucoma after taking a multiple dietary supplement for one week. The authors believe the sulphonyl component in MSM may have been responsible (Hwang et al., 2013).

There are no published trials to support the use of MSM by athletes or the general population for delayed-onset muscle soreness or acute soft tissue injuries.

In summary, there is a lack of high-quality evidence for many of the beneficial claims for MSM as a nutritional supplement. There is some limited evidence for the potential benefit of MSM in the symptomatic relief of osteoarthritis, but no definite recommendations can be made on current evidence.

Competing interests   None

MULTIPLE TRANSPORTABLE CARBOHYDRATES (MTC)

Asker Jeukendrup

Since the 1980s it has been known that carbohydrate intake during exercise can improve exercise performance lasting two hours or longer (see section on carbohdyrates). Soon after this discovery, it was established that not all carbohdyrates are equal and carbohydrates ingested during exercise may be utilised at different rates (Jeukendrup, 2010). Recently it was demonstrated that there is a dose response relationship between the amount of carbohydrate ingested and oxidized, and performance during prolonged exercise (Smith *et al.*, 2010, 2013). Therefore it is important to identify carbohydrate sources that are oxidised rapidly. Until a landmark publication in 2004 (Jentjens *et al.*, 2004), it was believed that carbohydrates ingested during exercise could be oxidised at a rate no higher than 1g/min (60g/h), independent of the type of carbohydrate. This is reflected in guidelines published by the American College of Sports Medicine (ACSM) from 2007–2009 which recommended that, during exercise lasting more than one hour, athletes should consume carbohydrate at hourly rates of between 30 and 60g (Sawka *et al.*, 2007) or 0.7g/kg (Rodriguez *et al.*, 2009a). Even when carbohydrate was ingested at rates up to 3g/min (180g/h), the oxidation of the ingested carbohydrate did not exceed 1g/min (60g/hr).

Exogenous carbohydrate oxidation appears limited by the intestinal absorption of carbohydrates (Jeukendrup, 2010). It is believed that glucose uses a sodium-dependent transporter SGLT1 for absorption, which becomes saturated at a carbohydrate intake around 1g/min (or 60g/h). However, when glucose is ingested at this rate and another carbohydrate (fructose) that uses a different transporter is ingested simultaneously, oxidation rates well above 1g/min (1.26g/min) have been observed (Jentjens *et al.*, 2004). This was the first study that showed the effects of the so-called multiple transportable carbohydrates (MTC) on exogenous carbohydrate oxidation. At present only two different intestinal carbohydrate transporters have been identified (SGLT1 for glucose or glucose polymers and galactose, and GLUT5 for fructose). Interestingly, sucrose (a disaccharide of glucose and fructose), which is said to have its own disaccharide transporter, appears to behave more like glucose than glucose:fructose (Jentjens and Jeukendrup, 2005). Studies suggest that exogenous carbohydrate oxidation from sucrose is similar to glucose and does not reach the high oxidation rates observed with glucose and fructose (or other MTC).

With the knowledge that a single carbohydrate could only be oxidised at a rate of 1g/min, a series of studies was initiated in an attempt to find the combination that would result in the highest oxidation rates. In these studies, variable rates of carbohydrate ingestion as well as the combinations of carbohydrates were investigated. All studies confirmed that MTC resulted in higher (up to 75%) oxidation rates than carbohydrates that use the SGLT1 transporter only (for reviews see Jeukendrup, 2008, 2010). Combinations of maltodextrin and fructose, and glucose and fructose, or glucose plus sucrose and fructose seem to produce the most favourable effects (Jeukendrup, 2008, 2010; Jentjens and Jeukendrup, 2005; Wallis *et al.*, 2005).

Important from a practical perspective, such high oxidation rates can not only be achieved with carbohydrate ingested in a beverage but also as a gel (Pfeiffer *et al.*, 2010a) or a low fat, low protein, low fibre energy bar (Pfeiffer *et al.*, 2010b). In line with the evidence of a dose response relationship between carbohydrate intake and endurance performance, studies have demonstrated that MTC can result in improved performance over and above the performance-enhancing effect of a carbohydrate drink with one single carbohydrate (Currell and Jeukendrup, 2008; Triplett *et al.*, 2010). It has also been demonstrated that multiple transportable carbohydrates may have advantages in fluid delivery (Shi *et al.*, 1995; Jeukendrup and Moseley, 2010) and studies suggest less gastrointestinal discomfort. Recently published recommendations take these findings into account, acknowledging that there may be different carbohydrate needs for different durations of exercise as well as for different levels of athletes (Jeukendrup, 2011). MTC can be recommended at all durations but are most effective when the exercise is 2.5 hours or longer. In those conditions, carbohydrate intakes of up to 90g/h are recommended and these would only be oxidised to any significant degree if they are multiple transportable carbohydrates in which glucose makes up no more than about 60g (Jeukendrup, 2011). For more in-depth information, the reader is referred to two recent reviews on this topic (Jeukendrup, 2013, 2014).

Conflict of interest   Asker Jeukendrup heads up the Gatorade Sports Science Institute, a division of PepsiCo Inc. The views expressed here are entirely his own and do not reflect views or policy of PepsiCo Inc.

N-ACETYLCYSTEINE (NAC)

Michael B. Reid

N-acetylcysteine (NAC) is a reduced thiol donor that supports cellular resynthesis of glutathione, a major antioxidant in skeletal muscle and other human tissues. As reviewed elsewhere (Reid, 2008, and elsewhere in this book), glutathione buffers reactive oxygen species (ROS) produced by muscle. ROS levels increase substantially during strenuous exercise, overwhelming glutathione buffering and depressing contractile function. This contributes to the development of muscle fatigue. NAC opposes this process. By supporting glutathione resynthesis, NAC slows the rise of ROS activity in exercising muscle and delays fatigue.

This was first demonstrated in humans by our group (Reid *et al.*, 1994) in studies of tibialis anterior, an ankle dorsiflexor muscle, during repetitive electrical stimulation. Subsequent studies confirmed that NAC inhibits fatigue during volitional exercise tasks, for example, loaded breathing (Travaline *et al.*, 1997), and handgrip exercise (Matuszczak *et al.*, 2005). The studies of greatest physiological relevance were conducted by McKenna and colleagues who showed that NAC delays fatigue of trained athletes during strenuous cycling exercise (Medved *et al.*, 2004b). The cellular processes in fatiguing muscle that are modulated by NAC remain poorly defined. Emerging evidence suggests that NAC influences muscle metabolism (Trewin *et al.*, 2013), and does not alter myosin light chain phosphorylation or inorganic phosphate levels (Katz *et al.*, 2014). Despite performance benefits in the laboratory, several issues limit NAC use as an ergogenic aid. First, only pharmacological doses of 140–150mg/kg have been shown to limit fatigue. It is not known if lower doses are effective. Second, doses that delay fatigue are safe but can have uncomfortable side effects including nausea and diarrhoea (Ferreira *et al.*, 2011). Finally, NAC may have negative effects on athletic training. Data suggest that chronic antioxidant supplementation blunts the positive effects of transient oxidative stress, a signal that appears to be essential for muscle adaptation to exercise (Petersen *et al.*, 2012).

Thus, while the actions of experimental high-dose NAC administration are intriguing, it is too soon to conclude that NAC supplementation is beneficial for athletes. Future directions for research include studies to optimise NAC dosage, balancing efficacy versus side effects, and to evaluate novel thiol donors for their effects on fatigue.

Competing interests   None

NITRATE

Andrew M. Jones

Nitric oxide (NO) is an important physiological signalling molecule that can modulate skeletal muscle function through its role in the regulation of blood flow, muscle contractility, glucose and calcium homeostasis, and mitochondrial biogenesis and respiration (Stamler and Meissner, 2001). Until quite recently, it was considered that NO was generated solely through the oxidation of the amino acid l-arginine (see section on arginine), in a reaction catalysed by nitric oxide synthase (NOS) (Moncada and Higgs, 1993). It is now appreciated, however, that NO may also be produced by the reduction of nitrate to nitrite and subsequently of nitrite to NO (Duncan et al., 1995). This pathway may be particularly important in hypoxia. Nitrate and nitrite are present in the body via NO production through NOS but are also modulated through the diet. Nitrate in foods (particularly green leafy vegetables) can be reduced to nitrite by oral bacteria, leading to an increased plasma nitrite concentration which serves as a circulating 'reservoir' for NO production (Lundberg and Govoni, 2004).

Several recent studies have addressed the extent to which dietary nitrate supplementation might affect the physiological responses to exercise. Larsen et al. (2007) first showed that three days of sodium nitrate supplementation (0.1 mmol/kg/day) reduced resting blood pressure and the O_2 cost of sub-maximal cycle exercise. Subsequently, we have reported that enhancing NO bioavailability through supplementation of the diet with a natural foodstuff (nitrate-rich beetroot juice) reduces resting blood pressure and the O_2 cost of exercise, and improves exercise performance (Bailey et al., 2009, 2010; Vanhatalo et al., 2010; Lansley et al., 2011a). Bailey et al. (2009) found that four to six days of dietary nitrate supplementation (0.5 L of beetroot juice per day containing ~6 mmol nitrate) reduced the 'steady-state' O_2 cost of sub-maximal cycle exercise by 5% and extended the time-to-exhaustion during high-intensity cycling by 16%. In a subsequent study, Bailey et al. (2010) used ^{31}P-magnetic resonance spectroscopy to investigate the mechanistic bases of this phenomenon. It was observed that dietary nitrate supplementation resulted in both a reduced pulmonary O_2 uptake and a reduced muscle metabolic perturbation, enabling high-intensity knee-extension exercise to be tolerated for a greater period of time. These data imply that the reduced O_2 cost of exercise following dietary nitrate supplementation is related to a reduced ATP cost of muscle force production, perhaps consequent to reduced cross-bridge cycling or sarcoplasmic reticulum Ca^{2+}-ATPase activity (Ferreira and Behnke, 2011). It is also possible, however, that nitrate supplementation enhances mitochondrial efficiency: Larsen et al.

(2011) have reported that sodium nitrate reduced proton leakage and increased the mitochondrial P/O ratio.

The positive effects of nitrate supplementation on the O_2 cost of sub-maximal exercise can manifest acutely (i.e. 2.5 hours following a 6 mmol nitrate 'bolus') and this effect can be maintained for at least 15 days if supplementation at the same daily dose is continued (Vanhatalo et al., 2010). Because beetroot juice contains compounds other than nitrate that might also be bioactive, we have developed a nitrate-depleted beetroot juice as a placebo. This nitrate-depleted beetroot juice had no physiological effects relative to a control condition, whereas nitrate-rich beetroot juice reduced the O_2 cost of both walking and running and extended the time to exhaustion by 15% (Lansley et al., 2011a). The same group also investigated the influence of acute dietary nitrate supplementation on 4 km and 16.1 km time trial (TT) performance in competitive cyclists (Lansley et al., 2011b). Cyclists were able to produce a greater power output for the same rate of pulmonary O_2 uptake, resulting in a 2.7% reduction in the time to complete both TT distances. Similarly, Cermak et al. (2012a) found that six days of nitrate supplementation improved 10 km time-trial performance in cyclists. There is a suggestion that intermittent exercise performance might also be enhanced by nitrate ingestion (Bond et al., 2012; Wylie et al., 2013b).

Several recent studies have investigated the influence of nitrate supplementation on performance in highly-trained or elite subjects, with mixed results (Christensen et al., 2013; Boorsma et al., 2014; Hoon et al., 2013). In general, it appears that highly-trained athletes respond less positively than sedentary or recreationally-active subjects to nitrate supplementation. The reasons for this are currently obscure but are likely to be manifold and may include: higher baseline plasma nitrite concentration, higher habitual nitrate intake, more efficient mitochondria, better muscle oxygenation, differences in muscle fibre type distribution, and better NOS function. However, there is intriguing evidence that 20–30% of elite athletes manifest a lower sub-maximal O_2 uptake and improved performance following nitrate supplementation (Christensen et al. 2013; Boorsma et al., 2014). It is possible that some of the variability in the observed effects of nitrate supplementation on performance is related to the dose of nitrate administered (Hoon et al., 2014b). In a recent dose-response study, exercise tolerance was improved with 8 mmol but not 4 mmol of nitrate, but there was no further improvement when 16 mmol of nitrate was ingested (Wylie et al., 2013a). Nitrate supplementation has considerable promise as an ergogenic aid but the exact conditions under which it may be efficacious (e.g. subject population, duration and intensity of exercise, nitrate loading regimen) remain to be established.

Competing interests   None

NOOTKATONE

Satoshi Haramizu

Nootkatone [4,4a,5,6,7,8-hexahydro-6-isopropenyl-4,4a-dimethyl-2(3H)-naphthalenone], a kind of sesquiterpenoid, was first isolated from the heartwood of Alaska yellow cedar, *Chamaecyparis nootkatensis* (Erdtman and Hirose, 1962). Traceable amounts of nootkatone are found in major Citrus species such as grapefruit (*Citrus paradisi*), and a whole grapefruit contains approximately 100mg of nootkatone, mainly in the peel. Nootkatone is now available through technological advances such as chemical synthesis, biosynthesis and biotransformation. Nootkatone has a grapefruit-like flavour, tastes slightly bitter, and has an odour threshold of ~1mg/L water. Nootkatone is used as a flavouring compound.

A recent animal study demonstrated that 0.2% (wt/wt) nootkatone feeding for ten weeks improved swimming endurance (i.e. swimming time to fatigue) and that long-term intake of diets supplemented with 0.1% to 0.3% nootkatone significantly reduces high-fat and high-sucrose diet-induced body weight gain, abdominal fat accumulation, and the development of hyperglycaemia, hyperinsulinaemia and hyperleptineamia (Murase *et al.*, 2010). These beneficial effects of nootkatone might be due in part to enhanced energy metabolism through the activation of AMP-activated protein kinase in the muscle and liver (Murase *et al.*, 2010). These findings indicate that nootkatone is a potential candidate for ergogenic and anti-obesity compounds. A previous study indicated that consumption of half a grapefruit or grapefruit juice before meals, three times a day for 12 weeks reduces body weight and improves insulin resistance in metabolic syndrome patients, compared to placebo (Fujioka *et al.*, 2006). On the other hand, there are no reports on the effects of grapefruit, including nootkatone, on physical performance in humans. Therefore, further studies are required to clarify the efficacy of nootkatone as an ergogenic compound, especially for athletes.

Competing interests None

OCTACOSANOL AND POLICOSANOL

Mayur K. Ranchordas

Octacosanol ($CH_3[CH_2]_{26}CH_2O_{14}$), a high-molecular-weight, primary aliphatic alcohol is typically found in the natural wax extract of various plants and is commonly found in fruits, barks, leaves and whole seeds (Singh and Mehta, 2002; Taylor *et al.*, 2005). Octacosanol has been purported to possess several health benefits when ingested as a supplement including lowering cholesterol, cytoprotective effects and antiaggregatory properties (Taylor *et al.*, 2005). The majority of studies that have investigated the effects of octacosanol have used policosanol (wheat-germ oil extract), because it contains a natural mixture of primary alcohols isolated from sugar cane wax, and octacosanol is the main component of policosanol (Kato *et al.*, 1995; Saint-John and McNaughton, 1986).

Although several studies have investigated the effects of octacosanol and policosanol on hyperlipidaemia and hypercholesterolaemia, few have examined their effects on athletic performance. It has been suggested that policosanol reduces cholesterol by decreasing the cellular expression of hydroxymethylglutamyl coenzyme A reductase although the exact mechanism remains to be elucidated (McCarty, 2002).

A meta-analysis comparing the efficacy of plant sterols and stanols as well as policosanol in the treatment of coronary heart disease, as measured by a reduction in low-density lipoprotein cholesterol levels (LDL), found that policosanol was more effective than both plant sterols and stanols in reducing LDL levels and more favourably altered the lipid profile (Chen *et al.*, 2005b). In the 29 eligible studies, 12mg/day (range 5–40mg/day in 1,528 participants) was found to significantly reduce LDL levels and the LDL:HDL ratio. Moreover, policosanol was more effective in reducing total cholesterol, increasing HDL cholesterol and lowering triglyceride levels compared with placebo, plant sterols and stanols (Chen *et al.*, 2005a). Despite the positive findings of Chen *et al.* (2005b), meta-analyses of other studies have since not found policosanol to be an effective treatment for hypercholesterolemia (Berthold *et al.*, 2006; Dulin *et al.*, 2006; Greyling *et al.*, 2006). An early study that examined the effects of octacosanol on athletic performance found that 1,000 μg significantly improved grip strength and reaction time in response to a visual stimulus (Saint-John and McNaughton, 1986). Policosanol supplementation has also been examined in combination with omega-3. Fontani *et al.* (2009) gave 18 karateka competitors either 2.25g omega-3 fatty acids plus 10mg policosanol or a placebo for 21 days, and showed reduced reaction time (computer test) and increase in vigour as measured by POMS (Profile of Mood States) questionnaire, but effects could be attributed to the policosanol or the omega-3 fatty acids, or both.

Although supplementing with octacosanol and policosanol has been shown to have favourable effects on hypercholesterolaemia and hyperlipidaemia, more recent studies have found no positive effects. Research on athletic performance is lacking and remains unclear.

Competing interests   None

ORNITHINE

Kevin Currell

Ornithine is an amino acid which plays a key role in the urea cycle, facilitating the disposal of ammonia. Ammonia is produced during intense exercise and may be one of the causes of fatigue. There is some evidence that L-ornithine hydrochloride supplementation prior to high-intensity exercise may prevent fatigue and improve performance by modulating the metabolism of ammonia (Demura *et al.*, 2011). At present the evidence is far from conclusive with a need to conduct more research using valid measures of performance.

Bucci *et al.* (1990b) studied bodybuilders and suggested that ornithine supplementation could promote the secretion of growth hormone within humans. However, research has not been conducted to show that this may enhance the adaptation to training and ultimately lead to an improvement in performance.

One potential avenue of future research is ornithine-α-ketoglutarate. This has been shown to improve recovery of individuals from burns, trauma and in the post-operative state. It may also be a precursor of nitric oxide (Cynober, 2004). At present there is not enough evidence to support the use of ornithine in sport performance. However, further research should be conducted to investigate its use.

Competing interests   None

OXYELITE PRO

Ano Lobb

OxyElite Pro was a dietary supplement promoted for weight loss and as a pre-workout product that was widely available both in retail stores and on the internet. An independent analysis of seven DMAA supplements found that a serving of OxyElite Pro contained more than 8.5 times the concentration of DMAA than the average DMAA supplement (Austin *et al.*, 2014). OxyElite Pro was subsequently withdrawn from the market after being linked to two-dozen cases of acute hepatitis and liver failure (CDC, 2013; USFDA, 2014b). The suspected cause of those adverse events was the ingredient DMAA (see section on DMAA), which is included on the WADA Prohibited List (WADA, 2014b).

At least two small, short duration studies of OxyElite Pro (funded by the manufacturer) also found that even a few doses of the supplement appeared to elevate blood pressure (Farney *et al.*, 2012, McCarthy *et al.*, 2012). The manufacturer no longer markets a product named OxyElite Pro.

Competing interests None

PANGAMIC ACID

Louise M. Burke

According to vitamin expert and campaigner against nutrition quackery, Dr Victor Herbert (1979), pangamic acid was described as an ester derived from d-gluconic acid and dimethylglycine and apparently initially isolated from apricot kernels by biochemists Ernst Krebs senior and junior. They trade-named it 'Vitamin B15' in a 1943 patent application and promoted it as having a wide range of medicinal properties; it was also championed in the Soviet Union in relation to a variety of proposed benefits including enhancement of exercise performance. Only two peer-reviewed studies of pangamic acid supplementation and exercise appear to exist. In these, neither chronic supplementation with 6 × 400mg/day of a 'mixture of calcium gluconate and N,N-dimethylglycine' (Girandola *et al.*, 1980) nor 6 × 50mg/day of 'pangamic acid' (Gray and Titlow, 1982) were found to alter exercise metabolism or capacity compared with a control. These findings may be best explained by Herbert who summarised that not only does pangamic acid lack evidence as a vitamin, nutrient or therapeutic compound, but it has never been scientifically verified to exist as a compound at all. In 1976, the Food and Drug Administration of the USA issued a statement noting that it considers pangamic acid products to be unsafe and recommends they be seized, with injunctions against manufacturers. This was revised as recently as 1995 and remains in effect (FDA website).

Competing interests   None

PAPAIN

Sarah Chantler

Papain, a protease derived from papaya, was originally used as a meat tenderiser in South America due to its ability to break down tough meat fibres. This effect extended to its use in various topical creams for chronic wound cleaning or debridement of dead tissue as well as assisting those with enzymatic digestive issues.

Earlier studies in people with injuries showed improved recovery with protease supplementation, but this was not confirmed in a larger, more comprehensive trial that focused on recovery from ankle sprains in orthopaedic patients (Kerkhoffs, 2004). A subsequent series of four studies have evaluated papain, in combination with other proteases, in small samples of male athletes, specifically with regard to its effectiveness in attenuating delayed onset muscle soreness (DOMS) post eccentric exercise. Two of the studies were able to show better flexion in the tested limb post eccentric load (Beck et al., 2007), which was hypothesised to be mediated by regulation of leukocyte activity and inflammation (Buford et al., 2009). Two further studies showed an improvement in contractile function (Miller et al., 2004), and subjective pain and tenderness ratings (Udani et al., 2009), but not in biochemical measures of DOMS. Further interpretation of these studies is difficult as all four used a combination of papain with other proteolytic enzymes (e.g. bromelain, amylase, lysozyme, trypsin) or other substances (vitamin C, curcumin). Furthermore, the supplementation period varied from four (Miller et al., 2004), up to 30 days (Udani et al., 2009), with dosages from 47.7 to 340mg of papain.

Therefore, although the use of papain or protease supplements in attenuating DOMS may show initial promise, further research in larger samples is needed.

Competing interests None

PEPTIDES

Nicholas A. Burd

Within the broad spectrum of the billion-dollar supplement industry are a range of protein and/or free form amino acid based supplements. Research substantiating the efficacy of these supplements is wide-ranging, from good evidence to support a reproducible anabolic effect of the ingestion of whey protein for the stimulation of muscle protein accretion (Burd *et al.*, 2011b), to no evidence for supplements like deer antler extracts which are purported to boost concentrations of the peptide hormone IGF-1. In recent times, a class of products that have become known as 'peptides' have gained unfavourable attention in sports for their use by athletes who believe they are gaining a competitive advantage.

Technically speaking, proteins are long chains of amino acids, while peptides are shorter chains of amino acids that can be produced synthetically, endogenously, or derived from food. It has been suggested that some naturally occurring food-derived peptides, such as the peptides that reside in milk proteins (such as whey and casein) and become active during proteolytic digestion, may offer health benefits (improved cardiovascular, digestive and immune function) independently of their role as a dietary source of amino acids (Nagpal *et al.*, 2011). More evidence is required to support or refute this claim. These peptides are not the concern of the sport authorities involved in the maintenance of the integrity in professional sport. Rather, attention has been focused on the use by athletes of a range of synthetic peptides which have apparently become commercially available (often via internet sites) under the guise of supplements. These products, which can be administered via a variety of methods (orally, intravenous, intranasal or transdermal cream, etc.), may exert anabolic effects and/or serve as masking agents for other drugs. A particular sub-set, the synthetic growth hormone-releasing peptides (GHRP) which include GHRP-6, hexarelin or CJC-1295, have been demonstrated to stimulate the release of GH from the pituitary gland thereby enhancing its endogenous production (Ghigo *et al.*, 1994; Teichman *et al.*, 2006). The synthetic GHRPs were specifically developed and intended for medical use in patients with intact or impaired pituitary function to mimic the pulsatile nature of endogenous GH release (Teichman *et al.*, 2006). In the case of CJC-1295, a single injection of this peptide has been demonstrated to induce an increase in serum GH concentrations that seems to persist for ~two weeks in healthy adults (Teichman *et al.*, 2006). GH therapy, however, is often administered in a single daily dose and results in a robust (supraphysiological) increase in systemic concentrations of GH that wanes over time.

Of course, the use of recombinant human form GH (rhGH) as an anabolic aid for clinically deficient individuals is well described (Gharib *et al.*, 2003). It has been reported that GH administration has an important role in the regulation of body composition by decreasing fat mass, with no effect on the net gain in muscle protein, in GH-deficient men (Salomon, 1989). However, evidence is lacking for rhGH administration alone or together with anabolic steroids or weightlifting programmes to enhance gains in muscle mass and strength in healthy adults (Taaffe *et al.*, 1994; Yarasheski *et al.*, 1993). Instead, there appears to be rhGH-induced stimulation of collagen protein synthesis in tendon and skeletal muscle in healthy adults (Doessing *et al.*, 2010) as well as increased body water retention (Yarasheski *et al.*, 1995). The anabolic effect on connective tissue may, at least partly, explain the use of GH by the athlete to accelerate recovery and/or injury prevention. Again, there is no firm evidence to support this claim.

It is important to note that there are well documented adverse consequences of GH therapy, e.g. carpal tunnel syndrome, fluid retention, diabetic-like symptoms (Yarasheski *et al.*, 1993). These harmful effects of GH administration are usually attributed to the high doses that are given to the patient (Schauster *et al.*, 2000). The high dose GH regimen is undoubtedly often used by the athlete as well. Interestingly, Lange *et al.* (2002) demonstrated that a single dose of GH administered prior to a bout of endurance exercise resulted in considerably higher blood lactate concentrations during the exercise bout in young adults. This outcome would not favour acute performance enhancement for an athlete wishing to gain a competitive advantage.

Beyond the discussion of supplemental GH to affect muscular adaptations, there is a consistent mistake made by athletes (and their coaches) that the natural robust exercise-induced rise in systemic GH concentrations after heavy weightlifting is of value to augment skeletal muscular adaptations. There is firm evidence that refutes this 'hormone hypothesis' for the support of gains in strength and lean mass after a programme of weightlifting in healthy adults (West *et al.*, 2010, 2012). Indeed, future research will need to underpin whether there are benefits towards GH on the connective tissue and/or lipolysis.

The use of synthetic peptides by athletes is likely to be a repeated theme in sport and thus drive the need of doping control centres to continue to evolve their analytical capabilities (Thomas *et al.*, 2010). Indeed, inroads are being made in this capacity, with the 'landmark' first analytical positive test for GH in 2010 (WADA, 2010), and the ability to store blood samples for at least eight years in WADA-sanctioned events may also prevent the athletes from cheating. In general, the available evidence, largely derived from studies that administer rhGH, suggests that the use of synthetic peptide hormones to elevate systemic GH concentrations is unlikely to result in a competitive advantage in healthy adults. The mass availability (via the internet suppliers, nutrition stores, medical practitioners, etc.) of synthetic peptides to the athlete combined with the lack of regulation of the supplement contents, underpins the importance of the sports scientists, coaches or medical practitioners to educate the consumer that this doping practice is ineffective and with unknown side effects. Synthetic peptides are included in various sections of the WADA Prohibited List (WADA, 2014b).

Competing interests   None

PHENYLALANINE

Daniel R. Moore

Phenylalanine is an essential amino acid (EAA) present in dietary protein, and in the artificial sweetener aspartame, with a minimum daily requirement of 39mg·kg^{-1}·d^{-1}, for example ~50g of egg protein for a 75kg athlete (Basile-Filho *et al.*, 1997). There is no available evidence to suggest phenylalanine requirements are enhanced in athletic populations and a balanced diet with adequate energy and protein would be sufficient to meet the metabolic demands for this amino acid. Increased blood phenylalanine concentrations that occur in untreated individuals with inborn errors of metabolism can lead to neural degeneration (Blau *et al.*, 2010); however, there is currently no upper tolerable limit for intake established for healthy individuals.

In addition to supporting increased rates of protein synthesis when ingested with the other EAA (Borsheim *et al.*, 2002), phenylalanine can be converted in the liver to the non-essential amino acid tyrosine, which is a precursor for the neurotransmitters dopamine and norepinephrine. Despite the implication that these neurotransmitters enhance exercise capacity at 30° (Watson *et al.*, 2005), their synthesis is generally uninfluenced by physiological variations in phenylalanine concentration (Fernstrom and Fernstrom, 2007). In fact, no studies investigating the supplemental effect of phenylalanine on exercise performance in either hot or at ambient temperatures have been reported. However, tyrosine supplementation (see section on tyrosine) has been utilised in an effort to enhance neurotransmitter synthesis directly during exercise as a means to improve performance. A study using a tyrosine and phenylalanine-free amino acid mix was shown to decrease exercise capacity in the heat (Tumilty *et al.*, 2013). This argues against the efficacy of phenylalanine for any potential benefits in athletic performance. There is currently, therefore, no evidence to suggest athletes require, or would benefit from, supplemental phenylalanine.

Competing interests   None

PHLOGENZYM AND WOBENZYM

Mayur K. Ranchordas

The active ingredients found in phlogenzym are the hydrolase trypsin, the endopeptidase bromelain and the bioflavonoid rutin. Trypsin is a digestive enzyme that is produced by the pancreas and secreted into the small intestine, where it hydrolyses proteins. Bromelain is a proteolytic enzyme obtained from pineapples, and rutin is a bioflavonoid found in many plants, fruits and vegetables, but the richest source is buckwheat. Similarly, wobenzym also contains trypsin, bromelain and rutin, but also includes the proteolytic enzyme papain, the endopeptidase chymotrypsin, and pancreatin which is an extract from the pancreas of animals that contains pancreatic enzymes.

Phlogenzym and wobenzym are commonly known as hydrolytic enzymes or systemic enzymes and have been purported to possess anti-inflammatory, fibrinolytic and analgesic properties as well as having positive effects on oedema. Studies investigating the efficacy of phlogenzym and wobenzym in the athletic population are lacking but several studies have investigated their effects on recuperation following injury, disease and health.

In a double-blind prospective, randomized study phlogenzym was compared to diclofenac in the treatment of activated osteoarthritis of the knee in 63 patients (Singer *et al.*, 2001). Phlogenzym supplementation for three weeks in doses of six tablets per day (540mg bromelain, 288mg trypsin, 600mg rutin) was found to be more effective than diclofenac in reducing pain over the three-week period, and phlogenzym was superior to diclofenac in reducing pain three weeks after supplementation had stopped (Singer *et al.*, 2001). In a similar study, phlogenzym supplementation was found to be just as effective and well tolerated as diclofenac in the management of osteoarthritis over three weeks of treatment (Tilwe *et al.*, 2001).

Results from studies investigating phlogenzym supplementation for the treatment of lateral ankle ligament injury are mixed. Two clinical trials have found positive effects (Hollmann, 1998; Van Dijk, 1994), but a separate larger study that recruited 721 patients found no positive effects (Kerkhoffs *et al.*, 2004). After injury, phlogenzym has been reported to decrease fibrin deposits and restore microcirculation in rabbit skeletal muscle (Neumayer *et al.*, 2006). Phlogenzym supplementation in conjunction with dietary counselling and acupuncture was more effective in treating rotator cuff tendinitis compared to an exercise group (Szczurko *et al.*, 2009). However, these findings should be interpreted with caution as the group that received phlogenzym also received diet counselling and acupuncture; therefore the significant improvement could have been attributed to other factors as there was no treatment group that solely received phlogenzym.

Although studies in the athletic population are lacking and findings have been mixed, the research investigating the effects of phlogenzym and wobenzym suggest that they could be used as an effective anti-inflammatory and analgesic. However, it should be noted that future research should also investigate potential mechanisms of action.

Competing interests   None

PHOSPHATE

Peter Peeling

Phosphate supplementation is suggested to have an ergogenic benefit for athletic performance via its effect on the metabolic pathway of energy production, acid-base regulation, myocardial function, and through changes in the erythrocyte levels of 2,3 diphosphoglycerate (2,3 DPG). A greater amount of 2,3 DPG results in a reduced affinity of haemoglobin for oxygen, thus creating a rightward shift in the oxygen dissociation curve (Benesch and Benesch, 1969). Previously, it was shown that a seven-day phosphate load (1g/day sodium phosphate spread into four doses) resulted in a ~25% increase in erythrocyte 2,3 DPG levels (Bremner *et al.*, 2002).

To date, acute phosphate loading protocols (three to six days) of oral phosphate supplements in various forms (sodium, calcium or potassium phosphate), provided in single or split doses that equate to approximately 3–4g per day have been investigated (Bredle *et al.*, 1988; Cade *et al.*, 1984; Folland *et al.*, 2008; Goss *et al.*, 2001; Kraemer *et al.*, 1995; Kreider *et al.*, 1990, 1992). The outcomes from such loading protocols are equivocal. Currently, there are a number of positive findings that show an enhanced maximal oxygen consumption: VO_{2max} (Cade *et al.*, 1984; Kreider *et al.*, 1990), improved anaerobic threshold (Kreider *et al.*, 1990, 1992), and greater time-trial/simulated race performances (Folland *et al.*, 2008) when oral sodium phosphate has been provided in split doses over a three- to six-day period. However, these performance enhancements have only correlated well with increases in 2,3 DPG levels in some instances (Cade *et al.*, 1984), and not others (Kreider *et al.*, 1992). Additionally, it should also be considered that a number of investigations have shown no performance improvements or changes in physiological capacities when supplementing with either sodium, potassium or calcium phosphate, or indeed with combination-buffer agents (Bredle *et al.*, 1988; Goss *et al.*, 2001; Kraemer *et al.*, 1995; Mannix *et al.*, 1990; West *et al.*, 2012).

Recently, West *et al.* (2012) showed in a relatively large sample size ($n=20$), that six days of sodium phosphate supplementation provided in a daily dose of 50mg/kg of fat-free mass in a cross-over repeated measures trial resulted in no significant improvements to VO_{2max} or the anaerobic threshold when compared to a placebo. It was, however, noted that 50% of participants experienced at least one acute episode of mild gastrointestinal (GI) distress during the sodium phosphate supplementation period, which may have impacted on their outcomes. Such incidence of GI distress has also previously been reported by Cade *et al.* (1984) and should therefore be thoroughly considered when using this supplement, due to the negative impact this may have on athletic performance.

Although in most instances the supplementation of various phosphate sources (sodium, calcium or potassium phosphate) in athletes is innocuous, the following should be noted: oral supplementation with phosphate may cause gastrointestinal distress, leading to cramping, diarrhoea and/or vomiting. In addition, excessive phosphate loading may place unnecessary strain on the kidneys and, as a result, any athletes with known kidney disorders should refrain from using this supplement.

Although it is likely that the equivocal outcomes shown in the current literature are in part due to differences in (a) the form of phosphate supplement provided, (b) the individual tolerance of the supplement, and (c) the exercise protocols implemented; it was recently proposed by Buck *et al.* (2013) that there may also be a gender difference that impacts on the efficacy of this supplement. Specifically, female athletes may not respond as well to sodium phosphate supplementation as their male counterparts (for review see Buck *et al.*, 2013). Regardless, it is evident that more research is required to establish the efficacy and best practice protocols for phosphate supplementation. Furthermore, when considered for athletic performance enhancement, this supplement should be tested in training in order to ascertain the individual's response, and any negative GI outcomes.

Competing interests   None

PHOSPHATIDYLSERINE

Nicholas A. Burd

Phosphatidylserine is a phospholipid that can be found in the brain and muscle cell membranes, and also in other bodily cell membranes. Dietary sources include organ meats and fish (Souci *et al.*, 2008). Phosphatidylserine supplementation is purported to improve cognitive function, prevent muscle soreness, and/or increase exercise capacity (e.g. time to exhaustion). Original work assessing the potential of phosphatidylserine supplementation to enhance mental/physical performance used phosphatidylserine derived from bovine cortex; however, the risk of transferring infectious disease makes this source no longer viable (Jorissen *et al.*, 2002; Kingsley, 2006). Instead, soy-derived phosphatidylserine, which is molecularly different from a bovine-derived source, has become a usable alternative (Jorissen *et al.*, 2002). The 'optimal' supplementation regimen for soy-derived phosphatidylserine remains to be truly defined, although typical daily doses range from 100–500mg. Nevertheless, ergogenic effects on performance have been reported to occur at higher daily doses (i.e. ~800mg/day) (Kingsley, 2006).

Overall, there is limited evidence that supplementation with soy-derived phosphatidylserine will increase exercise performance/capacity, decrease post-exercise cortisol responses, or improve mood state in healthy athletes (Kingsley, 2006; Jäger *et al.*, 2007; Wells *et al.*, 2013). Moreover, the removal of bovine-derived phosphatidylserine for human consumption prevents the opportunity to compare the results from studies of the bovine product with soy-derived sources. The uncertainty that exogenous phosphatidylserine sources are, in fact, incorporated into cellular membranes means that there are more questions than answers with regard to the potential ergogenic effects of plant-derived phosphatidylserine supplementation on cognitive function and/or performance.

Competing interests None

PINITOL

Sarah Chantler and Karlien Smit

Pinitol (D-pinitol) is a 6-carbon sugar-like molecule that can be found in legumes, leafy vegetables and citrus fruits. It is a derivative of methylated inositol, and therefore is similar in structure. Initial studies examined its ability to mimic insulin, and research considered the effects of pinitol in type 2 diabetics with regard to improving insulin sensitivity or glucose uptake. While one study of obese men and women with impaired glucose tolerance found no effect of daily supplementation with 20mg/kg of pinitol supplementation for 28 days compared to a placebo (Davis *et al.*, 2000), another study using 600mg of soybean-derived pinitol twice daily showed an improvement in controlling postprandial increases in blood glucose (Kang *et al.*, 2006) and reducing cardiovascular risk in Korean type II diabetics (Kim *et al.*, 2004). However, these studies were unclear on the exact mechanism for the increase in insulin sensitivity.

In athletes, pinitol's functionality was hypothesised to assist with creatine uptake in resistance training, via the increase in blood glucose uptake or via increased creatine retention. However, a clinical trial in 24 resistance-trained men found no extra benefit during a four-week supplementation period over and above that of creatine supplementation alone (Kerksick *et al.*, 2009). Therefore, until further research elucidates the mechanism in the insulin and glucose pathways and/or shows a positive physiological, practical or performance outcome, pinitol's use in sport remains theoretical.

Competing interests   None

PLANT STEROLS

David S. Senchina

Plant sterols are also known as phytosterols (or phytostanols when saturated). Phytosterols are typically produced from a cycloartenol precursor which makes their synthesis different from animal sterols (zoosterols) which are derived from a lanosterol precursor. Various phytosterols can be found in other sections of this book alphabetized by their respective names, including γ-oryzanol, octosanol and policosanol, pycnogenol, resveratrol, and supplements containing *Cissus quadrangularis* (see also 'Hydroxycut') and wheat germ oil. No direct ergogenic properties have been found from these phytosterols.

Sitosterol is the most abundant phytosterol in plants and consequently in Western diets. Ultramarathon runners supplemented with β-sitosterol capsules displayed fewer cellular markers of inflammation (particularly those related to neutrophils) after a race compared with placebo-treated controls, suggesting that phytosterols may mitigate the effects of acute, strenuous exercise on immunity (Bouic *et al.*, 1999). However, in a study of trained runners subjected to an exercise bout of increasing intensity until exhaustion, heart rate and blood lactate were uninfluenced by phytosterols (Timmons *et al.*, 2000). In a study of older sedentary adults, six months of endurance training reduced plasma cholesterol levels while increasing the absorption of phytosterols contained in a normal diet (Wilund *et al.*, 2009), suggesting that phytosterols may have beneficially regulated plasma lipids. A separate study of middle-aged and older-aged sedentary adults demonstrated that eight weeks of endurance training combined with sitosterol supplementation was associated with decreases in blood low density lipoproteins and triglycerides, but increases in high density lipoproteins, effects that were more strongly manifest when exercise and sitosterol therapies were combined (Varady *et al.*, 2004).

Current limited research suggests that β-sitosterol may mitigate the exercise-associated dysregulation of immune function and improve blood lipid profiles, though it has no direct ergogenic effects.

Competing interests   None

POTASSIUM

Nancy M. DiMarco

Potassium is the major intracellular cation in the body, with ~98% of the body's potassium stores located inside the cells. The concentration intracellularly is maintained at about 145mM. Potassium's major functions are to promote contractility of cardiac, smooth and skeletal muscle and influence the regulation of nerve conduction through the influx of sodium (Na^+) and efflux of potassium (K^+) on either side of the nerve terminal. The Na,K-ATPase, also known as the Na-K pump, is the primary active transporter system that maintains high K^+ and low Na^+ intracellular concentrations. The plasma membrane ATPase of all mammalian cells catalyzes the reaction: $ATP \rightarrow ADP + Pi$, with obligatory requirements for both Na^+ and K^+ and Mg^{++} required for the dephosphorylation of ATP.

There are some theories that support a purported benefit of K^+ supplementation by athletes. They stem from: 1) The known efflux of K^+ from the muscle cell during exercise, particularly high-intensity exercise (McKenna, 1992), and 2) the loss of K^+ as a sweat electrolyte. However, neither of these situations appears to require, nor to respond to, K^+ supplementation. The K^+ efflux from the muscle cell represents a temporary electrolyte shift that is effectively unconnected to altering body K^+ stores, and its role in developing fatigue associated with high-intensity or long duration exercise is unclear. Although sweat-prompted losses and a resultant deficit of K^+ have been suggested as a cause of exertional muscle cramps in athletes, the relative proportion of sweat potassium loss (compared to sodium and chloride) is minimal and the potential for a measurable sweat-induced K^+ deficit is unlikely (Bergeron, 2003). This is reinforced by the fact that there is no difference in serum K^+ concentration in ironman triathletes with/ without muscle cramps (Sulzer *et al.*, 2005). Moreover, a sports drink containing 25mM K^+ and 60mM Na^+, did not have an additive effect on restoring hydration over a drink containing Na^+ (Maughan *et al.*, 1994). Accordingly, potassium is a minor electrolyte in sweat and does not appear to require specific replacement during and/or after exercise.

The adequate intake (AI) of potassium from the diet for adults age 14 to 70 years in the USA is 4.7g/d; but the reported average intake is only ~2.5g/day (National Academy of Sciences, 2004). However, potassium should be consumed as a regular component of the diet rather than as a supplement. Foods containing more than 300mg K^+/serving include: banana, potato, orange juice, avocado, lima beans, cantaloupe, peaches, tomato, chicken, salmon, tuna, turkey and unsalted nuts. Also, some carbohydrate-electrolyte drinks provide higher amounts of K^+ (90mg) than others (10–30mg) per 8 fl oz (~240ml). The consumption of very high levels of supplemental forms of K^+ might result in hyperkalaemia which could lead to cardiac arrhythmias and even cardiac arrest. Furthermore, individuals with kidney failure or compromised kidney function or other chronic clinical conditions should seek clinical advice before taking any K^+ supplement or consuming potassium-rich foods.

Competing interests   None

PREBIOTICS

Nicholas P. West

Prebiotics are non-digestible polysaccharides that selectively stimulate the growth or activity/ies of one or more species of gut bacteria and that confer a health benefit on the host (Barile and Rastall, 2013). These supplements purportedly yield beneficial health effects via the symbiotic relationship that exists between bacteria inhabiting the gastrointestinal (GI) tract, known as the microbiome, and their human host. Clinical and mechanistic research has strongly implicated the microbiome in health and disease. Prebiotics increase the abundance of commensal bacteria in the gut by providing nutrients as a source of fuel. Naturally occurring food sources with a prebiotic effect include barley, banana, oats, wheat, soyabean, asparagus, leek, chicory, garlic, artichoke and onion. Various studies have shown that, at dosages above 2.5g, a dosage far higher than occurs in natural foods, the most common prebiotics, fructooligosaccharides (FOS) and galactooligosaccharides (GOS), increase the abundance of lactic acid bacteria (Barile and Rastall, 2013; Mekkes *et al.*, 2014). The fermentation of these starches by GI bacteria releases metabolic by-products, including short-chain fatty acids (SCFAs: butyrate, propionate and acetate), vitamins and lipid metabolites. These fermentation by-products modulate various aspects of the immune system and host metabolism (Macfarlane and Macfarlane, 2011). Non-digestible polysaccharides are thus an important dietary nutrient requiring more investigation.

Illness during training and competition may negatively affect performance, and research shows that athletes experiencing higher illness rates over a competition season tend to perform more poorly than their healthier peers (Pyne *et al.*, 2005). Preventing illness during training and competition is therefore a high priority for athletes. Any effects of supplementation with prebiotics on athletic performance are most likely to be indirect and associated with the maintenance of good health and, subsequently, the ability to train and compete optimally.

Findings from population cohorts suggest possible benefits of prebiotic supplementation in athletes. Prebiotic supplements have had beneficial effects in reducing gastrointestinal and respiratory illness symptoms. A study on student, investigating the effects of 2.5g and 5g of galactooligosaccharide (GOS) supplementation for eight weeks around examination time found that supplementation with GOS was associated with lower GI illness symptom scores, while 2.5 g of GOS was generally associated with reduced cold and flu severity scores (Jain *et al.*, 2009). Another GOS study at a dose of 5.5g daily in healthy volunteers undertaking international travel reported substantial reductions in the incidence and duration of diarrhoea (Drakoularakou *et al.*, 2010). These findings suggest that prebiotics may be a useful prophylactic strategy for athletes during competition stress and international travel.

Prebiotics may also influence host metabolism, which may have a range of implications for athletes. A key function of the microbiota is energy harvest from non-digestible starches, which due to the increased availability of energy may alter energy balance and body composition. In the absence of changes in dietary intake, transplantation of microbes from obese mice to lean mice increases fat mass in lean animals. Human investigations suggest microbial composition differences between obese and non-obese individuals may contribute to the increased body mass in some individuals. Diet plays an important role in shaping the microbiota, with high-fat and high-calorie diets promoting a microbial composition that favours body mass accumulation. Fibre added to a high-fat diet increased metabolisable energy but reduced it in low-fat diets (Baer et al., 1997). This suggests that dietary modification of the microbiota can alter calorific content of the diet. For athletes with high energy requirements, an increased extraction of energy may assist with meeting the demands of their sport. However, for athletes meeting weight restrictions or looking to minimise body fat, increased metabolisable energy may be detrimental in relation to managing physique goals.

Evidence supports a role for the use of prebiotic supplementation to alter lipid and glucose metabolism, the production of intestinal hormones and to reduce inflammation. Consumption of 16g per day of FOS by ten healthy adults in a randomized, double-blind placebo-controlled trial found that prebiotic consumption reduced appetite and increased plasma gut peptide concentration (Ostler et al., 2002). This effect may be of interest for energy-restricted athletes. Another study found that consumption of 23mg of cocoa flavonols per day for four weeks by 22 healthy volunteers reduced levels of plasma triacyglycerol and the inflammatory maker C-reactive protein (Graham et al., 1991). The potential role of prebiotics in exerting an anti-inflammatory effect is of particular interest to endurance athletes, who can suffer from increased gut permeability, which may result in chronic low grade inflammation. The effect of persistent low grade inflammation is metabolic dysregulation. Prebiotics are showing promise in attenuating the loss of gut barrier function and chronic low grade inflammation. SCFAs, in particular butyrate, are essential for gut barrier integrity as the primary energy source for colonocytes and have an anti-inflammatory influence on immune cells. Further to this, inflammatory control is' linked to exercise adaptation and overtraining (Ziemann et al., 2013), suggesting a role for the anti-inflammatory effect of prebiotics.

Further research is required in various athlete populations on the various types of prebiotic supplements, dosage, timing (pre- or post-exercise) and underlying mechanisms before definitive guidelines on supplementation can be issued.

Conflict of interest The author has been the recipient of commercial funding for research and consultation services from Chr Hansen A/S, Danisco Sweeteners Oy, Probiotec Pharma Pty Ltd, the Commonwealth Scientific and Industrial Research Organisation and the Australian Institute of Sport.

PROBIOTICS

Michael Gleeson

Probiotics are food supplements that contain live microorganisms which when administered in adequate amounts can confer a health benefit on the host (WHO/FAO, 2002). There is now a reasonable body of evidence that regular consumption of probiotics proven to survive gut transit can modify the population of the gut-dwelling bacteria (microbiota) and influence immune function (Borchers *et al.*, 2009; Kopp-Hoolihan, 2001; Matsuzaki, 1998; Mengheri, 2008; Minocha, 2009). However, it should be noted that such effects are dose, species and strain dependent. Probiotics modify the intestinal microbiota in such a way that the numbers of beneficial bacteria increase and, usually, the numbers of species considered harmful are decreased. Such changes have been associated with a range of potential benefits to the health and functioning of the digestive system, as well as modulation of immune function.

Probiotics have several mechanisms of action. By their growth and metabolism, they help inhibit the growth of other bacteria, antigens, toxins and carcinogens in the gut, and reduce the potentially harmful effects. In addition, probiotics are known to interact with gut-associated lymphoid tissue, leading to positive effects on the innate, and even the acquired immune system. There is now evidence that the improvement of protective responses by probiotics extends beyond the gut to distal mucosal sites. There is clear evidence from animal studies that regular probiotic ingestion can influence responses in the respiratory tract and improve protection against bacterial and viral pathogens via modulation of lung macrophage and T cell numbers and functions (Forsythe, 2014; Lehtoranta *et al.*, 2014; Marranzino *et al.*, 2012).

Studies have shown that probiotic intake can improve rates of recovery from rotavirus diarrhoea, increase resistance to enteric pathogens, and promote anti-tumour activity (Matsuzaki, 1998; Mengheri, 2008; Minocha, 2009). Some evidence suggests that probiotics may be effective in alleviating some allergic and respiratory disorders in young children (Forsythe, 2014; Kopp-Hoolihan, 2001). In recent years it has become evident that some probiotics, particularly *Lactobacillus (L.)* and *Bifidobacterium* strains, when ingested on a daily basis in doses of 10^8–10^{10} colony-forming units, can reduce upper respiratory tract infection (URTI) incidence in adults (Berggren *et al.*, 2011; de Vrese *et al.*, 2005; Guillemard *et al.*, 2010; Hao *et al.*, 2011; Lehtoranta, 2014; Winkler *et al.*, 2005). Currently, there are insufficient data on other probiotic species, or combinations of different species and strains, to predict positive health outcomes confidently.

Studies in athletes

Although there are few published studies of the effectiveness of probiotic use in athletes, there is growing interest in examining their potential to help to maintain overall general health, enhance immune function or reduce URTI incidence and symptom severity/duration (Gleeson and Thomas, 2008; West et al., 2009).

A randomized, double-blind study provided 141 marathon runners with either *L. rhamnosus* GG or placebo daily for a three-month training period before a marathon race (Kekkonen et al., 2007). There were no differences in the number of URTI or gastrointestinal symptom episodes. However, the duration of gastrointestinal symptom episodes in the probiotic group was shorter than in the placebo group during training (2.9 versus 4.3 days) and during the two weeks after the marathon (1.0 versus 2.3 days). In a double-blind, placebo-controlled, cross-over trial in which healthy elite distance runners received *L. fermentum* or placebo daily for 28 days with a 28-day washout period between the first and second treatments, the probiotic group ($n=20$) suffered fewer days of respiratory illness and lower severity of respiratory illness symptoms (Cox et al., 2010). The probiotic treatment also elicited a two-fold greater increase in whole-blood culture interferon (IFN)-γ production compared with placebo, which may be one mechanism underpinning the positive clinical outcomes. In another study of athletes who presented with fatigue, impaired performance and a deficit in blood CD4+ (T-helper) cell IFN-γ production compared with healthy control athletes, this apparent T cell impairment was reversed following a one-month course of daily *L. acidophilus* ingestion (Clancy et al., 2006).

In a study on the effect of a *L. casei* supplement on URTI, immunological and hormonal changes in soldiers participating in three weeks of commando training followed by a five-day combat course, no difference in infection incidence between groups receiving daily probiotic or placebo was reported (Tiollier et al., 2007). The major finding was a significant decrease in salivary immunoglobulin A (IgA) concentration after the combat course in the placebo group, with no change over time in the probiotic group. A randomized, placebo-controlled trial in 64 university athletes reported a lower incidence of URTI episodes during a four-month winter training period in subjects receiving daily *L. casei* Shirota compared with placebo, and this study also reported better maintenance of salivary IgA in the probiotic group (Gleeson et al., 2011). Importantly, in both athlete and non-athlete populations, falls in salivary IgA have been associated with increased URTI incidence (Walsh et al., 2011b). Another study using *L. fermentum* reported reduced URTI incidence among male but not female athletes during 11 weeks of training (West et al., 2011b). A recent large scale, randomized, placebo-controlled trial involving 465 physically active men and women reported fewer URTI episodes (relative risk ratio 0.73) in those who ingested daily a *Bifidobacterium animalis* subspecies *lactis* Bl-04 compared with placebo over a 150-day intervention period (West et al., 2014). Although most studies to date have examined probiotic effects in recreationally active individuals or endurance athletes, a recent study on elite rugby players provides evidence that beneficial effects of probiotics in reducing URTI incidence, but not severity, may extend to team games players (Haywood *et al.*, 2014).

From the research reviewed here, one cannot reach a definite conclusion that probiotics might benefit sportspeople. As with other supplements for which health claims are made there is a concern of bias in the literature, with a stronger likelihood of publication of studies with positive, as opposed to negative, outcomes. Nevertheless, there is now sufficient understanding of the mechanism of action of certain probiotic strains, and enough evidence from trials with highly physically active people to signify that this is a promising area of research with mostly positive indications at present. To date most studies of probiotic interventions in athletes have been relatively small scale; consequently some large scale, double-blind, placebo-controlled trials are needed to confirm any possible probiotic benefits for athletes.

Competing interests   None

PROHORMONES

Richard Baskerville and Douglas S. King

The term prohormone refers to synthetic analogues of anabolic steroids. In supplement form they are marketed to the bodybuilding community and elsewhere, as the dietary means to improve muscle strength, body composition and general wellbeing, whilst avoiding the legislative restrictions that surround anabolic steroids within UK, European and US law.

The term strictly refers to any post-translational peptide that is cleaved by convertases into a bioactive hormone. The use within commercial dietary supplements refers to androgenic precursors of testosterone which become enzymatically activated after ingestion and colloquially also refers to the non-precursor testosterone analogues, 1-testosterone and prostanzanol.

Didehydroepiandrosterone (DHEA) and its metabolites, androstenedione (DIONE) and androstenediol, with their 19-nor equivalents, form the main group of testosterone precursors. All are capable of conversion to testosterone but also have their own androgenic activity although weaker than testosterone itself. This is principally due to their rapid excretion via first-pass metabolism in the liver, but also because peripheral testosterone production is minor compared to that in the testes and may even suppress testicular function itself. As a result, prohormone supplements do not necessarily increase either plasma testosterone levels or the performance improvements one would intuitively expect. Females, however, derive a much larger androgen contribution from peripheral conversion and may experience significant testosterone elevations following prohormone ingestion (Leder *et al.*, 2002).

Via an alternative pathway these precursors can also be converted to oestrogenic steroids, potentially causing adverse effects such as gynaecomastia and liver dysfunction. To counteract these effects, some regular users of prohormones consume them for one month in three, allowing restoration of normal liver function within each period, known as a 'cycle'.

Regular users often combine or 'stack' differing prohormones of differing oestrogenicity within each cycle, augmented with N-acetyl cysteine to prevent liver dysfunction. In addition, selective oestrogen receptor modulators, or aromatase inhibitors, are taken to mitigate oestrogenic effects, along with androgenic herbal compounds to counteract periods of lowered mood state between cycles. None of these practices are evidence-based or within routine medical practice and may result in significant clinical harm.

Despite these sophisticated anecdotal regimens and marketing claims, research often demonstrates only modest or no enhancement in performance from prohormone consumption, but confirms the risk of adverse effects for both prohormones and their adjuncts.

A cohort study of 50 men aged 35–65 years included 200mg/day of androstenedione during a 12-week resistance training programme (Broeder *et al.*, 2000). This showed a significant 16% increase in total testosterone levels after one month of use but a return to pre-study levels by week 12, by endogenous negative feedback mechanisms via luteinising hormone. The major fate of the ingested prohormones appears to be aromatisation, since blood oestrogen levels were increased by nearly 63%. There was no enhancement in muscle strength during resistance training above placebo. However there was an 11% increase in the LDL-cholesterol/HDL-cholesterol lipid ratio, independent of dietary and body composition changes, corresponding to a significant increase in cardiovascular disease risk.

The last major review of the literature (Brown *et al.*, 2006) concluded that testosterone precursors do not augment the muscle size and strength gains of resistance training alone, and that their use may predispose to serious health risks.

However, a randomized controlled trial of 17 men taking a DHEA analogue within an exercise programme demonstrated an 8.6% improvement in maximal strength above placebo ($P<0.05$), but there were also multiple adverse changes in lipid profiles and liver function tests (Granados, 1985).

Whilst previous literature is only suggestive of real changes in body composition and performance, there is stronger evidence of objective harm via multiple mechanisms (Brown *et al.*, 1999; King *et al.*, 1999; Leder *et al.*, 2000, 2001). Because of the evolving number of compounds within this class, and their widespread use in society, further research with larger scale trials should be undertaken.

UK law legislates prohormones under Schedule 4 of the Misuse of Drugs Act 1971, and the current list of 54 'class C' substances includes both prohormones and anabolic steroids in recognition of their biochemical similarity, thus closing a previous loophole. Similar restrictions apply under the Anabolic and Steroid Control Act (2004) in US law. A worrying development is the continued appearance of new compounds outpacing updates in legislation. Despite these limitations, this legal framework provides an important role in supporting the efforts of the IOC and WADA in reducing the use of prohormones in professional sport.

In summary, there is reasonably strong evidence of a lack of anabolic or ergogenic effects in supplement form at supraphysiological doses. There is also strong evidence of dose and time-related widespread adverse effects resulting in several negative health consequences. Prohormones are classified as an androgenic/anabolic steroid and included on the WADA Prohibited List (WADA, 2014b).

Competing interests None

PROLINE

Malcolm Watford and Linda M. Castell

Proline is not considered essential in adult humans although early work demonstrated a potential benefit of proline when arginine was limiting. Proline is readily available in dairy, meat and eggs, and most plant proteins. Proline can be synthesized by two pathways, one arising from ornithine and arginine, and one from glutamine and glutamate (Watford, 2008). Although the glutamate pathway is considered to be the major route it is not known how much body proline is derived from the diet or made *de novo*. Proline and hydroxyproline (formed post translationally) comprise approximately 25% of the amino acids in collagen and thus proline is important in skin, bone, cartilage, tendons, ligaments and connective tissues (Barbul, 2008). Proline is degraded via proline oxidase (dehydrogenase) to glutamate or ornithine (Newsholme and Leech, 2010; Watford, 2008; Wu *et al.*, 2011) and the final stages include polyamines, arginine and entry into the tricarboxylic cycle (TCA). Proline is an osmoprotectant, a source of superoxide (in the immune system), and plays a role in sensing both energy availability and maintaining protein homeostasis. Hydroxyprolines are present in proteins other than collagen where they play a role in oxygen sensing while hydroxyproline, released from protein degradation, is an antioxidant.

Given the importance of proline in growth and wound repair, including the muscle hypertrophy of training, it has been proposed that proline may be conditionally essential. Indeed, proline has been marketed as a supplement for bodybuilders and weightlifters, and for recovery after strenuous exercise. However, while circulating proline concentrations decrease during burn injury, dietary supplementation with proline has no effect on plasma proline levels in such patients. Very few studies have looked directly at proline supplementation (Watford, 2008), although in patients with gyrate atrophy, supplements of up to 488mg.kg^{-1}.d^{-1} are well tolerated. It is, however, not possible to make any claims about the safety or even effectiveness of proline supplements due to an almost complete lack of data (Garlick, 2004; Watford, 2008). Nogusa *et al.* (2014) observed an increase in time to exhaustion in mice given combined supplementation of carbohydrate, alanine and proline cf. maltodextrin alone. An alternative approach to increase proline availability would be to provide proline precursors (glutamine, ornithine, arginine; see relevant sections in book) as dietary supplements but again there is little evidence that these are effective in increasing proline synthesis (Barbul, 2008).

Competing interests MW receives research funding from Ajinomoto.

PROTEIN

Stephan van Vliet and Nicholas A. Burd

Arguably one of the most debated topics in sports nutrition revolves around optimal protein consumption for athletic performance. Various studies have shown that the type, amount and timing of protein ingestion may be of relevance to maximize skeletal muscle recovery and the long-term adaptation, e.g. hypertrophy, increased strength or fatigue-resistant muscles (Cermak *et al.*, 2012b). Skeletal muscle mass is regulated by changes in muscle protein synthesis (MPS) and muscle protein breakdown (MPB), which ultimately define the overall net muscle protein balance. A positive net muscle protein balance is required to maximise skeletal muscle recovery and the longer term adaptation. From the standpoint of athletic performance, skeletal muscle protein turnover is important to repair any damaged/dysfunctional proteins and to facilitate adaptations in the contractile (e.g. myofibrillar) and/or energy-producing (e.g. mitochondrial) proteins of skeletal muscle. Performing an acute bout of either resistance (Biolo *et al.*, 1995; Phillips *et al.*, 1997) or endurance exercise (Sheffield-Moore *et al.*, 2004) stimulates skeletal muscle protein turnover, with MPS being the major variable that improves net muscle protein balance during post-exercise recovery.

However, it is important that dietary protein is consumed in the post-exercise recovery period to shift the net muscle protein balance into the positive and ultimately optimize recovery (Biolo *et al.*, 1997; Tipton *et al.*, 1999). What is noteworthy is that an acute bout of resistance exercise has been shown to sensitize the muscle to the anabolic properties of dietary protein-derived amino acids for ~24 hours (Burd *et al.*, 2011) and this sensitivity is likely to persist for an even longer duration (e.g. 48 hours) in the recovery period (Phillips *et al.*, 1997). Thus, the importance of protein consumption extends well beyond the initial hours after resistance exercise. While such evidence is not available with regards to endurance athletes, the value of protein ingestion in the late recovery period (> 24 hours) is likely to be of equal importance after an acute bout of endurance-type exercise. For example, di Donato *et al.* (2014) have recently shown that an acute bout of endurance exercise elevated the skeletal muscle myofibrillar and mitochondrial protein synthetic response for a prolonged period of time (> 24 hours) in the absence of food ingestion. It is reasonable to assume that protein ingestion in this extended window of anabolic opportunity will also further potentiate the muscle anabolic response when compared to the non-exercise state in endurance athletes.

The specific skeletal muscle adaptation that occurs depends on the type of exercise (e.g. resistance versus endurance exercise) that is chronically performed

(Wilkinson *et al.*, 2008). Specifically, the regular performance of resistance exercise will lead to an increase in muscle hypertrophy and strength (Cermak *et al.*, 2012b). The adaptation after endurance training may be more directed towards an increase in skeletal muscle oxidative capacity, e.g. mitochondrial-related proteins, angiogenic proteins, glucose transporters, etc. (Wilkinson *et al.*, 2008). It should be noted, however, that adaptations in skeletal muscle are not completely divergent. For instance, high-intensity resistance exercise stimulates early increases in the myofibrillar and mitochondrial protein synthetic response in untrained adults (Wilkinson *et al.*, 2008). A stimulation of all the major protein sub-fractions in skeletal muscle is also observed after an acute bout of endurance exercise (Burd *et al.*, 2011b; di Donato *et al.*, 2014; Wilkinson *et al.*, 2008). Overall the evidence suggests that, regardless of the type of exercise performed (e.g. resistance, endurance or concurrent exercise), the regular consumption of dietary protein during recovery from exercise is fundamental to maximize the acute skeletal muscle adaptive response.

Recently, researchers have manipulated various nutritional factors, such as the amount, type and timing of dietary protein ingestion, in order to describe their effects on muscle protein metabolism. In particular, scientists have applied sophisticated stable isotope amino acid tracer methodology combined with collecting muscle samples to provide detailed information towards the dietary protein needs of skeletal muscle tissue. This protocol is an improvement on nitrogen balance methods which determine a minimal dietary protein requirement for whole body proteins. Nitrogen balance methods have suggested that daily protein requirements for all athletes are ~1.2–1.7g/kg/d. While such recommendations of overall daily protein intake provided easy guidance for athletes, it is becoming increasingly clear that the muscle protein synthetic response to protein intake is short-lived, four to five hours (Moore *et al.*, 2009; Atherton *et al.*, 2010b), and that it changes on a meal-to-meal basis throughout the day (Areta *et al.*, 2013). Therefore, individualized meal-based recommendations achieving a regular spread of protein intake over the day are more likely to maximize net muscle protein balance than generic recommendations to achieve a certain daily protein target.

Using direct measurements of the dietary protein requirements of skeletal muscle tissue, an ingested protein dose-response curve of muscle protein synthesis has been established. Specifically, the ingestion of ~20g of high-quality protein maximized the post-exercise muscle protein synthetic response in 80 kg athletes (Moore *et al.*, 2009; Witard *et al.*, 2014b). Moreover, these studies demonstrated that the ingestion of greater amounts of protein (~40g) in a meal resulted in the excess dietary amino acid being shifted towards oxidation and/or urea synthesis. These data suggest that the ingestion of protein amounts above ~20g are used for energy production or excreted rather than used for synthesis of muscle proteins. The ingested protein dose-response relationship of muscle protein synthesis has not yet been determined during recovery from endurance exercise. However, some studies have shown that protein ingestion immediately after endurance exercise enhanced muscle protein synthesis rates during recovery (Breen *et al.*, 2011; Lunn *et al.*, 2012; Levenhagen *et al.*, 2002). In addition to stimulating post-exercise myofibrillar and mitochondrial protein accretion, the need for post-exercise protein ingestion with endurance exercise may also be necessary to replace the exercise-induced amino acid oxidative loss. For example, prolonged endurance exercise (> one hour) can result in ~10 % of the total energy needs being provided by amino acids (Tarnopolsky, 2004). The amino acids used for oxidation may largely be supplied by the breakdown of skeletal muscle proteins (Howarth *et al.*, 2010). Given all this, the evidence suggests that ~20g of dietary protein (or ~0.25g protein/kg per lean body mass) should be consumed after endurance exercise to maximize the muscle protein synthetic response. It is certainly possible that the distance/duration of endurance exercise (e.g. middle distance vs. marathon) may be an important consideration as the consumption of greater amounts of dietary protein may be required after longer distance exercise to counteract the increased amino acid oxidative loss. However, further work is required to define the dose-response curve of muscle protein synthesis to ingested dietary protein after an acute bout of endurance exercise.

The ingestion of ~20g of high quality dietary protein immediately after exercise is likely to meet the direct needs of skeletal muscle tissue during recovery from exercise. However, a truly optimal intake of dietary protein will also serve to facilitate proper remodelling of the bone and connective tissue (Phillips *et al.*, 2012a) to enhance immune function (Witard *et al.*, 2014a) and support gut health (Moore *et al.*, 2014). Witard *et al.* (2014a) have recently shown that dietary protein intakes of 3g protein/kg/day further improved the immune response when compared to the ingestion of 1.5g protein/kg/d. However, further work is required to confirm if higher dietary protein intakes are warranted to meet the needs of these other bodily amino acid consuming processes. Regardless, the consumption of slightly higher amounts of protein per meal would only be beneficial if the athlete is meeting the requirements for fat and carbohydrates.

There is substantial evidence which demonstrates that protein ingestion immediately after exercise is an effective strategy to support the muscle protein synthetic response during recovery. Indeed, the provision of protein immediately prior to an acute bout of resistance exercise has been shown to improve the post-exercise net muscle protein balance (MPS > MPB) (Tipton *et al.*, 2007). However, this strategy may predispose susceptible athletes to gastric distress during acute training, and pre-exercise protein feeding does not appear to provide any extra benefit to augment post-exercise muscle protein synthesis further when compared to ingestion of protein immediately after exercise. However, protein ingestion ~two to four hours before the training bout does not attenuate the increase in muscle protein synthesis during recovery from exercise (Witard *et al.*, 2009, 2014b). These data provide support for the recommendation for an athlete to consume ~0.25g protein/kg per lean body mass in a meal every three to four hours to maximize daily net muscle protein balance. This concept was recently confirmed in a well-designed study (Areta *et al.*, 2013).

The type of dietary protein consumed is likely to be another important consideration for the athlete to maximize the muscle protein synthetic response throughout exercise recovery. Animal-derived proteins, such as milk and beef, have been shown to result in greater increases in the muscle protein synthetic response when compared to the ingestion of isonitrogenous amounts of soy protein after resistance exercise (Wilkinson *et al.*, 2007; Phillips, 2012b). Importantly, it was shown that the ingestion of milk immediately after resistance exercise resulted in greater gains in lean mass when compared to the ingestion of a soy beverage containing equal amounts of protein (Hartman *et al.*, 2007). The greater anabolic potential of milk protein may be attributed to its high leucine by total amino acid content, milk-derived bioactive peptides (Nagpal *et al.*, 2011), and/or the transfer of microRNAs (miRNAs) into circulation that ultimately may serve as an anabolic signal to skeletal muscle tissue (Melnik *et al.*, 2013).

Recent work suggests that the whey portion of milk protein is of particular importance for the stimulation of the postprandial muscle protein synthetic response. For example, Tang *et al.* (2009) demonstrated that whey protein ingestion resulted in a greater stimulation of muscle protein synthesis rates when compared to isonitrogenous amounts of soy and casein. Whey protein is characterized by its accelerated dietary protein digestion and amino acid absorption kinetics which results in a 'fast' appearance of leucine into circulation (Pennings *et al.*, 2011) (see section on leucine in this book). Leucine has been shown to initiate mRNA translation in an insulin-independent manner and thus is a major anabolic driver of postprandial muscle protein anabolism (Kimball *et al.*, 2001). However, other animal-derived protein sources are also high in leucine, and other essential amino acids are required for the synthesis of fully functional bodily proteins. For example, egg (Moore *et al.*, 2009), beef (Phillips, 2012b) and milk (Wilkinson *et al.*, 2007) are all effective dietary protein sources for the athlete to consume to support muscle protein accretion after exercise. To date, there are very few data available on the impact of plant-derived protein sources to stimulate postprandial muscle protein anabolism (Wilkinson *et al.*, 2007; Tang *et al.*, 2009; Yang *et al.*, 2012b). Therefore, it is difficult to conclude whether the vegetarian athlete is at a true disadvantage for optimizing skeletal muscle repair and recovery.

It is common practice for athletes to use protein supplements to meet their daily dietary protein requirements. Popular protein supplements include animal-derived sources (e.g. whey protein, casein protein and isolated beef protein) and plant-derived protein sources (e.g. soy, pea, hemp protein). These protein supplements are often produced in isolated powder form, thereby offering an increased level of convenience for the athlete. There have been recent reports that some commonly consumed protein powders may be contaminated with other non-nutritional components including heavy metals and substances that are banned under anti-doping codes (Consumer Reports, 2010a, 2010b). As such, it is important for the athlete to ensure that protein powders are sourced from reputable companies, and in an attempt to reduce the risk of inadvertently consuming banned substances, the powders have been subject to third party auditing programmes.

In conclusion, dietary protein is required to stimulate postprandial muscle protein synthesis and facilitate the skeletal muscle adaptive response to prolonged exercise training. The type, timing and amount of dietary protein consumed immediately after exercise has been shown to modulate the muscle protein synthetic response differentially. In particular, the consumption of ~0.25g protein/kg per lean body mass per meal is sufficient to maximize the post-exercise muscle protein synthetic response in young men. It remains to be firmly established whether the consumption of slightly elevated amounts of dietary protein are required to satisfy the requirements of other processes requiring amino acids that will ultimately optimize immune function, gut health and/or remodelling of connective tissue. However, the increase in dietary protein requirements to meet these needs is probably modest. A balanced distribution pattern of dietary protein intake throughout the day (i.e. five to six isonitrogenous meals) is recommended to maximize net muscle protein anabolism and minimize amino acid oxidative losses. However, the consumption of protein immediately after exercise has the most anabolic potential. Finally, the ingestion of high quality protein sources that are easily digested and contain high amounts of essential amino acids is the most potent for stimulation of post-exercise muscle protein synthesis rates.

Competing interests   None

PYCNOGENOL

Jason C. Siegler

Pycnogenol (also referred to commonly as picnogel or pycnogel) is a combination of active bioflavonoids produced from the bark of the *Pinus maritime* pine tree. Pycnogenol supplementation has been reported to have a wide array of health benefits, including improved cognitive function, endothelial function, blood pressure regulation and venous insufficiency. Pycnogenol also may act as an anti-inflammatory agent (Rohdewald, 2002; Maimoona *et al.*, 2011). In most instances, reference is made to pycnogenol as a powerful antioxidant due to the proportionally high levels of procyanidins within the compound (Grimm *et al.*, 2004).

Recommended doses of pycnogenol range widely and depend upon the treatment aim. For example, to combat chronic venous insufficiency, recommended doses range from 150–360mg/day, whereas others have recommended approximately 75–90mg/day to prevent oxidative tissue damage (Maimoona *et al.*, 2002; Saliou *et al.*, 2001). In the majority of clinical trials, the duration of supplementation is generally two to three months. Side effects of pycnogenol supplementation are minimal.

At present, there is very little published research related to sports performance on this supplement. One study has reported a ~10% improvement in performance of a sprint distance triathlon (750m swim, 20km bike and 5km run) in a group of amateur athletes after four weeks of pycnogenol supplementation at 150mg/day (Vinciguerra *et al.*, 2013). However, very little data are provided in reference to study control measures, performance indicators, athlete characteristics and training regimens. Another study (Bentley *et al.*, 2012) has reported an approximate 16% improvement in time to failure during a cycling task at 95% peak power output after acute, oral administration of 360mg of pycnogenol in 150mL of the sport supplement Lactawayâ (extrapolated from a statement provided by the authors indicating Lactawayâ to contain 2.4g of pycnogenol L^{-1}). Although both studies suggest a possible performance benefit of pycnogenol supplementation, further evidence is required in order to determine the efficacy of pycnogenol as a performance-enhancing supplement.

Competing interests None

RESVERATROL

Markus Laupheimer

Resveratrol is a natural polyphenolic flavonoid antioxidant which may provide numerous health benefits like the prevention of cancer, cardiovascular disease and ischaemic injuries, as well as enhanced stress resistance (Baur and Sinclair, 2006; Markus and Morris, 2008). It is a freely available food supplement and is found in the seeds and skins of grapes, red wine, mulberries, peanuts and rhubarb (Baur and Sinclair, 2006; Markus and Morris, 2008).

Interest in sports medicine arose after animal studies assessed endurance performance of mice and found dose-dependent increases in exercise tolerance, improved motor skills and increased number and activity of mitochondria in muscle cells. Resveratrol-treated mice had a significantly higher maximum VO_2 rate, suggestive of an increased oxidative capacity. Resveratrol intake increases the ratio of oxidative to non-oxidative type muscle fibres and increases muscle strength in resveratrol-treated mice (Lagouge et al., 2006). The resveratrol effects also seem to be dependent on the length of intake, as one of the actions proposed is a gene switch (Murase et al., 2009).

To look at the effects of resveratrol on physical fatigue and exercise performance in mice, Wu et al. (2013) supplemented male mice for 21 days with 0, 25, 50 and 125mg/kg/day of resveratrol, and showed a dose-dependent decrease in serum lactate, ammonia and creatine kinase, and an increase in glucose, plus an increase in grip strength and exhaustive swimming time in the resveratrol group.

There are no established doses for resveratrol, but Kennedy et al. (2010) showed in humans that resveratrol administration with doses of 250mg and 500mg resulted in a dose-dependent increase in cerebral blood flow during task performance, and enhanced oxygen extraction. Recently, seven healthy male athletes were given 600mg/day resveratrol or a placebo, seven days immediately before a marathon, but failed to show an effect on inflammatory response or delayed onset muscle soreness after the marathon (Laupheimer et al., 2014).

Doses of 1,600mg per day in a 70kg participant are regarded as safe (Baur and Sinclair, 2006; Lagouge et al., 2006; Markus and Morris, 2008), even long-term (Juan et al., 2002; Kennedy, et al., 2010). Resveratrol as a food supplement in sports medicine has not received much attention despite strong basic scientific evidence that this substance could have multiple indications related to high performance sports, and therefore requires further studies to confirm the similar effects in humans.

Competing interests None

RHODIOLA ROSEA

Mayur K. Ranchordas and David S. Senchina

Rhodiola rosea is an herb from the Crassulacae family and is also known as arctic root, rose root and golden root. It grows in the mountainous and arctic regions of North America, Europe and Asia (Brown *et al.*, 2002). Though belonging to a completely separate botanical family, supplements from *Rhodiola* species are purported to have many of the same ergogenic outcomes attributed to ginseng, with a supposed source of bioactivity being a subclass of glycosides (in this case, rosavins). It is purported that *Rhodiola* possesses several ergogenic properties such as increasing physical and mental performance (Abidov *et al.*, 2003) and enhancing cognitive and neural function (Spasov *et al.*, 2000). Also, members of genus *Rhodiola* have a high polyphenol content, including quercetin, and so may also play a role in free radical mitigation (see section on antioxidants). It has been described as an adaptogen because of its cardioprotective effects (De Sanctis *et al.*, 2004).

Although the majority of research investigating the effects of *Rhodiola rosea* has been conducted in the animal model, there have been several studies done in humans. The dosages investigated in humans have ranged from 100–600mg/day. The most recent dedicated review concluded that studies of *Rhodiola* in athletes are equivocal (Walker and Robergs, 2006). Studies investigating its effects on exercise performance have been mixed. *Rhodiola* supplementation in doses of 100mg/day for 20 days and one acute dose of 200mg/day were found to improve endurance exercise capacity by 6.5% and 5.0% respectively (Maslova *et al.*, 1994; Spasov *et al.*, 2000). However, other studies have found no positive effects on VO_2peak, peak power, lactate threshold (de Bock *et al.*, 2004), or on ventilatory threshold (Earnest *et al.*, 2004). In one study of submaximal exercise, athletes given a single dose of *Rhodiola* (3mg/kg) demonstrated a lower heart rate response during submaximal cycling (Noreen *et al.* 2013). Studies investigating *Rhodiola* supplementation on neural and cognitive performance have also produced mixed results. Doses of 100–555mg/day have found positive effects on cognition (Colson *et al.*, 2005; Darbinyan *et al.*, 2000; Spasov *et al.*, 2000) and perceived effort during submaximal exercise (Noreen *et al.* 2013), but other studies have found no effect using doses of 200mg/day either acutely or for five weeks (Maslova *et al.*, 1994). As *Rhodiola* contains phenylopopropanoids, phenolic compounds and flavonoids, some studies have found that supplementation can increase antioxidant levels (Shevtsov *et al.*, 2003), decrease muscle damage markers (Nieman *et al.*, 2007a; Parisi *et al.*, 2010) and mitigate free radicals. By contrast, another study found no effect on muscle damage markers after a marathon (Shanely *et al.*, 2014).

Based on the available literature, it remains unclear whether *Rhodiola* supplementation, in doses of 100–600 mg/day, can enhance either mental and/ or exercise performance. However, there is some evidence that *Rhodiola* does possess antioxidant properties. Further tightly controlled studies in well-trained athletes need to be conducted in order to determine any performance-enhancing effects.

Competing interests None

RIBOSE

Ylva Hellsten

Adenosine 5′triphosphate (ATP) is the only directly usable source of energy for muscle contraction. At high exercise intensities the rate of ATP utilization can exceed that of its regeneration from other energy sources, and ATP levels in the muscle cells decrease. Most of the degraded ATP remains within the muscle as inosine monophosphate (IMP) which, after exercise, is used for resynthesis of ATP. However, a fraction of the IMP is degraded and lost from the muscle as purines. If intense exercise sessions are repeated, there may be an accumulated loss of ATP through the release of purines, whereby ATP stores in the muscle cells are reduced. The ATP lost from muscle may be replenished by *de novo* synthesis with a belief that D-ribose availability is a rate-limiting factor.

Experimental studies have shown that ribose supplementation does not lower the loss in nucleotides with repeated intense exercise bouts but allows for a faster recovery of ATP levels within 72 hours after termination of exercise training, most likely due to an improved rate of *de novo* ATP synthesis (Hellsten *et al.*, 2004). However, despite a higher level of ATP after ribose supplementation, there was no effect on intense intermittent exercise performance (Hellsten *et al.*, 2004). Accordingly, other studies examining the effect of ribose on performance during intense intermittent exercise (Berardi and Ziegenfuss, 2003; Eijnde *et al.*, 2001; Kerksick *et al.*, 2005; Kreider *et al.*, 2003) and rowing (Dunne *et al.*, 2006) have also not been able to demonstrate improved performance in humans.

Ribose supplementation up to ~40g/day, often split into two to three doses/day have been examined, with reports of minor adverse effects but solid evidence for potential short- or long-term side effects is lacking. In conclusion, although ribose supplementation appears to improve the rate of *de novo* synthesis of ATP in muscle, existing scientific evidence does not support the use of ribose as an ergogenic aid in young healthy individuals.

Competing interests   None

ROYAL JELLY

Joseph Lockey

Royal jelly is secreted by worker bees to feed young larvae to produce a queen bee: it contains a source of amino acids, fatty acids, carbohydrate and B-vitamins, and has long been used as a dietary supplement in alternative medicine. It contains royalectin, a protein that triggers the differentiation of honeybee larvae into queens through a growth factor-mediated signalling cascade resulting in increased body size (Kamakura, 2011). Guo *et al* (2007) gave 6g/day of royal jelly for four weeks to 15 volunteers, leading to improved plasma lipid profiles. However, Morita *et al.* (2012) failed to detect such a benefit in 61 volunteers taking 3g/day for six months. Instead they found that royal jelly led to increased red blood cell numbers, raised haematocrit, improved glucose tolerance and increased concentration of serum testosterone. There was no significant change in mean corpuscular volume. The authors suggest that royal jelly therefore either stimulated erythropoiesis or prolonged erythrocyte lifespan, most likely as a result of increased testosterone levels.

Little, however, is known about royal jelly in the context of exercise. Chupin *et al.* (1988) used sublingual doses of royal jelly, apparently combined with other components, on athletes undergoing rehabilitation in Irkutsk. It was not possible to deduce which components might have been responsible for the apparent improvements observed in the athletes' general wellbeing. Kamakura *et al.* (2001) reported a possible beneficial effect of fresh royal jelly (it degrades in storage) in mice, on recovery from swimming to exhaustion. No other studies on royal jelly *per se* in exercise have been found, and there is little or no evidence to suggest that it might be of use to athletes. Furthermore, case reports document that royal jelly may cause anaphylaxis (Katayama *et al.*, 2008), haemorrhagic colitis (Yonei *et al.,* 1997) and asthma (Thien *et al.,* 1996).

Competing interests   None

SELENIUM

Nathan A. Lewis

Selenium (Se) is a trace element essential for human health, and deficiency is rare. Its essentiality is achieved through the functioning of 25 known selenoproteins in the form of selenocysteine, with enzymatic activities being assigned to 12 of them (Hoffman and Reeves, 2009). Selenium is most well known as an antioxidant through its incorporation into the selenoprotein glutathione peroxidase (GPx), of which there are several forms. Se deficiency gives rise to cardiomyopathy, skeletal muscle myopathy, osteoarthropathy, reduced immune function, certain cancers and viral disease (Rayman, 2012).

Selenium's role in health and disease is complex, and is linked to numerous genetic variations for specific selenoproteins. Single nucleotide polymorphisms within selenoprotein genes affect the efficiency of synthesis, activity and concentrations of selenoproteins, and thus risk of disease. It has been recommended all future selenium studies should control for genotype (Rayman, 2012).

Skeletal muscle constitutes the main body pool of Se, comprising 50% of total body Se (Ashton *et al.*, 2009). The assessment of whole blood, plasma and red blood cell (RBC) Se provides a less invasive method for assessment of skeletal muscle Se content (Behne *et al.*, 2010). Full expression of plasma GPx has been observed at a plasma Se concentration of $>1.14 \, \mu mol/L$ (Duffield *et al.*, 1999).

The Se content of soil varies considerably depending on geographical locations (Rayman, 2012). Se is found in: meat and offal, seafood, cereals, nuts; milk, dairy, fruit and vegetables are particularly low.

Selenium toxicity occurs at intakes $>900 \, \mu g/d$, and deficiency at $<19 \mu g/day$ (Ashton *et al.*, 2009). Average European intakes are $40 \mu g/d$, $75 \mu g/day$ in the UK (Department of Health, 2001); this contrasts with US intakes of $93 \mu g/day$ in females and $134 \mu g/day$ in males (Rayman, 2012). In a large cross-sectional study (118 athletes), 23% of male athletes and 66% of female athletes had Se intakes below two-thirds of the French RDA, $<90 \mu g/day$ (Margaritis *et al.*, 2005).

Adequate Se is essential for immune system function (Hoffman and Reeves, 2009; Broome *et al.*, 2004). Se supplementation in subjects with low plasma Se ($<1.2 \, \mu mol/L$) increases GPx activity in T-lymphocytes, augments T-cell-mediated immune responses to an oral vaccine, and results in more rapid clearance of the poliovirus and a reduced number of viral mutations (Broome *et al.*, 2004). Se status may be important in those athletes who experience an increased frequency of upper respiratory tract illness.

Margaritis *et al.* (1997) found no effect on endurance training adaptations when supplemental Se alone was provided to endurance athletes. Other exercise studies examined the effect of different Se-containing antioxidant cocktails (90–200μg/day) on several parameters, pre- and post-exercise. Triathletes improved performance and VO_{2max} over eight weeks training and two weeks taper, whether receiving a selenium-ACE supplement or a placebo (Margaritis et al., 2003). Nevertheless, compared with placebo, the Se-ACE® supplement increased resting plasma GPx, lymphocyte CD4 count and reduced oxidative stress in response to the duathlon. Other protocols which showed no performance benefits included Se supplementation for six weeks in trained cyclists (MacAnulty et al., 2010) and two weeks in untrained females (Lamprecht et al., 2009). Antioxidant and Se supplement studies demonstrated increased lipid peroxidation (Martinovic et al., 2011); one observed no effect on performance (Lamprecht et al., 2009), another reported a reduction in post-exercise markers of protein and lipid oxidation, using eccentric exercise in untrained females (Goldfarb et al., 2005). All studies reported increases in either measures of plasma or whole blood antioxidant 'status', or actual antioxidant vitamins in the antioxidant groups. The cocktails combined minerals (zinc, manganese, selenium) antioxidant nutrients (beta-carotene, vitamins C, E, A, co-enzyme Q10) and essential fatty acids, EPA and DHA (see relevant sections).

No firm conclusions can be drawn regarding an effect of selenium supplementation *per se* on athlete health, immunity and performance. However, a plasma GPx of $> 1.14\ \mu mol/L$ may be associated with optimal Se status and, in well-trained athletes, a combination of Se, vitamins A and E in doses achievable through food intake, may benefit endogenous antioxidant defences, namely GPx activity.

Competing interests   None

SERINE

Mhairi Keil

Serine is a non-essential amino acid that is either obtained by *de novo* synthesis from the glycolytic intermediate 3-phosphoglycerate, through the conversion of the amino acid glycine, or through the absorption of dietary proteins and phospholipids. Serine is incorporated into a number of different proteins including enzymes, proteases and kinases, which are ubiquitous in the body, and are involved in numerous physiological processes including immune and inflammatory responses (Pham, 2008; Meyer-Hoffert and Wiedow, 2011). L-serine metabolism provides the formyl group for purine synthesis and methyl group for pyrimidine synthesis, and is therefore involved in the production of genetic material and cell replication. Interestingly, the D isoform is found in high concentrations in the brain (Hashimoto *et al.*, 1992), playing an important role as a neurotransmitter in the central nervous system, CNS (Darra *et al.*, 2009; Ding *et al.*, 2011). L- and D-serine have been implicated in brain and CNS development. Research has demonstrated how serine deficiency results in severe neurodevelopment abnormalities (Yoshida *et al.*, 2004) and has also been linked with the pathophysiology of neuropsychiatric disorders (Nishikawa, 2011). Deficient levels of serine are only likely to occur in patients with decreased biosynthesis of serine production (Yang *et al.*, 2010b). Conversely, high levels of D-serine have been reported in the spinal cord of individuals with amyotrophic lateral sclerosis, where it is thought to cause motor neurone degeneration (Sasabe *et al.*, 2012). For a review on serine and its role in the brain and CNS, readers are referred to Tabatabaie *et al.* (2010) and Martineau *et al.* (2014).

The body can synthesise sufficient serine to meet its physiological requirements. As a result, there is currently no published research to support exogenous consumption of serine in the form of a nutritional supplement. Thus, there is currently no evidence to suggest that additional serine can improve cognitive and/or athletic performance.

Competing interests None

SMILAX (SARSAPARILLA)

David S. Senchina

The plant genus *Smilax* includes several hundred species from the lily order that are distributed globally and commonly known as greenbriar or sarsaparilla (also spelled 'zarzaparilla' and often pronounced 'sasparilla'). The bark and parts that grow below ground (rhizomes and roots) from these plants are used by many traditional cultures to produce root beer, food or various herbal medicines. Smilax supplements are often produced from *Smilax aristolochiifolia* (syn. *S. medica*), *Smilax officinalis* and *Smilax regelii* and are rich in a category of plant sterols called saponins including sarsasapogenin (sarsapogenin), smilagenin (a derivative of sapogenin), sitosterol and stigmasterol. Plant sterols as a group are covered elsewhere in this book (see section on plant sterols).

Bodybuilders consume Smilax supplements for their purported anabolic effects (Bucci, 2000), mistakenly perceiving sarsaparilla sterols to be prohormonal compounds that can be converted into testosterone by the human body to subsequently enhance metabolism, muscle mass, power and performance. These claims, however, have been disproved (Grunewald and Bailey, 1993; Kreider *et al.*, 2010). Other benefits attributed to Smilax supplements include an increase in endurance or energy, enhanced recovery, reduction in body fat (Grunewald and Bailey, 1993) and improved immune function (Kreider *et al.*, 2010). Documented side effects include stomach upset and kidney problems (including increased urination) and possible interactions with other supplements or drugs (Bucci, 2000; Deuster *et al.*, 2004). Typical daily doses for Smilax supplements are 5–10ml of extract or 1–4g of dried belowground parts (Deuster *et al.*, 2004). There is presently no evidence of ergogenic benefits from Smilax supplementation and its use is discouraged.

Competing interests   None

SODIUM

Susan M. Shirreffs

Sodium is a cation with an atomic weight of 23. It is an essential nutrient and although it is commonly found in the diet as sodium chloride (NaCl), many other anions are partnered with it in foods, food ingredients and supplements. An example of these is the use of sodium bicarbonate as a buffer, as described elsewhere in this publication (see section on sodium bicarbonate). Typical daily sodium intake varies greatly between individuals depending on the composition and quantity of food intake, with processed foods (where salt is used as a preservative and flavour enhancer) being a major contributor to intake. Most major health organisations recommend that daily sodium intake for adults should not exceed about 1,500–2,300mg (4–6g/day of salt) because of the association between high intakes and hypertension (EFSA, 2005), although this is more pertinent for those individuals that are 'salt sensitive'. High blood pressure is strongly associated with cardiovascular disease and may also be linked to other health problems, such as renal disease. Average daily salt intake for adults in Europe is about 8–12g/day for men and 6–10g/day for women, but this varies between countries (EFSA, 2005).

Sodium is the main electrolyte in the extracellular fluid, present in concentrations averaging around 140mmol/l, and it can be lost in significant amounts during sweating, with normal sweat sodium concentration in the range of 15–80mmol/l. Therefore, when thermally induced sweating occurs, the typical response is a loss of water in excess of sodium, relative to the extracellular fluid concentration, which causes an increase in the extracellular sodium concentration. (See section on electrolytes elsewhere in this book.) Plasma sodium concentration is a key determinant of plasma osmolality, and therefore of plasma volume, and thus plays a key role in the regulation of body water balance.

Sweat rates and sweat composition vary greatly, depending on exercise intensity and duration, environmental conditions and individual physiology. Football players typically lose about 3–5g of salt in a 90 min training session, but some individuals may lose 10g or even more (Shirreffs et al., 2006). During periods of intensive training in warm environments, daily salt intakes of some individuals may therefore need to exceed the recommendations aimed at the general population. After sweat-induced water and sodium loss, replacement of sodium is a pre-requisite for maintenance of replaced water losses and euhydration (Shirreffs and Maughan, 1998). When sodium is consumed in rehydration drinks, plasma volume and osmolality is better maintained and the effect has been attributed to the presence of sodium in the drinks. Systematic investigation into the mechanisms of post-exercise rehydration showed that the ingestion of large volumes of plain water after exercise-induced dehydration resulted in a rapid fall in plasma osmolality and sodium concentration, leading to a prompt and marked diuresis caused by a rapid return to control levels of plasma renin activity and aldosterone concentration. Therefore, the replacement of sweat losses entirely with plain water will, if the volume ingested relative to sweat loss is sufficiently large, lead to haemodilution. The fall in plasma osmolality and sodium concentration that occurs in this situation stimulates urine output, and has potentially more serious consequences such as hyponatraemia. The anion accompanying sodium for hydration effectiveness has not been systematically studied to date, and much of the information available to date is based on sodium consumed in the form of sodium chloride.

Hyponatraemia, a serum or plasma sodium concentration below the lower limit of the normal reference range (normally 135 mmol/l), has been reported to occur in some participants in long duration endurance events. It is typically associated with excessive drinking behaviour that leads to weight gain during exercise, with low body weight, with female gender, with slow running or performance pace and event inexperience. The condition is generally asymptomatic and harmless but, if severe, it may be fatal due to osmotically-induced water shifts that lead to brain swelling and encephalopathy. By contrast, as noted above, the normal response to exercise and sweat loss is a contraction of plasma volume and an associated hypernatraemia. Hyponatraemia can generally be avoided by limiting water intake during exercise so that weight gain does not occur. It should be noted, though, that mild and transient asymptomatic hyponatraemia may also be relatively common in the general population.

Competing interests   None

SODIUM BICARBONATE AND SODIUM CITRATE

Lars R. McNaughton and Adrian W. Midgley

Sodium bicarbonate ($NaHCO_3$) or sodium citrate ($Na_3C_6H_5O_7$), collectively recognised as 'buffers', are substances permitted for use by the WADA code that can potentially provide the body with improved resistance to the fatigue caused by changes in acid-base balance. Water has a neutral pH of 7.0 but human arterial blood at rest typically has a pH of approximately 7.4, making it slightly alkalotic. However, after strenuous exercise the pH may fall to ~7.1, while muscle pH decreases to an acidic ~6.8. The ingestion of these buffers increases blood pH and resting buffering capacity, allowing it to counteract more of the H+ ions produced by the muscle during high-intensity exercise in which anaerobic glycolysis provides a large contribution to ATP production. In this way, exercise may continue for a longer time before fatigue occurs.

Although earlier hypotheses proposed that the buffering occurred in the extracellular space following the efflux of H+ from the muscle cell, more recent work has questioned this underpinning mechanism. Raymer *et al.* (2004) compared blood and muscle pH perturbation, via ^{31}P-MRS, after ingestion of 300mg/kg $NaHCO_3$ using incremental forearm exercise to exhaustion. They reported an attenuation of intracellular acidosis during alkalosis when compared to control. This work, as well as the recent work of others, has proposed instead that the intracellular perturbation may have been minimized by increased Na^+/H^+ or monocarboxylic transporters, or a strong ion difference.

High-intensity exercise

Studies on high-intensity running in the 1980s suggested that $NaHCO_3$ supplementation ('bicarbonate loading') could enhance the performance of 400–800 m track events (Goldfinch *et al.*, 1988). An ergogenic benefit in 200m freestyle swimming performance after $NaHCO_3$ ingestion has also been reported (Lindh *et al.*, 2007). Indeed, several reviews have concluded that there is support for the effect of bicarbonate loading on sustained high-intensity sporting events lasting one to seven minutes (Burke, 2013; McNaughton *et al.*, 2008). A meta-analysis (Carr *et al.*, 2011a) of 38 studies found that the typical loading dose (300mg/kg taken ~two to three hours pre-event) achieved a possibly moderate performance enhancement of 1.7% (90% CL ± 2.0%) in a single one-minute sprint in males. This effect was increased by ~0.5% for larger doses or for events involving further sprints, and decreased by the same amount for females, untrained subjects or longer/lower intensity events. Citrate was found to be less effective: over 16 studies, a typical dose of 0.5g/kg/BM (body mass) had an unclear performance effect of 0.0% (±1.3%). Meanwhile, a different meta-analysis of 40 studies concluded that the effect size of bicarbonate loading was moderate (0.36) with effects being larger in untrained people (Peart *et al.*, 2012).

Prolonged continuous exercise

The efficacy of bicarbonate loading has been examined in other sporting activities in which there is a dependence on anaerobic glycolysis. A $NaHCO_3$ dose of 300mg/kg was used in a randomized controlled trial on ten well-trained male cyclists undertaking one hour maximal effort cycle ergometer time trial (McNaughton *et al.*, 1999b). The cyclists performed, on average, 13% and 14% greater total work with $NaHCO_3$ than control and placebo, respectively. More recently, however, the same dose was found to have no effect on a cycling protocol lasting ~60 min (Stephens *et al.*, 2002).

Prolonged intermittent exercise

Sporting events involving the repetition of sprint efforts might benefit from enhanced buffering (Burke, 2013). Bicarbonate loading was trialled in a group of recreational team sport participants during repeated sprints (5 × 6s) or multiple effort bouts (Bishop *et al.*, 2004). No differences were reported in total work or % fatigue, but improvements in sprints 3–5 were observed, along with significantly higher post-test muscle lactate values, attributed to a high rate of glycolytic flux. In a 30-min intermittent cycling protocol, elevated pH and lactate levels and an improved sprint performance were observed after $NaHCO_3$ ingestion (Price *et al.*, 2003). Furthermore, a study on amateur boxers found they were able to land more punches when given $NaHCO_3$ versus placebo in a randomized crossover trial against the same partner (Siegler and Hirscher, 2010). However, another study failed to find evidence of improved repeated sprint ability in college wrestlers (Aschenbach *et al.*, 2000).

Recovery and training support

Some researchers have investigated whether buffering agents can improve recovery from exercise, with implications for training as well as performance. Siegler *et al.* (2007) suggested that athletes could improve recovery from high-intensity supra-maximal cycling, by using pre-exercise alkalosis and a passive recovery technique. In support of this, Edge and co-workers (2006) studied the effects of chronic loading with bicarbonate (400mg/kg) prior to interval training sessions (3/week) over an eight-week training block in moderately trained female athletes. The bicarbonate supplemented group showed substantially greater improvements in both lactate threshold (26% vs. 15%) and time to exhaustion (164% vs. 123%) than a placebo group.

Individuality of responses and side-effects

The typical bicarbonate loading protocol involves the acute pre-exercise intake of 300mg/kg of $NaHCO_3$ using either common household 'bicarb soda' or specially prepared pharmaceutical products made to treat the discomfort associated with urinary tract infections. However, consuming large amounts of bicarbonate or citrate in the hours prior to exercise can cause gastrointestinal discomfort/ upset and performance impairment rather than provide benefit (Saunders *et al.*, 2014). Alternative protocols include a serial loading protocol with a progressive intake of 600mg/kg/d, split into several doses, over several days prior to an event (Rossi *et al.*, 2006). A systematic investigation (Carr *et al.*, 2011b) found the best protocol to optimise blood alkalosis and reduce the occurrence of gut problems was consumption of bicarbonate capsules spread over 120–150 min before exercise and, if practical, at the same time as consuming a carbohydrate-rich meal and some fluid. Meanwhile, Siegler and colleagues (2012) found that GI upset was lessened if exercise occurred 180 min after ingestion, although this may not coincide with peak pH. Further research is needed but practical use of bicarbonate loading requires individual trialling and fine-tuning of protocols.

Short-term high-intensity exercise (~8min), and possibly high-intensity longer duration performance, can benefit from the ergogenic effects of these buffers. Loading sequences and timing of pre-exercise doses tend to be different in most studies, leading to confusion regarding effectiveness of the various buffering substances. More work continues to be undertaken to examine the efficacy of such buffers.

Competing interests   None

SPIRULINA

Adam J. Zemski

Spirulina is a microalgae belonging to the cyanobacteria class, with nutritional supplements (tablets, flakes and powders) typically being produced from the cultivation of two species *Arthrospira platensis* and *Arthrospira maxima*. Although spirulina's taste can prevent it from becoming a popular stand-alone food item, it is now being incorporated into more everyday products, such as desserts, corn chips, soups, salad dressings, confectionary and even beer (Small, 2011). Several cookbooks specifically dedicated to spirulina have been published. It is also used as a feed supplement in the aquaculture, aquarium and poultry industries. Spirulina was primarily recognised as being rich in proteins, essential amino acids and essential fatty acids, but recently has attracted attention due to its content of phytochemicals with antioxidant and hypolipidemic properties (Dang and Chow, 2010).

Claims for general health benefits from spirulina intake are centuries old (Dang and Chow, 2010), including that it possesses anti-cancer, antiviral, antibacterial, metalloprotective and immunostimulant properties (Hoseini *et al.*, 2013). However, the numerous claims of medical benefits are largely based on animal studies, the results are at times contradictory, and spirulina has not been established to be useful in treating most human illnesses in comparison with current standard treatments (Small, 2011; Hoseini *et al.*, 2013).

Claimed ergogenic benefits relate to antioxidant defence and favourable changes in substrate utilisation during exercise. Indeed, moderately trained runners who received four weeks of spirulina supplementation (6g/day) showed increased fat utilisation, reductions in markers of antioxidant stress and increased endurance at high-intensity exercise (95% VO_{2max}) following two hours of sub-maximal running, compared to a similar trial following supplementation with egg protein placebo (Kalafati *et al.*, 2010). Similarly, enhancements in basal antioxidant status and time to fatigue during an incremental exercise test were claimed when untrained students consumed 7.5g/day of spirulina for three weeks (Lu *et al.*, 2006).

Although these results are of interest, limitations of the current literature include the failure to study well-trained individuals, failure to standardize or identify active ingredients, general issues related to monitoring antioxidant status (Powers *et al.*, 2010b) and the lack of protocols related to sports performance. Additionally, little is known about the interaction of microalgae with the properties of food. Although spirulina is generally considered safe for human consumption, concerns related to spirulina supplements include contamination with heavy metals or toxins produced by blue-green algae. As such, no more than 15g per day is recommended for consumption (Small, 2011). It may join the list of other antioxidant-rich food sources and extracts that require further investigation of potential benefits to exercise performance, along with mechanisms to explain them.

Competing interests None

SUCCINATE

Martin J. Gibala

Succinate is an intermediate of the tricarboxylic acid (TCA) cycle, which is the central common pathway involved in the oxidation of carbohydrates and fats for energy. The regulation of TCA cycle flux is complex, but one potential factor involved is the total concentration of TCA cycle intermediates (TCAI). It has been proposed that 'expansion' of the TCAI pool in skeletal muscle during exercise is crucial in order to permit high rates of oxidative energy delivery; while this theory is controversial (Bowtell *et al.*, 2007), it has led to speculation that TCAI supplementation may improve physical performance.

To the author's knowledge, no study has directly investigated the ergogenic effect of succinate supplementation *per se*. However, Brown *et al.* (2004) used a randomized, double-blind crossover design to evaluate whether a commercial supplement that contained succinate and dozens of additional compounds including other TCAIs and precursor amino acids would improve performance in trained male cyclists. Subjects ingested a supplement that provided 1,000mg of succinate or an iso-energetic carbohydrate placebo for three weeks in conjunction with their normal training, and prior to an acute exercise trial that consisted of cycling at 75% of maximal oxygen uptake. The treatment did not alter whole-body substrate oxidation or selected blood metabolites during exercise or improve cycling time to exhaustion, compared to placebo.

Investigators have used a variety of other interventions in order to manipulate the size of the TCAI pool in human skeletal muscle (Bruce *et al.*, 2001; Dawson *et al.*, 2003; Gibala *et al.*, 2002). These studies have revealed no obvious relationship between the total muscle content of TCAI (including succinate) and the capacity for oxidative energy provision. There is little direct evidence to support the hypothesis that the size of the TCAI pool in human skeletal muscle is causally linked to mitochondrial respiration or exercise capacity. Thus, in the absence of an established mechanism, the underlying rationale for succinate supplementation for exercise performance is questionable.

Competing interests   None

SUCROSE

Ros Quinlivan

Sucrose is a disaccharide, i.e. two linked monosaccharide (single sugar) molecules, which is broken down during digestion by the enzyme sucrase located in the intestinal microvilli, into the monosaccharides glucose and fructose; it has a glycaemic index of 64. Sucrose is odourless and has good palatability; it is not as sweet as fructose but is sweeter than glucose, and in solution it is colourless and very stable with a long shelf-life. Sucrose (table sugar) normally comes from sugar beet and cane, but is also found naturally in all fruits and vegetables, and even most herbs and spices. As a sweetener it has acquired a bad reputation for being associated with obesity, insulin resistance and dental caries.

However, when consumed in moderation as a sport supplement it can have a positive effect on peak performance (see sections on carbohydrate and MTCs). There is much evidence for the use of carbohydrate ingestion before, during and after prolonged strenuous exercise to increase fuel availability for muscle and central nervous system (Jeukendrup, 2004). Carbohydrates, both sugars and starches, with moderate to high glycaemic index, such as glucose (high) and sucrose (moderate), are absorbed rapidly, providing a readily available source of carbohydrate and so are viewed as effective sources, particularly for intake during exercise (Jeukendrup, 2004; Maughan *et al.*, 2010). The two monosaccharide components of sucrose are absorbed by differing mechanisms: glucose is absorbed by a sodium co-transporter SGLUT-1 and rapidly enters the blood stream, while fructose is absorbed by glucose transporter 5 (GLUT5) and has to be converted to glucose by the liver before being available for muscle metabolism (Jeukendrup, 2004; Shi *et al.*, 1997). Therefore the bioavailability of sucrose as an energy source is greater than by ingesting fructose or glucose alone (Shi *et al.*, 1997). Because lower concentrations are required, there is less risk of gastro-intestinal slowing and stomach upset (Jeukendrup, 2004). While sucrose ingestion at rest can lead to a rebound hypoglycaemia from a surge in insulin release, evidence suggests that serum insulin levels actually fall within minutes of starting exercise and remain low for the duration of activity (Shi *et al.*, 1997). Hypoglycaemia during prolonged exercise is more likely to occur as a consequence of glycogen depletion and is a cause of fatigue which can be prevented by sucrose ingestion before and during exercise (Jeukendrup, 2004; Maughan *et al.*, 2010).

Competing interests None

TAURINE

Lawrence L. Spriet

Taurine is a sulphur containing β-amino acid (2-aminoethanesulphonic acid) that is conditionally classified as an indispensable amino acid (Huxtable, 1992). It is the most abundant free amino acid in heart, brain, leukocytes and skeletal muscle (Huxtable, 1992), but is not incorporated into protein within skeletal muscle (Graham *et al.*, 1995). It has been suggested to be involved in a wide range of cellular processes including: regulation of cell volume, Ca^{2+} -dependent excitation-contraction processes, antioxidant defence from stress responses, modulation of nerve excitement potential, and several metabolic effects related to improved glucose tolerance, insulin sensitivity and substrate uptake, storage and oxidation in skeletal and cardiac muscle (Huxtable, 1992).

Rodent studies have shown that taurine supplementation increases muscle taurine content (Goodman *et al.*, 2009; Yatabe *et al.*, 2003), and prolonged exercise of varying durations causes a decline in skeletal muscle taurine content (Matsuzaki *et al.*, 2002). In addition, changes in taurine concentrations have been correlated with muscle function: when muscle taurine was decreased, contractile ability declined (Hamilton *et al.*, 2006) and, when it was increased, muscle force production improved (Goodman *et al.*, 2009). Lastly, the knock-out of taurine transporters has been associated with low muscle taurine levels and severe impairment of skeletal muscle exercise capacity (Warskulat *et al.*, 2004). A recent study by Dutka *et al.* (2014) used mechanically skinned human skeletal muscle fibres and examined the effects of taurine exposure on sarcoplasmic reticulum (SR) Ca^{2+} accumulation and contractile apparatus properties in type I and II fibres. Taurine concentrations of 10 or 20 mM (but not 5 mM) increased the rate of Ca^{2+} accumulation by the SR in both fibre types, but did not affect maximum Ca^{2+} accumulation. Taurine had little or no effect on the responsiveness of the Ca^{2+} release channels, the Ca^{2+} sensitivity of the contractile apparatus or the maximum Ca^{2+}-activated force in either fibre type. The taurine effect on SR Ca^{2+} accumulation required prolonged taurine exposure and lasted for some time after removal of the taurine, leading the authors to speculate that the effects were due to taurine acting inside the SR (Dutka *et al.*, 2014). This work demonstrated that manipulating the taurine availability can affect contractile processes in human skeletal muscle, but other evidence discussed below suggests that altering the *in vivo* muscle taurine content through dietary means is currently not at hand (Galloway *et al.*, 2008).

Taurine is currently claimed to be a functional ingredient in several commercialized 'energy' drinks (~1,000–2,000mg taurine per serving), with many manufacturers claiming that taurine is ergogenic for many types of exercise. However, scientific evidence to support these claims does not exist (Campbell *et al.*, 2013), as most studies have examined the metabolic, cognitive and performance effects of taurine supplements in combination with many additional ingredients which have been shown to be ergogenic (e.g. caffeine and carbohydrate) or have not utilized appropriate placebo control beverages (Geiss *et al.*, 1994; Ivy *et al.*, 2009; Gwacham and Wagner, 2012; Nelson *et al.*, 2014b). Therefore, a role for taurine alone to improve exercise performance and/or alter metabolism in humans has not been demonstrated.

Recent studies have examined the plasma taurine kinetics following a single acute dose of taurine, as well as the chronic effects of seven days of taurine supplementation on skeletal muscle taurine content and substrate metabolism during two hours of submaximal cycling (Galloway *et al.*, 2008; Rutherford *et al.*, 2010). Acute supplementation with ~1.7g taurine caused a 13-fold increase in plasma taurine at two hours and remained elevated for at least four hours. A second 1.7g taurine dose increased the plasma taurine even higher and it stayed elevated again for at least four hours. However, seven days of taurine supplementation (~5g/day) did not increase the taurine content before exercise or alter skeletal muscle taurine content or substrate utilization during two hours of submaximal exercise (Galloway *et al.*, 2008). The effects of an acute dose of taurine (~1.7g) given one hour before 90 min of submaximal cycle and subsequent endurance time-trial performance and whole-body metabolism in well-trained cyclists was also studied (Rutherford *et al.*, 2010). Acute taurine ingestion had no effect on time-trial performance compared with the control trial. In a third trial, telling subjects they were receiving taurine in their pre-exercise drink, when they did not (placebo), was also not ergogenic. Taurine also had no effect on the normal physiological and mental responses to exercise such as heart rate and rating of perceived exertion as compared with control and placebo trials (Rutherford *et al.*, 2010). Acute taurine ingestion did produce a significant 16% increase in total whole-body fat oxidation during 90 min of submaximal exercise prior to the time trial (Rutherford *et al.*, 2010), although this was not evident in the previous study (Galloway *et al.*, 2008).

In conclusion, despite large increases in plasma taurine following the acute ingestion of a large oral dose of taurine, it does not enhance endurance performance in well-trained athletes and does not accumulate in skeletal muscles when consumed chronically (5g/day for seven days). These data suggest that supplemental taurine is not ergogenic in human subjects.

Competing interests None

THEOBROMINE AND THEOPHYLLINE

David S. Senchina

Theobromine and theophylline are methylxanthine alkaloids originally identified from the chocolate or cocoa plant *Theobroma cacao* L. (Malvaceae (syn. Sterculiaceae)), but subsequently identified in tea, cola, guarana and many other plants. Theobromine and theophylline are isomers of one another and paraxanthine. All three are structurally similar to caffeine and metabolites of caffeine in the human body, though paraxanthine much more so. Theobromine and theophylline are found in energy- or metabolism-enhancing foods, beverages and sports supplements where they may work as stimulants. Pure theophylline is widely prescribed as an anti-asthmatic and is under investigation as a treatment for other cardiorespiratory diseases.

Theophylline is a purported ergogenic aid, though studies both support and refute this capacity. One study found no effect of theophylline (serum concentrations 10–20mg/l) on VO_{2max}, muscle or lung measures, or reaction time in non-asthmatic athletes, concluding it was not ergogenic (Morton *et al.*, 1989). In contrast, two other groups dosed athletes with 4.5mg/kg theophylline/body mass and reported improved time-to-exhaustion when athletes cycled either at 80% of their VO_{2max} or intermittently (1 min cycling at 120% VO_{2max} alternating with 3 min rest) and concluded it was ergogenic (Greer *et al.*, 2000; Pigozzi *et al.*, 2003). Although a more thorough review exists elsewhere (Senchina *et al.*, 2012b), these examples demonstrate why the potential ergogenic effects of theophylline are still being questioned. Similar studies of theobromine could not be found. Body mass and exercise are known to influence the metabolism of both compounds (Arnaud, 2011) and, given current reports, it is likely that both may act additively or synergistically with other compounds (Senchina *et al.*, 2012b). For example, theophylline is known to augment the effects of ephedrine, another stimulant (see section on ephedra). Within *in vitro* or non-exercise *in vivo* contexts, both theobromine and theophylline have proven anti-inflammatory actions at cellular and molecular levels. These effects have not been demonstrated in exercise studies, partially due to the use of multi-component preparations and the lack of reporting on individual alkaloids, ergo no firm statements about the effects of theobromine and theophylline on athlete immune function can be made currently (Senchina *et al.*, 2014).

The past (IOC and WADA) and present (USA NCAA) restrictions on high doses of caffeine intake by athletes in competition have created some discussion on whether theobromine and theophylline should also be regulated. Anti-doping agencies have never placed restrictions on the use of these compounds, though one research team argued during the period when urinary caffeine concentrations were restricted to $<12\mu g/ml$, that urinary levels of $5\mu g/ml$ for theophylline and a theophylline/paraxanthine ratio of 0.50 should be used for doping standards (Delbeke and de Backer, 1996). Quantities of theobromine and theophylline in commercially available products are probably too low to elicit any ergogenic benefits when such products are consumed in typical or even tolerable quantities (Senchina *et al.*, 2012b), and pure theophylline is only available by prescription in many countries. Available data suggest that current policies regarding these compounds should be maintained but not cemented.

Competing interests   None

THREONINE

Nicholas A. Burd and Naomi Cermak*

Threonine is a nutritionally essential amino acid that has no metabolic precursor and thus must be obtained through the diet. Dietary threonine requirements for healthy adults are $15mg \cdot kg^{-1} \cdot d^{-1}$. Foods that contain high amounts of threonine are cottage cheese, fish, chicken, sesame seeds and lentils. Relative to other amino acids, threonine is a major component of the protein core in the intestinal mucous. Animal studies show that manipulating dietary threonine intake can affect whole body and skeletal muscle protein metabolism. Specifically, low intakes of threonine have been demonstrated to reduce skeletal muscle and splanchnic tissue protein synthesis rates (Wang et al., 2007). As such, chronically consuming low intakes of dietary threonine, or any other essential amino acid, will impair tissue growth and function. Moreover, it has been shown that threonine supplementation has a positive effect upon immune function in pigs, mice and poultry (Defa et al., 1999; Li et al., 2007).

From a human performance perspective, there is no evidence to suggest that threonine supplementation will offer an ergogenic effect when consumed above daily dietary requirements. Indeed, threonine can be broken down into molecules that play a role in energy metabolism, and its suggestive role in the immune response may imply a beneficial effect on human performance. However, more definitive data would be required to promote threonine supplementation to athletes as an ergogenic aid.

Competing interests   None

*Tribute to Dr Naomi Cermak

On December 14, 2013, Naomi Cermak passed on after battling stage 4 melanoma for nearly 13 months. Even though she was only 31 years old she had accomplished so much in her short life. As a competitive athlete and academic scholar she pursued her dreams with passion and perseverance. Her intelligence, drive and passion for research in sports nutrition made her one of the upcoming principal investigators and leaders in the field. She is greatly missed.

Luc van Loon, 2014

TRIBULUS TERRESTRIS

David S. Senchina

Tribulus terrestris (caltrop, puncturevine) grows in southern Asia and is consumed primarily by anaerobic athletes for its purported strength-enhancing capacities. Steroidal saponins (glycosides) are the purported bioactive compounds, believed to increase testosterone production thereby increasing muscle mass and strength. A recent study of young male rugby players who supplemented with *T terrestris* for five weeks (60% saponins by content) showed no effect of supplementation on strength, fat-free mass or urinary testosterone/epitestosterone levels (Rogerson *et al.*, 2007). This study is representative of the few others on the topic; considering this and other studies, one recent review concluded that *Tribulus* supplements should be considered neither safe nor beneficial (Pokrywka *et al.*, 2014). *Tribulus* supplements have also been found contaminated with substances banned by the World Anti-Doping Agency (de Hon and Coumans, 2007).

Competing interests None

TRYPTOPHAN

Takanobu Yamamoto and Linda M. Castell

Tryptophan (MW: $C_{11}H_{12}N_2O_2$) is an essential amino acid which contains an indole functional group and, uniquely, binds to albumin in the blood. Fatty acids bind competitively to albumin, and their mobilisation during exercise leads to tryptophan becoming unbound and thus to an increase in the plasma concentration of free tryptophan. Tryptophan is a precursor of 5-hydroxytryptamine (5-HT, also known as serotonin) which is involved in sleep and fatigue. Lieberman *et al.* (1983) observed that administration of tryptophan to humans increased subjective drowsiness and fatigue. An increase in tryptophan is thought to lead to an increased rate of synthesis of 5-HT and kynurenic acid.

Performance can be affected by central fatigue (emanating from the brain), which is linked to muscle fatigue (peripheral). The suppression of voluntary movement due to fatigue is a result of modulation of motor-neuron pathways in both the central and peripheral nervous systems. This is known to be triggered by tryptophan (Greenwood *et al.*, 1975; Yamamoto *et al.*, 2012). In addition, tryptophan is metabolized to the kynurenic pathway. Excessive brain tryptophan has been observed to lead to increased brain kynurenic acid in central fatigue as a result of chronic sleep disorder. This suggests that tryptophan and kynurenic acid may produce an amplified effect in central fatigue (Yamamoto *et al.*, 2012; Yamashita and Yamamoto, 2014). Branched chain amino acids (BCAA, see section on BCAA) bind competitively to the same port of entry across the blood-brain barrier as tryptophan. Coppola *et al.* (2013) observed that administration of BCAA in rats not only lowered exercise-induced fatigue but also reduced the higher concentration of kynurenic acid in the brain.

Tryptophan is best known for being prescribed to alleviate depression, probably because of its effects on sleep patterns. However, it has also been purported to have a beneficial effect on athletes. Two studies reported that 600mg tryptophan/day was linked with an increase in exercise duration (Segura and Ventura, 1988) or performance (Javierre *et al.*, 2010): the authors suggested that tryptophan ingestion might dampen the sensation of pain, thus enabling athletes to exercise for longer periods. However, Stensrud *et al.* (1992) repeated the 1988 study and found no beneficial effects of oral L-tryptophan on running performance. More recently, Stepto *et al.* (2011) studied football players undertaking reactive motor skills and agility protocols before and after fatiguing exercise. The intervention consisted of tryptophan-depleting and tryptophan-containing supplements ingested three hours before the trials. The participants also performed a baseline test in which no supplements were consumed. The tryptophan-depleted group showed a small improvement in reactive motor skills; however, there was a small performance decrement in the group which ingested tryptophan. In rats, where tryptophan uptake in the brain was suppressed via pre-treatment with 2-amino-2-norbornanecarboxylic acid (BCH), diminished central fatigue and improved running performance were observed (Yamamoto and Newsholme, 2000).

Some readers may be aware that L-tryptophan was removed from the market for several years from 1989, after deaths due to eosinophilia-myalgia. However, it was eventually established that the problem was contamination in the manufacturing process of one company. For a few years those wishing to prescribe tryptophan were careful to obtain it from other sources; its prescription to patients has again become more widespread.

Tryptophan availability has been observed to be important in immune function; however, this has not been studied in the context of exercise. There is currently no credible evidence that tryptophan supplementation has any beneficial effects on athletes. Indeed, as discussed at the start of this review, tryptophan is known to be a key substance in the initial reactions leading to fatigue and perception of fatigue. Thus, it seems more likely that tryptophan supplementation and a consequent increase in the plasma concentration of tryptophan might lead to premature fatigue in, for example, endurance events.

Competing interests   None

TYROSINE

Romain Meeusen and Bart Roelands

Tyrosine (4-hydroxyphenylalanine) is an amino acid that can be synthesized in the body from phenylalanine. Tyrosine shares a common transport molecule with large neutral amino acids at the blood-brain barrier; therefore an increase in the tyrosine ratio causes an increase in brain tyrosine which would lead to an increase in brain dopamine (DA) and noradrenaline (NA) concentration. Since both DA and NA play a key role in a variety of stress-related behaviours, it is not surprising that tyrosine has been the focus of considerable military interest for its cognitive 'anti-stress' effects.

A series of pre-clinical animal studies clearly indicate that tyrosine reduces many of the adverse effects of acute stress on cognitive performance in a wide variety of stressful environments. Although it has been difficult to demonstrate conclusively that tyrosine has beneficial effects in humans, in part due to ethical concerns, most of the evidence suggests that tyrosine is useful as an acute treatment to prevent stress-related declines in cognitive function. After finding that tyrosine supplementation promoted working memory updating, specifically in the demanding but not the easier condition of the N-back task (subjects were required to decide whether each stimulus in a sequence matched the one that appeared 'n' items ago), Colzato et al. (2013) suggested that tyrosine selectively targets cognitive control operations. This further suggests that tyrosine can replete cognitive resources when more control is needed. Tyrosine affects the same neurotransmitter systems as the amphetamines and related drugs, which are potent performance-enhancing compounds, although they have many side effects (Yeghiayan et al., 2001).

Results from studies examining acute tyrosine supplementation are not that straightforward. Different studies did not show benefits either on prolonged exercise capacity (Strüder et al., 1998) or performance (Chinevere et al., 2002) in temperate conditions. In the heat the outcomes are conflicting. Tumilty et al. (2011) showed that supplementing tyrosine one hour pre-exercise was associated with an increased cycling time to exhaustion in the heat (30°C). However, when the exercise mode was changed to a self-paced time trial at 30°C, there was no influence of the same dose of tyrosine (Tumilty et al., 2014). Furthermore, Watson et al. (2012) were not able to detect any effect of tyrosine supplementation on cycling time to exhaustion, nor on any cognitive markers when exercise was undertaken in the heat. More research is necessary to demonstrate any potential exercise and cognitive performance-enhancing effect of tyrosine.

Competing interests None

VALINE

Adrian B. Hodgson

Valine is a branched chain amino acid (BCAA), together with leucine and isoleucine; all are also essential amino acids (EAA) as they are not endogenously synthesised. While BCAA have been extensively studied (see section on BCAA), valine, in isolation, has received less attention. Valine has a number of important regulatory roles in the human body. Valine is involved as a precursor for succincyl-CoA anaplerosis in the tricarboyxlic acid (TCA) cycle (Gibala, 2001) and was hypothesised to contribute towards delaying the decrease in TCA intermediates and thus local muscle fatigue during prolonged and high-intensity exercise (Gibala *et al.*, 1999).

However, the ingestion of valine, in combination with the other BCAAs, does not alter the TCA cycle pool expansion during exercise (Gibala *et al.*, 1999). By contrast, BCAA have been shown to be effective in stimulating muscle protein synthesis following resistance exercise. However, in isolation, when valine was added to C2C12 myotubes, the anabolic signalling to mTORC1 was inferior when compared to leucine and other EAA (Atherton *et al.*, 2010a), suggesting the ingestion of all BCAA or complete EAA is required to generate a maximal anabolic response. Additionally, as reviewed elsewhere in this book, BCAA may have a role in reducing central fatigue. Valine alone has been shown to support the central fatigue hypothesis by attenuating the exercise-induced rise in tryptophan and 5-hydroxytryptamine in the hippocampus of rats (Gomez-Merino, 2001).

At present, there is little evidence, especially in humans, for the use of valine as an ergogenic aid in isolation from other BCAA and EAA.

Competing interests None

VANADIUM

Richard Baskerville

Vanadium is a trace element that is probably an essential nutrient, although deficiency states in humans have not been described and its precise biological role is yet to be fully defined. It is commonly found in mushrooms, green beans and cereals, with the usual dietary daily intake around 10–60 μg (Barceloux, 1999).

Vanadium has been taken in the form of vanadyl sulphate (VOSO4) for muscle development in weight training athletes at doses up to 60mg/day, to enhance muscle growth and body composition (Kreider, 1999). There is little evidence to support this practice. Of five studies using vanadyl sulphate supplementation, all failed to demonstrate a significant effect on anthropometry and/or body composition. The only study to demonstrate an improvement in performance was probably because the treatment group had a lower baseline fitness than the controls (Kreider, 1999). However, the cationic species of vanadium $(VO^{(2+)})$ does interact with muscle tissue actin at specific binding sites, altering protein conformation and function. The significance of this is unclear, but suggests some biological basis behind claims for vanadium effects on muscle (Ramos *et al.*, 2011).

At supraphysiological levels, *in vitro* and animal studies indicate that vanadate and other vanadium compounds exert measurable biological effects (Rehder, 2012). Effects on glucose transport activity and pancreatic β-cell function, via phosphatases and kinases, are currently the subject of research into antidiabetic therapeutics (Smith *et al.*, 2008). The role of vanadium as a transcription modulator of genes in oxidative stress and oncogenesis has also been described (Willsky *et al.*, 2006; Manna *et al.*, 2011) in studies investigating anti-cancer agents.

Vanadium in sulphate form has low toxicity or side effects (Barceloux, 1999). One study into adverse effects of vanadium failed to find any haematological or biochemical changes in 31 athletes taking 0.5mg/kg/day of vanadyl sulphate (Fawcett *et al.*, 1997).

In summary it appears that vanadium compounds are biologically active but not in areas associated with supplement consumption by weightlifting athletes.

Competing interests None

VITAMINS A, C AND E

David S. Senchina and Samantha J. Stear

Vitamins are a diverse set of chemicals that the human body is unable to make so need to be supplied in adequate amounts by the diet. They are required in very small quantities, μg or mg per day, but are essential for many processes carried out by the body. Vitamins are not chemically related, but one of the easiest ways of classifying them relates to their solubility in fat or water. The fat-soluble vitamins are A, D, E and K and the water-soluble vitamins are the B group of vitamins and vitamin C. This classification helps provide some indication of food sources, function and distribution in the body, and potential toxicity (see Figure 23).

Vitamins A, C and E are being discussed together because all three have antioxidant properties, though they differ in many other respects (see Figure 24). Individual reviews on vitamins B, D and K follow next in this book. Recent research has focused on these vitamins' antioxidant prospects because exercise induces free radical (ROS, reactive oxygen species) release which leads to cellular damage, fatigue and overtraining. Literally hundreds of studies on antioxidant vitamin supplementation and exercise have been published (see section on antioxidants). In the representative sample reviewed here, vitamin A was given as β-carotene, vitamin C as ascorbic acid and vitamin E as α-tocopherol.

Systematic training causes the body to develop adaptations naturally to the increase in exercise-induced ROS (Finaud et al., 2006), but it has been hypothesised that antioxidant vitamin supplementation may provide additional benefits (Bloomer, 2007). Studies both validate and refute this possibility.

	Fat-soluble vitamins Vitamins: A, D, E and K	Water-soluble vitamins Vitamins: B group and C
Risk of deficiency	Very low-fat diets and conditions where fat absorption is impaired	Diets lacking in variety
Stability in foods	Robust to heat and light	Varies; often unstable when exposed to heat and light
Storage in body	Can be large and long-term	Often small; so frequent regular intakes are required
Risk of toxicity	High	Low; as high intakes are usually excreted in urine

FIGURE 23 Characteristics of vitamin groups

	Vitamin A	Vitamin C	Vitamin E
Also known as	Retinol	Ascorbic acid	Tocopherol
Solubility	Fat	Water	Fat
Males 15–50+	700 µg/d (UK RNI) 900 µg/d (USA DRI)	40 mg/d (UK RNI) 75–90 mg/d (USA DRI)	4 mg/d (UK AI) ★ 15 mg/d (USA DRI)
Females, 15–50+	600 µg/d (UK RNI) 700 µg/d (USA DRI)	40 mg/d (UK RNI) 65–75 mg/d (USA DRI)	3 mg/d (UK AI) ★ 15 mg/d (USA DRI)
Functions	Antioxidant. Cell division and growth, bone and epithelia maintenance, vision	Antioxidant. Bone and cartilage maintenance, hormone synthesis, immune function, metabolism. Haemoglobin and red blood cell production. Helps absorption of iron from plant foods	Antioxidant. Immune function. Promotes normal growth and development
Dietary sources	Liver and offal, oily fish, dairy products, margarine, spinach, broccoli, carrots, red peppers, tomatoes, dark green and orange vegetables	Citrus fruits, berries and currants (e.g. strawberries and blackcurrants), kiwifruit, broccoli, green peppers, cabbage, spring greens and potatoes	Vegetable oils, wheatgerm, nuts, seeds, margarine, egg yolk, avocado
Body storage	Liver	Not stored	Adipose tissues

FIGURE 24   Properties of vitamins A, C and E★

Dietary recommended intakes are provided for UK RNI (recommended nutrient intake) and USA DRI (dietary recommended intake) for the general population aged 15–50+ years, for males and females (Department of Health, 2001; USDA/NAS, 2012).

★   Note: UK does not specifically provide a RNI for Vitamin E, since requirements depend on PUFA (polyunsaturated fatty acid) intake which varies widely. Instead they provide an estimated adequate intake (AI) for men and women.

In one study nine sedentary and nine active young males received 50mg/day vitamin A, 1,000mg/day vitamin C and 800mg/day vitamin E for two months and performed a treadmill ergometer VO_{2max} test before and after the treatment period (Senturk et al., 2005). Before supplementation, sedentary, but not trained, participants exhibited exercise-induced increased white blood cell and granulocyte levels and increased erythrocyte aggregation and deformability; after supplementation, these phenomena did not occur. Both sedentary and trained participants showed elevated erythrocyte lipid peroxidation after the VO_{2max}

test pre-supplementation but not post-supplementation. This study suggests that vitamin A, C and E supplementation augmented the already increased antioxidant capacity found in trained individuals. Adolescent male basketball players receiving 500mg/day vitamin C and 150mg/day vitamin E during intense training for 35 days, had higher plasma vitamin A (retinol), vitamin C and vitamin E, concomitant with elevated erythrocyte antioxidant glutathione (GSH-Px and GSH) compared with controls (Naziroğlu *et al.*, 2010).

By contrast, Yfanti *et al.* (2012) provided 21 sedentary young adult males with 500mg/day vitamin C and 400 IU/day vitamin E for 16 weeks, during endurance training for 12 weeks starting in week five. They observed a decrease in plasma IL-6 concentration in response to an acute exercise bout (cycle Pmax test) before training, but the same effect did not occur after training. Plasma IL-6 was higher in the supplemented/trained group than the placebo/trained group, indicating that either the supplement only worked in the sedentary condition or it attenuated the effects of training. Theodorou *et al.* (2011) supplemented 14 young adult males with 1g/day vitamin C and 400 IU/day vitamin E during seven weeks of resistance training and found no differences in acute exercise-induced plasma GSH or other markers of antioxidant capacity and redox status compared with similarly trained but non-supplemented controls.

Maximal performance parameters and muscle biopsy-determined glycogen, citrate synthase and β-hydroxyacyl-CoA activity levels were no different in antioxidant vitamin supplementation versus non-supplemented groups (Yfanti *et al.*, 2010). Roberts *et al.* (2011) gave eight active males 1g/day vitamin C for four weeks concomitant with aerobic training and found no impact on running performance. Gomes and colleagues (2011) reported that ten well-trained young adult male runners given either 500mg/day vitamin C plus 100 IU/day vitamin E or placebo for two weeks in a crossover design showed no differences in 8 km time-trial performance. Intriguingly, this latter study used an environmental chamber that simulated a hot, humid, ozone-polluted environment for the time trials and also reported that total plasma vitamin C and vitamin E concentrations were higher, whereas plasma and nasal lavage CC16 (Clara cell protein; a marker for lung cell damage) levels were lower in the vitamin C and E supplemented group versus placebo group (Gomes *et al.*, 2011). Braakhuis (2012) has suggested that those studies dosing athletes with vitamin C at 1g/day or greater, demonstrate negative effects on performance more often than benefits.

It is premature to draw any conclusions regarding the effectiveness or lack of antioxidant vitamin supplementation in athletes (see section on antioxidants). Experimental parameters (including subject, exercise and dosing characteristics) are variable across studies, rendering it difficult to make direct comparisons. Regardless of this, athletes who consume well-balanced meals should be receiving adequate supplies of vitamins A, C and E (Lukaski, 2004). It has been suggested that athletes would not be likely to receive any additional benefits from exceeding recommended daily intakes, RDI (Nikolaidis *et al.*, 2012), and that additional supplementation may only be necessary in cases of extreme, prolonged physical exertion under adverse environmental conditions (Gomes *et al.*, 2011; Halsey and Stroud, 2012). Nevertheless, multivitamin supplements are readily available to athletes, vary widely in their vitamin doses, and often contain vitamins at RDI or greater levels (35–300% RDI). Toxicity via over-supplementation is more likely to occur with the fat-soluble vitamins (vitamins A, D, E and K). Excess antioxidant vitamins may be detrimental to athletes when they interfere with normal levels of ROS-mediated intracellular signalling, disrupting redox balance and interfering with normal muscle cell function (McGinley *et al.*, 2009) and performance. Current data suggest that vitamin A, C and E supplementation, in the doses used across studies, either improved or had no effect on physiologically relevant markers of antioxidant capacity and either decreased or had no effect on performance outcomes.

There is no question that athletes experience increased oxidative stress as a result of their activity levels, but the issue of whether or not athletes need higher dietary antioxidants than less active counterparts remains under debate. There are hypotheses as well as data to support a beneficial use, a neutral outcome in people who are already achieving intakes at recommended levels from dietary sources, and even a detrimental effect on training adaptations. Athletes consuming a balanced diet commensurate with their caloric needs, including vegetables, fruits and whole grains, are likely to be receiving adequate levels of antioxidant vitamins. For those athletes 'erring on the side of caution', food-based sources of antioxidant vitamins may be preferable to supplement-based sources because the possibility of toxicity is lower when foods are utilised. Although daily multivitamin supplements are generally regarded as safe, over-supplementation may result in disrupted redox balance or diminished performance. Further studies may help clarify which of these outcomes is the most likely, given the various scenarios of training, environment and diet in which athletes may find themselves.

Competing interests   None

VITAMIN B

Mayur K. Ranchordas and Shelly Meltzer

The B-vitamins are water-soluble vitamins that play crucial roles in energy metabolism, in synthesis of new cells, red blood cells and in cell repair. There are eight B-vitamins: thiamine (B1), riboflavin (B2), niacin (B3), pantothenic acid (B5), pyridoxine (B6), biotin (B7), involved in energy-producing pathways, folic acid (B9), and cobalamin (B12) involved in synthesising new cells, red blood cells and in cell repair. The richest sources of B-vitamins are unprocessed foods such as whole grains, green leafy vegetables, nuts, dairy products and animal foods such as meat and eggs, but in many countries foods such as cereals and bread are fortified with these vitamins.

It has been reported that inadequate intake and deficiencies in B-vitamins could impair athletic performance (van der Beek *et al.*, 1988, 1994) and there is also the notion that requirements may increase with heavy exercise training (Telford *et al.*, 1992; Woolf and Manore, 2006). Studies examining dietary intakes of B-vitamins in athletes have found that males typically report higher intakes than females because of their overall higher energy intake (Hawley *et al.*, 1995; Martinez *et al.*, 2011). Female athletes on an energy-restricted diet and/or who exhibit disordered eating practices have lower intakes of riboflavin, folate and pyridoxine (Manore, 1994, 2000; Beals and Manore, 1998; Woolf and Manore, 2006). In semi-professional adolescent swimmers, a poor intake of fruit and vegetables has been associated with an inadequate dietary intake of folic acid (Martinez *et al.*, 2011).

Results from studies on the status of B-vitamins are mixed. Some studies reported adequate cobalamin status in athletes (Woolf and Manore, 2006) but others demonstrated altered cobalamin metabolism in recreational athletes compared with non-exercising controls (Herrmann *et al.*, 2005). Similarly, poor pyridoxine and folate status in athletes has been documented in some studies (Fogelholm, 1992; Fogelholm *et al.*, 1993b; Beals and Manore, 1998; Herrmann *et al.*, 2005). In a recent study, swimmers did not sufficiently increase their energy intake to meet their increased energy expenditure requirements, and their blood thiamin concentrations decreased significantly, yet the concentration of riboflavin was unchanged, suggesting that intense training affects thiamin but not riboflavin requirements (Sato *et al.*, 2011). The effects on performance *per se* were not determined.

Similarly, several researchers have shown that exercise modifies pyridoxine metabolism with one study reporting losses of 1mg during a marathon race (Rokitzki *et al.*, 1994); however, there are no studies on the effects of pyridoxine supplementation on performance. When adequate status is present, supplementation of single B-vitamins (for example, thiamine or folate) does not appear to enhance exercise performance (Webster *et al.*, 1997; Matter *et al.*, 1987). However B-vitamin deficiencies do not usually occur in isolation and may be why single vitamin depletion studies fail to detect performance effects.

Therapeutic benefits of folate and cobalamin supplementation in exercising populations have been demonstrated. High folate and cobalamin intakes in conjunction with regular exercise may reduce plasma homocysteine concentrations which, in turn, can lower the risk factor for cardiovascular disease (Crozier *et al.*, 1991). Several recent studies have demonstrated that 10mg folic acid for four to six weeks significantly improved brachial artery flow mediated dilation in eumenorrheic (Hoch *et al.*, 2009b) and amenorrheic runners (Hoch *et al.*, 2010) and in professional ballet dancers (Hoch *et al.*, 2009a), however the investigators caution that optimal dosage still needs to be determined in a larger cohort, supplemented for a longer time, before this should be considered as a therapeutic intervention for athletes opposed to estrogen supplementation (Hoch *et al.*, 2010).

Athletes and female athletes in particular, who eliminate certain food groups such as dairy, milk or fruit and vegetables, restrict energy intake, and engage in disordered eating practices, are at a greater risk of developing inadequate status of B-vitamins. Regular exercise training may increase the requirements for some B-vitamins such as thiamin and pyridoxine; however, further research is necessary to establish whether this is the case for folate and cobalamin (Woolf and Manore, 2006). According to current evidence, when adequate intakes and status of B-vitamins are present, further supplementation does not enhance exercise performance.

Further well-controlled studies are required to investigate the effects of B-vitamin supplementation on exercise performance in athletes, and on physical activity and health, against a background of both adequate and inadequate status.

Competing interests   None

VITAMIN D

D. Enette Larson-Meyer

It is well recognised that vitamin D plays an important role in calcium regulation and bone health. Emerging evidence, however, suggests that vitamin D is also important in immune and inflammatory modulation and skeletal muscle function. With such roles, vitamin D has the potential to impact the health, training and performance of athletes, necessitating an updated understanding of the vitamin D status of athletes and appropriate guidelines for managing sub-optimal status.

Vitamin D synthesis and sources

Although vitamin D is considered a 'vitamin', required amounts can be obtained entirely from cutaneous synthesis via exposure to ultraviolet-B (UVB) radiation in sunlight (Holick, 2007; Hossein-Nezhad and Holick, 2013). Cutaneous synthesis of vitamin D, however, is dependent on factors including time of exposure, season, latitude, cloud cover, smog, skin pigmentation, sunscreen coverage and age. Vitamin D is not synthesised during the winter at latitudes greater than 35° north or south because insufficient UVB photons reach the earth's surface during these months (Holick, 2007; Hollis, 2005).

Vitamin D is also obtained in the diet from limited natural and fortified sources (Figure 25). Dietary vitamin D includes vitamin D3 (cholecalciferol), derived from animal sources, and vitamin D2 (or ergocalciferol), derived from UVB exposure of fungi and yeast ergosterols (Holick, 2007; Hossein-Nezhad and Holick, 2013). Both forms are readily absorbed (~50% bioavailable), except in individuals with malabsorptive disorders (Basu and Donaldson, 2003).

Vitamin D status of athletes

It is well recognised that suboptimal vitamin D status (see definitions, Figure 26) is widespread among the general population worldwide. Among athletes, the prevalence of deficiency varies by sport, training location (Larson-Meyer and Willis, 2010), lifestyle habits and skin colour (Hamilton *et al.*, 2010; Pollock *et al.*, 2012; Shindle *et al.*, 2011). 25(OH)D concentrations are generally lower in the winter and among athletes who train predominantly indoors, but serum concentrations can also be low among outdoor athletes who train in the early morning or late afternoon. For example, a high prevalence of vitamin D deficiency has been observed in gymnasts training in East Germany (Bannert *et al.*, 1991) and Finland (Lehtonen-Veromaa *et al.*, 1999), with 37% to 68%

Recommended dietary allowance (Adults*)	Australia and New Zealand: 200 IU Nordic countries: 300 IU United Kingdom: 200 IU United States and Canada: 600 IU World Health Organisation: 200 IU
Dietary sources	Fatty fish (salmon, mackerel, sardines, tuna); irradiated mushrooms; fortified milk; egg yolk; some brands/types of margarine, yogurt, soy milk, fruit juice and ready-to-eat cereal; egg yolks
Signs and symptoms of deficiency	Elevated parathyroid concentration, decreased bone density; bone pain; increased bone fracture risk; muscle weakness and discomfort; atrophy of type II fibres, abnormal growth in children (Note: Many symptoms of deficiency mimic those of fibromyalgia and chronic fatigue syndrome)
Signs and symptoms of toxicity	Elevated serum calcium; fatigue; constipation; back pain; forgetfulness; nausea; vomiting. Complications of prolonged elevated serum calcium include soft tissue calcification, hypertension and abnormal heart rhythm

FIGURE 25 Vitamin D: recommended dietary allowance, dietary sources and signs and symptoms of deficiency and toxicity

* Note: Adult requirements generally include adults 18 or 19 years and older; requirements are higher in most countries in adults older than 65 to 70 years.

of these athletes having serum 25(OH)D concentrations under 10–15 ng/mL (25–37.5 nmol/L). Similarly, 91% of Middle Eastern sportsmen training in Qatar were found to have serum 25(OH)D concentrations under 20 ng/mL (50 nmol/L), indicating high rates of deficiency (Hamilton et al., 2010). In contrast, a low prevalence of insufficiency/deficiency and better overall status has been documented in several groups of US college athletes with as few as 0 to 12% exhibiting deficient or insufficient status in the autumn (Halliday et al., 2011; Lewis et al., 2013). The one study that evaluated frequency of optimal status found that 15% to 76% maintained optimal status at different points during the season with the best status observed in autumn (Halliday et al., 2011). Although the most probable reason for suboptimal vitamin D status is limited (or insufficient) UVB exposure, poor vitamin D intake may contribute. Studies have found that athletes do not meet the recommended dietary allowance (RDA) for vitamin D of most countries, as summarised in Figure 25 (Helle and Bjerkan, 2011; Larson-Meyer and Willis, 2010; Sonneville et al., 2012). Indeed, one study found that only 5% of US college athletes consumed the US RDA of 600 IU of vitamin D from food alone (Halliday et al., 2011).

Vitamin D status and overall health

Evidence increasingly suggests that suboptimal vitamin D status is linked to increased risk for many chronic and autoimmune diseases including hypertension, diabetes, cardiovascular disease, osteoarthritis and cancer (Holick, 2007; Hossein-Nezhad and Holick, 2013), and possibly also acute illnesses and injury (Larson-Meyer and Willis, 2010). Poor vitamin D status and/or low dietary intake has been linked to increased risk for stress fracture (Ruohola et al., 2006; Sonneville et al., 2012), upper respiratory tract infection (Halliday et al., 2011; He et al., 2013; Laaksi et al., 2007), elevated concentrations of systemic inflammatory markers (Willis et al., 2012) and delayed recovery following orthopaedic surgery (Barker et al., 2011). Elevated systemic inflammatory markers may prove to be important in the development and progression of over-training syndrome and/ or chronic injury. A few studies have found that vitamin D supplementation and/or UVB exposure improves these health outcomes. For example, in female naval recruits, eight weeks of supplementation with 800 IU vitamin D plus 2,000mg calcium reduced stress fracture incidence by 20% compared to placebo treatment (Lappe et al., 2008). In non-athletic post-menopausal women, one-year supplementation with 2,000 IU vitamin D (as part of a randomized-control trial for osteoporosis prevention) nearly abolished reported incidence of colds and flu compared to control (Aloia and Li-Ng, 2007). An older German treatment study found that UVB irradiation via a central sun lamp for six weeks resulted in a reduction in chronic pain due to sports injuries (Spellerberg, 1952). Another recent study in UK professional dancers found that four-month supplementation with 2,000 IU vitamin D/day reduced the occurrence of injury (Wyon et al., 2014).

Vitamin D status and athletic performance

Muscle pain and weakness are well-documented but frequently forgotten symptoms of severe vitamin D deficiency (Figure 25) that improve upon repletion (Holick, 2007). Recent animal and *in vitro* studies have found that vitamin D is important for calcium handling across the sarcolemma and expression of proteins involved in muscle contraction (Barker et al., 2011). Whether such muscle pain or weakness is common in athletes to a level that would deter performance is not yet established. Currently only a handful of studies have evaluated vitamin D status and performance in athletes (Close et al., 2013a, 2013b; Dubnov et al., 2013). Of these studies, two have found improved performance markers after oral supplementation. One in previously deficient elite English soccer players found that supplementation with 5,000 IU/ day for eight weeks improved 10-metre sprint and vertical jump performances but not 30-metre sprint time or squat ability (Close et al., 2013a). The other in professional UK dancers found that supplementation with 2,000 IU/day for four weeks improved quadriceps strength and power and vertical jump performance (Wyon *et al.*, 2014). Provocative evidence from the Russian and German literature at the turn of the twentieth century also suggests that UVB exposure positively affects athletic performance (Cannell *et al.*, 2009). These studies, however, were not conducted using the rigorous scientific standards employed today.

Assessment and recommendations for supplementation

Vitamin D supplementation may benefit the health and performance of many athletes but should not be routinely recommended without assessment. Serum 25(OH) D concentration, the best indicator of vitamin D status (Holick, 2007; Hollis, 2005; Hossein-Nezhad and Holick, 2013), should first be evaluated along with anthropometric measurements (including body fat estimation), dietary intake, and lifestyle and environmental factors that potentially impact status (Larson-Meyer and Willis, 2010). Both body fat and body size are important to consider because they are inversely correlated with vitamin D status. This is due to either sequestration (Holick, 2007; Larson-Meyer and Willis, 2010; Heller *et al.*, 2014) or volumetric dilution (Drincic *et al.*, 2012) of ingested or cutaneously-synthesised vitamin D by the larger fat mass. This potentially increases supplemental dose in larger or fatter athletes.

Following assessment, recommendations for achieving/maintaining optimal vitamin D status can be individualised to the athlete's current serum 25(OH) D concentration, diet, belief system and, if present, clinical symptoms (Figure 25) (Larson-Meyer and Willis, 2010). Habitual exposure to arms, legs and back several times a week for five minutes (for fair-skinned individuals) to 30 minutes (for darker-skinned individuals) at close to solar noon without sunscreen (Holick, 2007; Hossein-Nezhad and Holick, 2013) usually leads to sufficient vitamin D synthesis in summer months.

Individuals with limited sun exposure require supplementation with at least 1,500–2,000 IU/day vitamin D to keep 25(OH)D concentrations in the sufficient (Holick *et al.*, 2011), but not necessarily optimal, range. Higher supplemental doses may be required in those with little sun exposure, regular sunscreen use, dark-pigmented skin and/or excess adiposity. Athletes who live or train at latitudes above/below 35 to 37° north or south should consider vitamin D supplementation during winter, rainy or cloudy seasons even if they maintain adequate stores during sunnier seasons. Regular consumption of vitamin D-fortified foods is not likely to result in sufficient status in the absence of UVB exposure (Cannell and Hollis, 2008).

Although specific guidelines for supplemental vitamin D are not yet established, a rule-of-thumb is to increase supplemental vitamin D by 1,000 IU over three to four months for every 10 ng/mL elevation in 25(OH)D desired (Cannell and Hollis, 2008). Thus, a 'normal-weight' athlete with a serum 25(OH)D concentration of 20 ng/mL would require an additional 2,000 IU daily to increase stores to 40 ng/mL in three to four months. Higher doses than estimated using this rule-of-thumb may be needed to improve status in some athletes; these include those with larger body size, excess adiposity or very low starting serum 25(OH)D concentration. Genetic differences also influence response to supplementation (Fu *et al.*, 2009). Supplemental vitamin D can be taken either daily or as a larger bimonthly or monthly dose (i.e. 50,000 IU/ month ~1667 IU/day).

To replenish stores more rapidly, athletes with deficient status may benefit from short-term, high-dose 'loading' regimens under supervision of a physician. Examples of high-dose regimens include 50,000 IU/week for eight to16 weeks or 10,000 IU/day for several weeks (Cannell and Hollis, 2008; Holick, 2007). Increasing evidence suggests that supplementation with D3 is more effective than D2 at higher doses (Heaney *et al.*, 2011). Vitamin D2 supplementation was recently found to amplify muscle damage following eccentric exercise in athletes (Nieman *et al.*, 2014). Athletes who often believe more is better should be cautioned that daily supplementation with more than 10,000 IU could lead to toxicity.

Conclusion

Vitamin D plays an important role in a vast array of physiological functions; vitamin D deficiency could negatively affect the health and performance of athletes. Research suggests that certain athletes are at risk for suboptimal vitamin D status, which may increase risk for stress fractures, acute illness, elevated inflammatory markers and impaired recovery following orthopedic injury. Given these findings, regular vitamin D supplementation may be beneficial for some but not all athletes to help optimise health and athletic performance.

Competing interests None

VITAMIN K

Sarah L. Booth and Bronwen Lundy

Vitamin K is of interest to sports performance through its proposed role in either preventing or speeding healing from bone injury. Vitamin K is a co-enzyme involved in the γ-carboxylation of certain proteins in bone, including osteocalcin. Vitamin K is found in plant-based foods as phylloquinone (K1) and can be synthesised by bacteria as menaquinones (K2). Little is known about relative bioavailability and biological activities of the different forms of vitamin K. Current recommended dietary intakes for vitamin K are based on a diet that is sufficient to promote normal blood clotting. It is not known how much vitamin K is required for optimal bone health (Beulens *et al.*, 2013), but low vitamin K status has been linked with increased risk of hip fracture (Booth *et al.*, 2000; Cheung *et al.*, 2008). Reduction in the number of bone injuries or the time taken to recover from these could significantly enhance sports performance by reducing the loss of training time due to injury.

The impact of vitamin K on bone health has been examined mostly in post-menopausal women. In a 2006 meta-analysis (Cockayne *et al.*, 2006), vitamin K supplementation was assessed against bone loss and fracture risk. It was concluded that menaquinone supplementation may decrease fracture risk, and both phylloquinone and menaquinones reduced bone loss. However the authors cautioned that the low number and poor quality of studies available at the time of the analysis limited the validity of the conclusions (Cockayne *et al.*, 2006). Another meta-analysis concluded that supplementation with phylloquinone may improve bone density at the lumbar spine, but not at the femoral neck (Fang *et al.*, 2012). The strength of the conclusions was again limited by the large heterogeneity in findings. Supplemental doses of vitamin K studied in these analyses varied between 1–45mg/day, which are well above the current Australian Adequate Intake (AI) of 60–70 μg/day (Australian National Health and Medical Research Council *et al.*, 2006). In both meta-analyses, the majority of studies were undertaken in post-menopausal Asian women meaning this may not be applicable to other population groups, such as athletes, and individuals of different racial/ethnic groups.

Only a few studies have examined either dietary vitamin K intake or status and fracture risk in athletic populations. Iwamoto *et al.* (2010) assessed 71 professional baseball players for urinary markers of bone resorption; of these, nine were found to have high levels of the marker and were further assessed for dietary vitamin K intake and serum status of phylloquinone and menaquinones. While dietary vitamin K was found to meet the Japanese AI (Sasaki, 2008), serum status was found to be low in all nine players assessed. These players were also shown to have sub-optimal calcium intake and a low vitamin D status, thus it is unclear what relationship if any vitamin K status had on the raised bone resorption markers. Another study looking at 16 Japanese Shorinji Kempo athletes found a mean vitamin K intake of 149.5 ± 105.3 μg, which is lower than the designated AI; however, there was no relationship between vitamin K intake and fracture in this group (Sasaki, 2008).

A pilot for an intervention study (Craciun *et al.*, 1998) found that phylloquinone supplementation (10mg/day for four weeks) improved markers of bone formation in athletes. Five out of eight athletes were classed as deficient in vitamin K at baseline, with supplementation having a larger effect on bone markers in these athletes with low vitamin K status. It is unclear if this is representative of status in athlete populations generally. Braam and colleagues (2003) undertook a two- year study of phylloquinone supplementation (10mg/day) in 115 female runners, tracking menstrual status and bone loss, as measured by BMD. This study failed to find any benefit of supplementation, although limitations such as the low level of follow up (six-monthly contact) and absence of adherence measures are noted.

Given the mixed findings in the role of vitamin K in bone health generally, and the limited information available in athletic populations, further studies are required before it is routinely considered in the management of bone health in athletes.

Competing interests   None

WATER (OXYGENATED)

Louise M. Burke

Oxygenated water products, also marketed as super-oxygenated water, oxygenized water or 'Vitamin O', are claimed to contain three to 30 times the oxygen (O_2) content of normal tap water and to enhance health, vitality and sports performance. Manufacturers have been known to claim that at one time the O_2 level in our environment was at 38%, now it is at 21%, and thus we seemingly have only about half the oxygen that our bodies were apparently designed to run on in order to be in good health! However, in fact it is believed that although atmospheric O_2 levels may have peaked at 30%, this was 300 million years ago, with the earliest human ancestors evolving only around six or seven million years ago when O_2 levels would have been very similar to today's. Hence, the background provided by some manufacturers of these products is unlikely and the central issue of whether the gut can deliver a useful source of O_2 to the bloodstream is not supported by good evidence. Furthermore, the recommended doses of different products range from several drops to substantial volumes (e.g. 500ml).

Despite the uncertainty of the hypothetical basis of oxygenated waters, several studies have been undertaken to investigate the marketing claims targeting athletes. Results from published peer-reviewed literature involving the acute intake of oxygenated water products prior to exercise in normoxic conditions show a failure to increase VO_{2max} in recreational to moderately trained people (Hampson *et al.*, 2003; Leibetseder *et al.*, 2006; Wilmert *et al.*, 2002). Similarly, acute intake of a product was also unable to enhance O_2 use during submaximal cycling or performance of a subsequent time trial (McNaughton *et al.*, 2007). Indeed, when the O_2 content of the products used in the studies was measured, it was found to be higher than tap water but failed to meet the oxygenation levels claimed by the manufacturers (Hampson *et al.*, 2003; Leibetseder *et al.*, 2006). Finally, a three-day protocol of supplementation failed to achieve benefits to cycling time-trial performance undertaken under hypoxic conditions (Wing-Gaia *et al.*, 2005). The role of O_2 delivery to the muscles in determining the performance of many sports is clearly recognised, but it appears that oxygenated waters fail to improve on the capacity provided by the respiratory and circulatory system. Thus there is little to recommend the use of these products by athletes. In fact, the abstract of another review on this topic provides a succinct summary in the form of a single sentence, 'Ergogenic claims for oxygenated water cannot be taken seriously' (Piantadosi, 2006).

Competing interests   None

WEIGHT LOSS SUPPLEMENTS: GENERAL

Samantha J. Stear

Without doubt, physique, including body mass or composition, size and shape, has an important role to play in optimizing sports performance. Size does matter! Consequently various strategies, including dietary intervention, are employed in an effort to influence physique. Fundamentally, body weight (body mass) is lost when dietary energy (energy intake) is consumed at a level less than daily requirements (energy expenditure), with an energy deficit ~10–20% being both effective in producing loss and being tolerated over the longer term. However, although any strategy, including popular/fad diets, that reduces energy intake below expenditure will result in weight loss, most athletes need to achieve a more specific goal of promoting loss of body fat while maintaining lean body mass and optimizing sports performance. Therefore, athletes embarking on an energy-reduction programme should do so only under the guidance of a sports nutrition professional. This will ensure that intakes of important macronutrients and micronutrients are not detrimentally compromised and that energy intake is sufficient to support their training/competition needs. Although there is growing evidence of a positive role for dairy/calcium intake in assisting weight/ fat loss (Manore, 2012), this has not yet been extensively studied in the athletic population.

In the multibillion dollar supplement industry, 'weight loss' supplements contribute a significant proportion. A huge range of supplements claim to enhance sports performance by affecting body composition – either by increasing muscle mass and/or reducing body fat. Often, these 'weight loss', sometimes described as 'fat burner', supplements contain a number of ingredients, each with its own proposed mechanism of action, which include: increasing fat metabolism or energy expenditure; impairing fat absorption, increasing fat utilization as a fuel source during exercise. Supplements in the broad 'weight loss' category include: caffeine (including coffee, green tea, guarana and yerba maté); L-carnitine; chromium picolinate; CLA (conjugated linoleic acid); dairy/ calcium supplements; HMB (β-hydroxy- β-methylbutyrate); Hydroxycut; leucine; phenylalanine; protein supplements; and tyrosine. This list covers the most popular ingredients/supplements purported to aid weight loss, all of which are reviewed individually elsewhere in the book, though not all may have mentioned the 'weight loss' aspect due to lack of supporting evidence. To ensure this appraisal of weight loss supplements is complete, these ingredients/ supplements will be mentioned briefly here, alongside their reference from when they were previously reviewed for our A–Z nutritional supplement series in the *BJSM*. However, since caffeine and hydroxycut are of a herbal origin, they will be discussed further in the review that follows, on herbal weight loss supplements.

L-carnitine is synthesised from the amino acids lysine and methionine and is found naturally in the human diet, particularly in red meat and dairy products. It has been suggested that L-carnitine supplementation can increase fatty acid transport into mitochondria, leading to an increase in fatty acid oxidation and hence the proposed potential benefit for weight management, but further investigation is required (Broad *et al.*, 2005; Rogers *et al.*, 2009). Chromium picolinate, a complex of trivalent chromium (a trace mineral) and picolinic acid, which is better absorbed than dietary chromium, has been heavily marketed for both muscle building and fat loss, but the overwhelming majority of the data does not support these purported benefits (see section on chromium picolinate). Furthermore, it has been shown that chromium picolinate supplementation coupled with a training programme does not enhance body composition or performance variables beyond improvements seen with training alone (Clancy *et al.*, 1994; Trent and Thieding-Cancel, 1995; Walker *et al.*, 1998).

Conjugated linoleic acid (CLA), is a term for a series of structural and geometric isomers of linoleic acid. Studies investigating the role of CLA supplements in decreasing fat mass and/or increasing lean mass have been inconsistent with systematic reviews generally showing no effect or such a small effect that it is not clinically relevant (see section on CLA). Moreover, studies of CLA supplementation, either singularly or in combination with other potentially 'active' ingredients, in individuals who exercise have also produced mixed results.

There is now considerable evidence showing that during periods of energy restriction in exercising individuals, a higher protein intake can enhance fat-free mass (FFM) preservation (Bendtsen *et al.*, 2013; Murphy *et al.*, 2014). Therefore, athletes wishing to reduce fat mass while preserving FFM, should combine a moderate energy deficit (-500kcal d^{-1}) with some form of resistance exercise, whilst increasing their protein intake ($\sim$1.8–2.7g kg^{-1} d^{-1}). Furthermore, they should focus on the protein in post-exercise meals being from protein sources with high leucine content and rapid digestion kinetics such as whey protein (Murphy *et al.*, 2014).

In addition, some of the individual amino acids, namely leucine, phenylalanine and tyrosine, and a metabolite of leucine, HMB, have been specifically studied regarding their potential effect on weight/fat loss (see relevant sections in book). HMB is a metabolite of the essential branched chain amino acid leucine, with research providing some evidence that HMB supplements offer some assistance in reducing the breakdown of muscle protein, similar to the effect shown with leucine, and another essential amino acid, phenylalanine. Recent reviews suggest that HMB supplementation augments lean mass and strength gains associated with resistance training, but the results differ according to training status, with generally a minimal effect in untrained subjects to negligible effect in those more experienced (see section on HMB). However, tyrosine, an amino acid that can be synthesized in the body from phenylalanine, has not specifically been investigated in regard to its potential effect on weight loss.

In terms of weight loss, it is advisable to make informed dietary changes prior to reaching for supplements. As always, and particularly in the case of some of the herbs discussed next where the evidence is scant, athletes are strongly recommended to seek advice from a sports nutrition professional before considering using any supplements. Furthermore, as stressed throughout this book, it is essential to reiterate that any athlete who competes under the WADA code (World Anti-Doping Agency: www.wada-ama.org) needs to be extremely cautious about using supplements and should always work with a qualified professional on risk minimisation of supplement use. The ethical/legality issues of sport can be contravened either by deliberate use of over-the-counter compounds that are prohibited by such codes (e.g. prohormones and stimulants) or by inadvertent intake of these products due to contamination, fake or doping issues, with banned stimulants, such as ephedrine or sibutramine, being frequently found in weight loss supplements (see introduction chapter for further information on WADA and inadvertent doping).

Finally, there is also a vast array of herbs found in supplements including, but not limited to, those marketed for weight loss. The diversity of individual herbs as well as their simultaneous presence in some products, sometimes more than ten in one product, has become a minefield that both athletes and their sports medicine and science support staff find difficult to navigate. It is worrying how prolific these supplements have become, despite their tenuous, if any, link to a mechanism for weight loss and the lack of supporting scientific evidence (Senchina *et al.*, 2013b). The following review on herbal weight loss supplements includes a utilitarian and novel classification, originally developed for our A–Z of nutritional supplements series in the *BJSM* (Senchina *et al.*, 2013b), to help demystify and clarify the rationale behind the wide assortment of herbs used as the active ingredient(s) in multiple supplements, particularly in the seemingly fashionable supplements marketed as having 'thermogenic' properties.

Competing interests None

WEIGHT LOSS SUPPLEMENTS: HERBAL

David S. Senchina

Many weight loss supplements used by athletes contain herbs as active agents (see Figure 27) which can be vexing given their botanical, chemical and clinical diversity. This section uses a system originally developed for the *BJSM* 'Nutritional Supplement Series' (Senchina *et al.*, 2013b) for conceptualizing herbal weight loss supplements by putative mechanisms of activity based on each supplement's presumed bioactive compounds, which are mainly secondary metabolites (SM) and can be categorized into six main groups: alkaloids, flavonoids, polysaccharides, phenolics, terpenoids and other molecules. Most herbs in this review contain compounds from multiple SM categories.

Alkaloids are nitrogen-rich molecules derived from amino acid precursors: caffeine is a well-known example. Caffeine and similar molecules increase metabolism and consequently achieve a small increase in the body's rate of energy (calorie, kilojoule) expenditure. Although the physiological relevance of this effect is debated, such herbal weight loss aids are often described as 'thermogenic'. Examples of caffeine-rich herbs include coffee, green tea, guarana and yerba maté (see relevant sections in the book). Other alkaloid-rich herbs used for weight loss include bitter orange, black pepper, cayenne pepper, ephedra, ginger and Indian coleus (see relevant sections). Not all plants that contain alkaloids are considered weight loss aids (e.g. chocolate, which contains theobromine and theophylline; see section in book). Reviews have concluded that, of these, bitter orange, caffeine, ephedra, ginger and green tea supplements may be efficacious in weight loss (Sharpe *et al.*, 2006; Hasani-Ranjbar *et al.*, 2009; Poddar *et al.*, 2011), but isolated supplements of caffeine, ephedra and guarana may carry serious adverse event risks in the general population (Pittler *et al.*, 2005; Poddar *et al.*, 2011). Indeed, the sale of ephedra was banned by the FDA in 2004. Furthermore, it was included on the List of Banned Substances by the International Olympic Committee years prior to that and is currently prohibited for use in competition according to the WADA Prohibited List (WADA, 2014b). Research reports have suggested that multi-component green tea/black pepper/ cayenne pepper (Rondanelli *et al.*, 2013), and yerba maté (Andersen and Fogh, 2001) supplements may promote weight loss, but yerba maté supplements may carry adverse effects (Pittler *et al.*, 2005).

Terpenoids, also called isoprenoids, are lipids derived from five-carbon isoprene structures and include carotenoids, steroids and saponins. Terpenoids could conceivably work through several different mechanisms, though anorexiant and diuretic effects are most commonly reported. Weight loss herbs that presumably work through terpenoids include bearberry (kinnikinnick, uva ursi), bitter melon, dandelion, ginseng, gymnema, hoodia, Indian coleus, rhodiola, sarsaparilla (*Smilax*), Siberian ginseng and veldt grape, which contains *Cissus quadrangularis*, a frequent component of Hydroxycut (see relevant sections in the book). Recent reviews indicate bitter melon, ginseng, Siberian ginseng and veldt grape may be efficacious or have no effect on weight loss in the general population (Sharpe *et al.*, 2006; Hasani-Ranjbar *et al.*, 2009; Poddar *et al.*, 2011), but none have been flagged for adverse events. The supplement Hydroxycut, which contains multiple herbal and other products and varies in composition, is not recommended for use by athletes due to safety and efficacy concerns (see section on Hydroxycut). Hoodia has no evidence for or against it as a weight loss agent (Whelan *et al.*, 2010). One study in overweight women concluded that Indian coleus supplementation does not directly promote weight loss, but may help in weight management (Henderson *et al.*, 2005). In obese rodents, gymnema supplements stimulated weight loss (Luo *et al.*, 2007), whereas in diabetic rodents, bearberry supplementation maintained body weight, but decreased appetite and thirst (Swanston-Flatt *et al.*, 1989a), and dandelion had no effect (Swanston-Flatt *et al.*, 1989b). No studies could be located regarding sarsaparilla and weight loss.

Flavonoids are derived from phenylalanine precursors and include anthocyanins and quercetin (see section on flavonoids), and are found in herbs such as dandelion and elderberry. A mechanism by which they might assist weight loss is by reducing lipogenesis and/or increasing lipolysis. Elderberry, along with milk thistle, white willow, coffee and tea, also contain phenols (characterised by having both aromatic hydrocarbon and hydroxyl groups) such as tannins. From little information, reviews indicate elderberry, milk thistle and white willow have not convincingly demonstrated weight loss properties, yet none have perceived risk (Sharpe *et al.*, 2006; Hasani-Ranjbar *et al.*, 2009; Kidd, 2009).

Some weight loss aids presumably work through fibre (roughage). Fibre is comprised of polysaccharides that stimulate peristalsis through their laxative effects, may satiate appetite and may block fat absorption, thus contributing to weight loss. Fibre-rich weight loss herbs include guar bean, konjac and psyllium. Primary data conflict regarding their safety and efficacy. Two recent reviews concluded konjac and psyllium may be effective but carry some risk of adverse effects (Pittler *et al.*, 2005; Poddar *et al.*, 2011).

The 'other' category includes herbs that presumably work through the enzyme phaseolamin, like white bean, which may be efficacious in weight loss, and gambooge (*Garcinia* spp; not to be confused with the pigment 'gamboge'), which putatively works through hydroxycitric acid. Gambooge, formerly a common component of Hydroxycut was removed from that formulation around 2010 due to concerns about hepatotoxicity; several recent reviews conflict in

Common name	Scientific name	Organ used	SM group	Bioactive compound(s)	Comment
Bearberry, Kinnikinnick	*Arctostaphylos uva-ursi*	F,L	TER	Arbutin	?
Black pepper	*Piper nigrum*	F	ALK	Piperine	?
Bitter melon	*Momordica charantia*	F	TER	Momordicins	✓
Bitter orange	*Citrus aurantium*	F	ALK	Synephrine	?
Cayenne pepper	*Capsicum annuum*	F	ALK	Capsaicin, capsinoids	?
Coffee	*Coffea* spp.	F	ALK, PHE	Caffeine	✗
Dandelion	*Taraxacum officinale*	R	FLA, TER	Unknown	?
Elderberry	*Sambucus nigra*	F	FLA, PHE	Anthocyanins, lectins, quercetin	?
Ephedra, Ma Huang	*Ephedra sinica*	T	ALK	Ephedrine, pseudoephedrine	✗
Gambooge	*Garcinia gummi-gutta* (G. *cambogina*)	F	OTH	Hydroxycitric acid	✗
Ginger	*Zingiber* spp.	R	ALK	Gingerols, shogaols	✓
Ginseng	*Panax* spp.	R	TER	Ginsenosides	?
Green tea	*Camellia sinensis*	L	ALK, PHE	Caffeine, EGCG	✓
Guar bean	*Cyamopsis tetragonoloba*	S	POL	Galacatomannan	?
Guarana	*Paullinia cupana*	S	ALK	Guaranine	✗
Gymnema, Cowplant	*Gymnema sylvestre*	L	TER	Gymnenic acid	?
Hoodia	*Hoodia* spp.	R	TER	Steroidal glycosides	?
Indian Coleus	*Plecanthrus barbatus* (*Coleus forskohlii*)	R	ALK, TER	Forskolin	?

Konjac	*Amorphophallus konjac*	T	POL	Glucomannan	?
Milk thistle	*Silybum spp.*	L,S	PHE	Silybin	?
Psyllium	*Plantago spp.*	S	POL	Fiber, mucilage	?
Rhodiola	*Rhodiola rosea*	R	TER	Rosavin	?
Sarsaparilla	*Smilax spp.*	B,R	TER	Saponins	—
Siberian ginseng	*Eleutherococcus senticosus*	R	TER	Eleutherocides	?
Veldt grape	*Cissus quadrangularis*	T	TER	Steroids, carotenoids	?
White bean	*Phaseolus vulgaris*	F	OTH	Phaseolamin	?
White willow	*Salix alba*	B	PHE	Salicin, salicylic acid	?
Yerba maté	*Ilex paraguariensis*	L,W	ALK	Caffeine	?

FIGURE 27 Herbs commonly used as weight loss aids

Notes:

Designator 'spp' indicates that multiple species from the genus are employed commercially.

'Organ used' abbreviations: B, bark; F, fruit; L, leaf; R, rhizomes and roots; S, seed; T, stem; W, twigs.

'SM group' abbreviations: ALK, alkaloid; FLA, flavonoid; OTH, other; PHE, phenolic; POL, polysaccharide; TER, terpenoid.

Symbols are based on information from cited sources.

✗ = No evidence for efficacy and/or potential safety or toxicity issues.

? = Little or no evidence for efficacy but no perceived harm.

√ = Moderate or strong supporting evidence and no perceived harm.

– = Lack of evidence prohibits a conclusion from being made.

their assessment of its potential risk and efficacy (Pittler *et al.*, 2005; Sharpe *et al.*, 2006; Poddar *et al.*, 2011).

Literature regarding herbal supplements and weight loss is patchy but suggests varying levels of efficacy and risk as summarized in Figure 27. However, it is important to note that many of these conclusions are based on isolated studies or small samples; the majority is conducted on obese (i.e. non-athletic) populations; and mechanisms are often speculative. On the other hand, some may confer additional health benefits: for example, polyphenols found in green tea and milk thistle may have anti-cancer, anti-inflammatory, antioxidant, or other immunomodulatory effects (Kidd, 2009; Senchina *et al.*, 2014), while elderberry may be an immunomodulator capable of binding and incapacitating the influenza virus (Senchina *et al.*, 2013a).

Additional herbs not covered in this review, but used for weight loss, include bladder wrack (*Fucus vesiculosus*), blood orange (*Citrus sinensis*), bromeliad (*Bromelia* spp), celery seed (*Apium graveolens*), fenugreek (*Trigonella foenum-graecum*), horsetail (*Equisetum* spp), passionflower (*Passiflora* spp), red grape (*Vitis vinifera*) and xanthan gum. As is the case with phaseolamin and hydroxycitric acid, other compounds from herbal sources have been used for weight loss (Cimolai and Cimolai, 2011), such as γ-oryzanol, nootkatone, and yohimbine (see relevant sections in the book). All warrant further scrutiny.

Competing interests None

WHEAT GERM OIL

Mayur K. Ranchordas and Samantha J. Stear

The wheat germ (*Triticum vulgare*, Gramineae), a by-product of the flour-milling industry, represents about 2.5–3.8% of the total seed weight. Wheat germ and the oil extracted from wheat germ contain significant quantities of bioactive compounds, and in particular are known to be the richest plant origin source of tocopherols, i.e. vitamin E (Leenhardt *et al.*, 2008), with the antioxidant activity of tocopherols being well documented. Wheat germ contains mainly α- and β-tocopherols (Leenhardt *et al.*, 2008), alongside other bioactive compounds such as: phytosterols; polycosanols (POC); thiamine (vitamin B1); riboflavin (vitamin B2); and carotenoids, particularly lutein and zeaxanthin (Brandolini and Hidalgo, 2012). Wheat germ is also a source of α-linolenic-rich PUFA (Yuldasheva *et al.*, 2010), and contains several minerals, principally potassium, magnesium, calcium, zinc and manganese.

The wheat germ contains about 10–15% lipids (oil), with oil extraction being primarily achieved by mechanical pressing or solvent extraction, which retrieve about 50% or more than 90% of total lipids, respectively (Brandolini and Hidalgo, 2012). Crude wheat germ oil (WGO) is usually dark-coloured and may have strong odour and flavour, depending on the oxidative conditions of the oil. To produce high quality, stable oils, undesirable compounds must be eliminated while retaining as much of tocopherols and other key nutritional compounds as possible. WGO is widely utilized for vitamin production (e.g. *a*-tocopherol) in medication and cosmetic industry as well as in food, animal-feed and as a biological insect control agent.

WGO has been purported to improve human physical endurance/fitness, an effect attributed to its high POC, specifically its high octacosanol (OC) content, alongside other marketed health benefits such as reducing plasma and liver cholesterol levels and possibly helping to delay effects of aging. Despite these claims, studies investigating the effects of WGO supplementation in humans, on exercise performance and health, are sparse. A study investigating the effects of phytosterols from wheat germ on cholesterol absorption in humans found that consuming a meal containing 80g of original wheat germ containing 328mg phytosterols resulted in less cholesterol absorption when compared with ingestion of phytosterol-free wheat germ (Ostuland *et al.*, 2003). This suggests that phytosterols found in wheat germ may have an important role in cholesterol metabolism. Another study recruited 32 patients with hypercholesterolaemia to examine the effects of two months of daily WGO supplementation or a placebo (maize oil) on oxidative stress (Alessandri *et al.*, 2006). Although no differences in serum lipid profile were observed in both groups, oxidative stress and platelet CD40L, a protein with inflammatory and prothrombotic properties, was reduced, suggesting that WGO supplementation had positive anti-inflammatory effects in patients with hypercholesterolemia (Alessandri et al., 2006).

Despite the lack of supporting evidence regarding a role for WGO in sports performance, WGO does provide an excellent source of vitamin E, with the high fat content of the wheat germ enabling its transport. The recommended dietary intake for vitamin E of 15mg/day could be reached through consumption of 100g of wheat germ – that's a pretty large handful! A more practical alternative source would therefore be WGO, being more concentrated in vitamin E than raw wheat germ.

Competing interests   None

WHEY PROTEIN

Nicholas A. Burd

Whey protein is a widely available dietary supplement that is often used to promote weight loss and/or support the maintenance, repair and synthesis of muscle proteins. Whey is the liquid portion of coagulated milk and represents ~20% of the total protein mass of milk. It is a high quality protein source that contains all the amino acids to synthesize fully functional bodily proteins (Tang et al., 2009). Compared with other dietary protein sources, the amino acid composition of whey is high in leucine (see section on leucine), an amino acid known to regulate mRNA translation in an insulin-dependent manner (Burd et al., 2013). Recent interest has also emerged with regards to specific whey-derived bioactive peptides that may have a positive impact on several bodily functions including cardiovascular, digestive or immune activities (Nagpal et al., 2011).

An innovative study using specifically produced intrinsically-labelled milk-proteins showed that the ingestion of whey resulted in accelerated dietary protein digestion and amino acid absorption kinetics, and an increased rise in postprandial plasma leucine concentrations when compared to the ingestion of other dietary protein sources, casein or hydrolysed casein (Pennings et al., 2011). The speed of dietary protein digestion/absorption and the subsequent pattern of plasma leucine concentrations after protein ingestion are often suggested to be key factors responsible for modulating the postprandial muscle protein synthetic response (Tang et al., 2009; Pennings et al., 2011; West et al., 2011a). Of course, the scenario in which these leucine characteristics has generally been investigated involves a postprandial phase in the absence of exercise in clinical or aging populations; more work is required to establish firmly whether they are of equal value in the post-exercise phase in healthy athletes (Pennings et al., 2011; Wall et al., 2013).

Some evidence suggests that ingestion of whey promotes greater satiety when compared to the ingestion of casein (Hall et al., 2003). It has been speculated that a rapid appearance of whey protein-derived amino acids into circulation stimulates the production of hormones involved in satiety and reduced appetite. Thus the ingestion of whey protein prior to meals may be a helpful weight management strategy. However, it has been demonstrated that whey protein supplementation during a nine-month exercise programme does not further enhance strength or changes in body composition in middle-aged overweight and obese adults (Weinheimer et al., 2012). In this case, the data showed that increasing habitual physical activity is the overriding variable affecting weight loss, and is a simple and effective lifestyle strategy to promote healthy aging and long-term weight maintenance.

Whey protein supplements (or food protein sources) appear to be safe to consume; there is no direct evidence that high intakes of protein (as commonly observed in athletes) are harmful to healthy kidneys (see section on protein). Moreover, whey protein ingestion appears to be a highly effective protein source for the stimulation of the postprandial muscle anabolic response (Tang *et al.*, 2009; Pennings *et al.*, 2011) and thus will support muscle health and performance.

Competing interests   None

WOLFBERRY (GOJI BERRY)

Richard J. Godfrey and David S. Senchina

Wolfberry and goji berry are interchangeable terms for the red fruits of either of the two boxthorn plants in the potato family, *Lycium barbarum* (syn. *Lycium halimifolium*) and *Lycium chinense*. Both are important herbal components of traditional Chinese medicine, where they are often referred to as *gou qi*. The berries (i.e. *fructus barbarum*, *fructus lycii*) are used for both food and medicine whereas root bark (*cortex lycii radicis*) is used solely for medicine (Potterat, 2010). These plants should not be confused with *Solanum lycocarpum*, variously known as wolf's apple, wolf's fruit or fruit-of-the-wolf, which contains toxic alkaloids. Wolfberry fruits are the plant component used most often in sports supplements and contain several purported bioactive molecules including carotenoids, flavonoids, vitamins including plentiful vitamin C, sterols and polysaccharides (Potterat, 2010). Bioavailability studies suggest that, when berries are extracted in milk as in traditional Chinese medicine, zeaxanthins (a subclass of carotenoids) are found in the bloodstream, peaking at six hours post-ingestion (Benzie *et al.*, 2006).

Many claims are made for the health benefits of wolfberries, including improved immune function, fertility, skin and eye health and even anti-aging. Robust peer-reviewed evidence for many of these effects is hard to find, although there do appear to be some reports of benefits in preventing diabetic retinopathy (Song *et al.*, 2012) and inhibiting prostate cancer progression (Luo *et al.*, 2009). Reports of allergy to wolf berries suggest the risk of sensitivity in some individuals (Carnés *et al.*, 2013), including of anaphylaxis (Monzón Ballarín *et al.*, 2011) and the potential for skin photosensitivity (Gómez-Bernal *et al.*, 2011).

In conclusion, there is some evidence that there may be a few health benefits in using wolfberries but potential side effects are possible. There is, however, little scientific evidence to justify commercial claims that wolfberry is a 'super food' and there is no evidence that it is of any benefit as an ergogenic aid for sports performance.

Competing interests None

YERBA MATÉ

Samantha J. Stear

Yerba maté tea (Mate), is made from an infusion of the dried leaves of the *Ilex paraguariensis* tree, which is widely consumed in South America, but also found globally as both a herbal tea beverage and an ingredient in formulated foods and nutritional supplements (Heck and de Mejia, 2007). Numerous active phytochemicals have been identified in yerba maté tea: the two most prevalent compounds are the polyphenols (chlorogenic acid) and the xanthines, caffeine and theobromine (Athayde *et al.*, 2000); followed by purine alkaloids (caffeic acid, 3,4-dicaffeoylquinic acid, 3,5-dicaffeoylquinic acid); flavonoids (quercetin, kaempferol and rutin); amino acids; the minerals, phosphorus, iron and calcium; and vitamins C, B1 and B2 (Heck and de Mejia, 2007). See elsewhere in the book for individual reviews. However, unlike other teas, particularly white, green and oolong and to a lesser extent black, yerba maté is a better alternative as it does not contain catechins (Heck and de Mejia, 2007; Chandra and de Mejia, 2004), which have recently been linked with liver toxicity.

Notably, the amount of caffeine in 150ml of yerba maté tea is approximately 78mg (Heck and de Mejia, 2007), which is similar to the amount found in a 250ml cup of coffee (see section on caffeine). Hence, the primary association with sports performance is due to yerba maté being a natural source of caffeine and its associated dose-dependent ergogenic properties (Spriet *et al.*, 2010; Schubert *et al.*, 2013), such as alterations to the central nervous system to change perceptions of effort or fatigue, described further in the review on caffeine. Yerba maté has been shown to be hypocholesterolaemic, hepatoprotective, a central nervous system stimulant, diuretic, antioxidant, of benefit to the cardiovascular system, and associated with both the prevention and increased risk of some types of cancers (Heck and de Mejia, 2007). Also, as reviewed in the section on herbal weight loss supplements, yerba maté, either on its own or in combination with other ingredients such as guarana and green tea, has been associated with weight loss (Senchina *et al.*, 2013b), primarily due to its caffeine content and its proposed effect on increasing energy expenditure and fat utilization as a fuel source (Spriet *et al.*, 2010; Outlaw *et al.*, 2013). However, as with many herbal supplements, the specific evidence for an effect on athletic performance is limited and cannot be attributed to yerba maté *per se*, with only a couple of studies to date, both using a commercial product (Outlaw *et al.*, 2013; Schubert *et al.*, 2013). There remains an increased risk of adverse effects using herbal supplements, particularly those containing multiple ingredients (Senchina *et al.*, 2013b).

Competing interests   None

YOHIMBINE

Richard J. Godfrey

Yohimbine is an alkaloid derived from the bark of the West African tree, *Pausinystalia yohimbe*, which can be bought over the counter as a herbal preparation. Traditionally, it has been used for erectile dysfunction and as an aphrodisiac.

Yohimbine is a monoamine oxidase inhibitor and an adrenergic α2 antagonist (Hedner *et al.*, 1992) and, as yohimbine hydrochloride, it is registered by the NIH as a treatment for impotency where tolerance for sildenifil (Viagra) is poor. Evidence for this use in humans is not compelling but has been demonstrated in rats (Saad *et al.*, 2013). Recent evidence suggests yohimbine may benefit type 2 diabetes by increasing blood flow to Islet cells (Sandberg *et al.*, 2013); furthermore, it has been used for some time to improve saliva flow for those with xerostomia (Bagheri *et al.*, 1997).

In sport, yohimbine is perceived to reduce body fat, mobilise lipid and enhance endurance. Accordingly, it is often used in bodybuilding and other aesthetic sports, as well as sports in which there is a significant aerobic component. However, research findings refute any ergogenic benefit for sport (Ostojic, 2006; Herda *et al.*, 2008). Care should be taken as yohimbine is known to cause agitation, anxiety, hypertension and tachycardia with the severity of these effects increasing with dose (Cimolai and Cimolai, 2011).

In conclusion, research findings do not support any ergogenic effect for yohimbine and there are acute, negative, nervous system effects which increase with increasing dose.

Competing interests   None

YUCCA

Markus Laupheimer

Yucca encompasses about 40–50 medicinally potent plant species that generally thrive in arid parts of southwestern USA and Mexico (Patel, 2012). Although the medical research into yucca is very limited, the most researched species is *Yucca Schidigera* (Mojave yucca), which is found in a variety of food supplements. Yucca has a reputed place in folk medicine for a variety of conditions with the most mentioned anti-inflammatory and anti-arthritic effects (Cheeke *et al.*, 2006). The yucca extract is widely used as an animal feed additive to increase growth rate, improve feed conversion efficiency and ease joint pains in horses and dogs (Cheeke *et al.*, 2006; Patel, 2012). Yucca also has been shown to have antioxidant, anti-cancer, antidiabetic, antimicrobial and hypocholesterolaemic properties (Bassarello *et al.*, 2007; Cheeke *et al.*, 2006; Patel, 2012). Steroidal saponins, resveratorol and yuccaol have been identified as active principles (Bassarello *et al.*, 2007; Cheeke *et al.*, 2006; Patel, 2012). Having identified this combination of substances, despite no scientific evidence, there has been an interest in yucca by the sports medicine community. Yucca saponins are precursors to cortisone. Yuccaols and resveratrol, which are mainly found in the yucca bark, are known to have a variety of actions, including inhibitors of NF-kB, and thus anti-inflammatory, antioxidants and free-radical scavengers (Cheeke *et al.*, 2006; Patel, 2012). In addition, resveratrol (see elsewhere in this book) has been shown to have an influence on muscle fibres, strength and possible ergogenic effects (Lagouge *et al.*, 2006; Murase *et al.*, 2009). Reseveratrol, on its own, or in the form of yucca extract, has several potential indications in sport and exercise medicine, which warrant further research efforts (Laupheimer *et al.*, 2013; Nieman *et al.*, 2014). Yucca extracts have acquired generally-recognised-as-safe (GRAS) status, so are FDA-approved for use in humans, but there are currently no established oral doses or recommendations (Cheeke *et al.*, 2006; Patel, 2012), and there is no evidence of an ergogenic benefit in sports performance.

Competing interests   None

ZINC

Patricia A. Deuster

The essential trace mineral zinc (Zn) serves multiple biological functions – catalytic, structural, regulatory and substrate (Andreini *et al.*, 2011) – in support of metabolic, endocrine, signal transduction, cellular control, protein stabilization and immune networks/pathways (Andreini *et al.*, 2011; Chasapis *et al.*, 2012). Overall, approximately 3,000 Zn proteins are encoded in the human genome (Andreini *et al.*, 2011) and Zn is a cofactor to more than 300 enzymes; these include superoxide dismutase, alkaline phosphatase and alcohol dehydrogenase (Andreini *et al.*, 2011; Chasapis *et al.*, 2012) in the liver, and carbonic anhydrase III (Vaananen *et al.*, 1982), AMP-deaminase (Stankiewicz, 1981), and the matrix metalloproteinases (Carmeli *et al.*, 2004) and in skeletal muscle. As one of the most widely distributed metals in the body, 85% of Zn resides in muscle and bones, 11% in skin and the liver, and the remaining in all the other tissues (Chasapis *et al.*, 2012). This clearly demonstrates the overall importance of Zn and would suggest that it may be important in physical performance. The best food sources of Zn are oysters, wheat germ, liver, beef, melon and squash seeds, and cocoa.

Improvement in physical performance or aspects of physical performance by administration of Zn can be demonstrated in one of three ways: 1) showing that providing Zn to persons who are Zn-deficient restores/improves performance; 2) demonstrating that providing Zn to healthy individuals with adequate Zn status improves some aspect of performance; or 3) showing that Zn supplementation counters a particular health risk that could compromise performance. Performance improvement in this case is considered as any of the following: enhanced endurance, increased strength and/or lean body mass, and/or higher aerobic capacity. The question is: does supplementation with Zn confer any clear benefits?

This review only deals with supplements that have provided zinc as a single ingredient, while the multi-component product, ZMA, is reviewed elsewhere in this book.

With regard to a Zn deficiency, the multiple functions of Zn suggest repletion should restore decrements in performance through a variety of mechanisms. One of the earliest mechanisms proposed was related to Zn's influence on testosterone and growth hormone (Hafiez *et al.*, 1989; Hamza *et al.*, 2012; Om and Chung, 1996). In both human and animal studies it has been clearly shown that a Zn deficiency can adversely affect plasma levels of testosterone, growth hormone (GH) and insulin-like growth factor 1 (IGF-1) (Hafiez *et al.*, 1989; Hamza *et al.*, 2012; Om and Chung, 1996; Chung *et al.*, 1986; Mansour *et al.*, 1989).

Specifically, Zn deficiency in rats is associated with lower plasma luteinizing hormone and testosterone concentrations, and alterations in steroid metabolism and sex steroid hormone receptors when compared to Zn-sufficient rats (Om and Chung, 1996). Moreover, administration of Zn to animals and humans with either Zn deficiency or retarded growth increased serum testosterone and IGF-1 levels (Hafiez et al., 1989; Hamza et al., 2012).

The studies in humans with Zn deficiency led investigators to evaluate whether administration of Zn would elicit/invoke biological increases in GH, IGF-1 and testosterone. To date, most studies indicate that supplemental Zn promotes growth and an anabolic environment only under conditions of Zn deficiency and has no effect on plasma testosterone T in Zn-sufficient and/ or normal growth humans (Koehler et al., 2009; Shafiei Neek et al., 2011). Shafiei Neek et al. (2011) showed that providing 30mg of Zn per day for four weeks had no effect on testosterone. However, other studies suggest that Zn supplementation may prevent exercise-related decreases in testosterone (Kilic, 2007; Kilic et al., 2006).

Killic (2007) and Kilic et al. (2006) reported that supplementation with Zn for four weeks prevented decreases in testosterone caused by fatiguing exercise. Surprisingly, they did not measure performance or show that maintaining serum testosterone conferred any performance benefit, despite stating that a physiological dose of zinc could benefit performance (Kilic, 2007; Kilic et al., 2006). The dose was not physiological, but was very high: 3mg/kg/day of Zn sulphate or ~85mg/day for a 70 kg person. This is a concern as it is twice as high as the Tolerable Upper Intake Level of Zn for adults (40mg/day, National Academies Press, 2001). In addition, doses/servings sizes over 100mg day are associated with health problems – headache, abdominal cramps and nausea – as well as resulting in a copper deficiency, which can cause anaemia, leucopaenia and neutropaenia (Leitzmann et al., 2003). None of these issues were addressed and the finding would have been pharmacological, rather than physiological.

In addition to Zn effects on anabolic pathways, others have suggested that Zn supplementation may improve blood rheology, in particular erythrocyte deformability and factors regulating blood viscosity (Khaled et al., 1997, 1999). However, the evidence for any clear performance benefit is weak, and the effects may be specific to those with a Zn deficiency, as determined by low serum Zn levels. Importantly, although inconsistent findings have been reported with regard to serum Zn concentrations in athletes (Konig et al., 1998; Fogelholm et al., 1991; Lukaski, 1989; Deuster et al., 1986, 1989), dietary intake of Zn is often below the recommended dietary allowance (RDA: 8 and 11mg/day for adult women and men, respectively (National Academies Press, 2001) in many athletes (Deuster et al., 1986, 1989) and other special populations, such as being associated with depression (Yary and Aazami, 2012).

Finally, Zn supplementation may mitigate performance decrements by mediating health barriers, such as the common cold (Hemila, 2011; Maggini et al., 2012; Prasad, 2009; Science et al., 2012; Stefanidou et al., 2006). Although the data are not strongly positive, several systematic reviews/meta-analyses have indicated that supplementation with Zn may provide more rapid relief from cold symptoms (Maggini *et al.*, 2012; Science *et al.*, 2012; Singh and Das, 2013) and/or shorten the duration of a cold (Hemila, 2011; Singh and Das, 2013) compared with placebo. However, in the USA, if a Zn product being marketed as a dietary supplement claims to be supportive in treating a common cold, it would be subjected to drug regulations and would require an Investigational New Drug Application.

In summary, although the biological actions and functions of Zn would lead one to predict it might serve as a performance enhancer, the scientific evidence is weak in the absence of a Zn deficiency. Perhaps new evidence noting otherwise may emerge but, as of 2013, taking a Zn supplement is unlikely to confer any performance benefit.

Competing interests   None

ZMA – ZINC MAGNESIUM ASPARTATE

Adrian B. Hodgson

ZMA is a popular nutritional supplement which regularly features in the nutritional supplementation regimens of many athletes. The original product was developed by Victor Conte, from the Bay Area Laboratory Co-operative (BALCO) sports nutrition company, who separately pleaded guilty to anti-doping violations. It is composed of Zn (~30mg/serving), magnesium (~450mg/serving) and vitamin B6 (~11mg/serving), with many other companies promoting their own versions with added proprietary blends that claim to improve uptake and activity of the multivitamins and minerals.

The rationale for the use of ZMA is that athletes have been reported to suffer from zinc and magnesium deficiency (Konig *et al.*, 1998). Studies conducted in clinical populations and animals have shown growth retardation, blunted testosterone and IGF-1(insulin-like growth factor-1) concentrations with zinc deficiency (Favier, 1992; Prasad *et al.*, 1981). Plasma magnesium concentrations have been shown to be associated with plasma cortisol concentrations (Golf *et al.*, 1984), which is believed to lead to inferior gains in muscle mass and strength following resistance training. Collectively this suggests that zinc and magnesium deficiency may have deleterious effects on skeletal muscle adaptations and exercise performance.

With this evidence in mind, Brilla and Conte (2000) investigated the hormonal and training responses following seven weeks ZMA supplementation in 23 US football players. The authors showed that plasma zinc and magnesium concentrations significantly increased following ZMA supplementation, which was also accompanied by a significant increase in plasma testosterone and IGF-1 concentrations. The athletes who received ZMA also improved muscle strength when compared to the placebo control group. However, it is important to highlight that the study was funded and conducted by Victor Conte who is the patent holder for ZMA and owner of the nutrition company, SNAC systems. Since then, only two studies have been conducted in athletes in an attempt to support the putative claims of Brilla and Conte (2000). Research by Wilborn *et al.* (2004) suggested that eight weeks of ZMA supplementation (with a similar protocol to that used by Brilla and Conte, 2000) combined with resistance training, failed to show significant differences in plasma zinc or magnesium concentrations, anabolic (testosterone, IGF1, growth hormone) or catabolic hormones (cortisol), gains in muscle mass and strength or cycling anaerobic capacity when compared to placebo. Koehler *et al.* (2009) also reported in a well-controlled study that 56 days of ZMA supplementation in physically active males (sourced from SNAC systems) did not alter plasma total testosterone, free testosterone or urinary excretion of testosterone metabolites.

There have been anecdotal reports, with no supporting data, suggesting ZMA as a possible aid to sleep quality. This notion seems to have originated from a study showing a causal relationship between magnesium deficiency and sleep quality in elderly individuals suffering from insomnia (Abbasi *et al.*, 2012). An extrapolation to ZMA, or to athletes, is therefore not appropriate.

At present, there is little evidence to support the use of ZMA as an anabolic nutritional intervention or to improve sleep quality. Future well-controlled studies are required to investigate its effects further.

Competing interests   None

IN PRACTICE

*Louise M. Burke, Samantha J. Stear and
Linda M. Castell*

'So, what's the bottom line on Product X: does it work or not?'

Sports dietitians/scientists/physicians are frequently confronted by this question, in forums ranging from athlete consultations to media interviews, and student lectures to dinner parties. There is an expectation of a single and emphatic answer, mirroring the certainty of the messages found in the marketing of many supplements and sports foods. Frustration and disappointment often ensue when the response contains uncertainty and is couched with caveats and qualifications. Yet, as this book demonstrates, particularly in the concluding chapter which provides an efficacy index of all products reviewed, rarely is the evidence about a supplement sufficient in the number or consistency of findings to enable a 'black or white' decision about its value to the health or performance of an athlete. Even when the judgement is made, however, caveats must then come into play since it is the application of the product to real life use rather than the product *per se* that creates the bottom line. This chapter provides an opportunity to consider issues of the application or supplement practice, against the backdrop of safety, efficacy and legality/ethics.

Conditions and protocols of use

The marketing of supplements and sports foods often focuses on the product or an ingredient with stark and often magical claims about the benefits it achieves. X enhances recovery! Shed body fat with Y! Z improves performance by 30%! Superfood! This message is understandable since the manufacturer wants you to purchase their product over a rival one, to maximize their consumer base by implying that the product is right for everyone, and to appeal to our natural laziness by suggesting that no effort or knowledge is necessary to achieve a benefit. The reality, even with substances that enjoy the greatest scientific support, is that a favourable outcome requires a combination of a large number of factors including the right athlete, the right product source, the right protocol of use, the right timing of use in the periodised training/competition calendar and the right type of sport/event/issue. All these factors must be built into the decision to justify the use of a product in the first place, as well as the actual implementation of its use.

The first factor that must be built into a supplementation plan is the alignment of the product with its correct scenario of use. This requires an understanding of the physiology and biochemistry underpinning the goals of the athlete's training and competition programme, including the periodisation of various issues according to the season, macrocycle, microcycle and individual session. For example, Figures 28 and 29 summarise a periodised approach to preparing for a marathon, showing the range of characteristics that a runner would try to achieve during training, then further enhance on race day (Stellingwerff, 2013). The implementation of this plan involves the integration of a range of nutritional strategies into the various phases of training and race execution, many of which might involve the acute, intermittent or chronic use of supplements or sports foods.

Within the individualized training scenario for any sport, an athlete may benefit from judicious use of supplements and sports foods that assist with manipulation of physique, reduce muscle damage or soreness, enhance rehydration, refuelling and protein synthesis following certain workouts, or reduce the risk of illness. In addition, he or she may find, expense notwithstanding, that sports foods often provide a valuable practical alternative to everyday foods in a busy lifestyle or during travel. Other supplement strategies may be undertaken to support good performance in workouts, or to experiment with, and fine tune, competition practices. The achievement of long-term sporting goals requires a sophisticated knowledge of training and nutrient interactions that can identify not only when to implement a particular nutritional strategy, but also when it should be withdrawn. In some cases, a strategy that may enhance one goal (e.g. acute recovery) may be at the expense of another (e.g. adaptation). For example, whereas early intake of carbohydrate enhances glycogen recovery after exercise, withholding it for several hours may prolong the period of enhanced cellular signalling which enhances synthesis of proteins favouring fat utilization as an energy substrate (Hawley and Morton, 2014). Furthermore, whereas antioxidant supplementation may reduce the damage associated with free oxygen radical production during exercise, it may also blunt adaptive responses to exercise that are mediated by these radicals (Peternelj and Coombes, 2011). Clearly, supplement use within the periodised nutrition plan requires expert knowledge and athletes are always encouraged to seek professional advice.

Competition use of supplements typically targets the specific physiological and biochemical factors that limit performance and cause fatigue. This specificity includes the sport, the event, the environment, the competition programme, the particular event pacing/tactics/work patterns on the day and the

Desired physiological adaptation	Type of training or environmental intervention	Potential nutrition or hydration intervention
↑ muscle glycogen contents.	Large volumes of upper aerobic power training (e.g.fartleks. tempos).	↑ CHO cycling via periodically training under low CHO availability and acute pre-race CHO loading.
↑ or maintain healthy hemo-globin content for optimal O_2-carrying capacity.	Minimize inflammatory responses by large volumes of aerobic training at intensities below lactate threshold: potentially use hypoxic environments to increase natural RBC production.	Optima] dietary iron and vitamin B_{12} intake.
↑ PV leading to ↑ SV and VO_{2max} and heat acclimation.	Periodic VO_{2max} training sessions (large durations of high quality of training intensity at or near HR....): training in a heat-stress environment.	Targeting mild to moderate dehydration during heat-stress training and ingestion of protein after heat-stress training
↑ buffering capacity or ↑ lactate or ventilatory threshold.	High-intensity anaerobic training to increase anaerobic capacity and lactate tolerance.	Chronic β-alanine supplementation.
↑ aerobic or mitochondrial genes, enzymes, transporters.	Large volumes of upper aerobic power training (e.g. fartleks. tempos) and lactate-threshold training.	Periodically training under low CHO availability and potentially L-camitine supplementation.
↑ intestinal CHO-transporter density and/or function.	Marathon race-pace-specific training in target marathon weather conditions to mimic race-specific GI blood shunting and GI stress.	↑ exercise-specific CHO fueling and overall dietary CHO intake over a several-week period.

↑ overall training load in a volume-dependent sport via optimized nutritional recovery practices.

↑ ratio of power to body mass to improve running economy via long-term management of energy expenditure vs. energy intake.

Abbreviations: CHO, carbohydrate; O_2, oxygen; RBC, red blood cell; PV, plasma volume; SV, stroke volume; VO_{2max}, maximal oxygen consumption; HR, maximal heart rate; GI, gastrointestinal.
Question mark indicates that more research is needed to fully validate initial findings.

FIGURE 28 Summary of nutrition and training interventions to achieve physiological adaptations underpinning marathon performance (Stellingwerff, 2013, with permission)

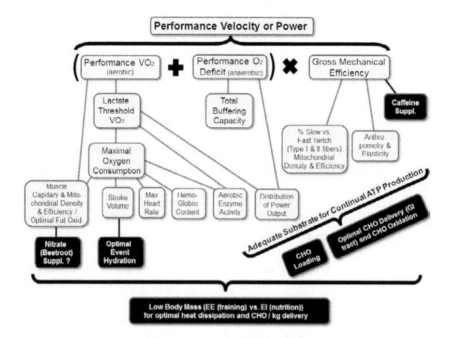

FIGURE 29 Summary of race day physiological and nutritional determinates of marathon performance (Stellingwerff, 2013, with permission)

Key: VO$_2$, oxygen uptake; CHO, carbohydrate; GI, gastrointestinal; EE, energy expenditure; EI, energy intake.

individual athlete – in some cases, a protocol that is suitable for one athlete in a race or match will be unsuitable for another, and will need to be modified for the same athlete in an identical competition in different circumstances. Clearly, if the use of supplement does not address a characteristic that is limiting for the performance of a specific athlete – either because the identified factor does not actually limit performance or the supplement protocol does not adequately address the factor – then an enhanced outcome cannot be expected.

The failure of a supplement or sports food to achieve a desired or expected outcome is often simply due to the failure of the athlete to implement an appropriate protocol of use. This may be because the athlete's supplement use is poorly informed or supervised. Athletes may fail to comply with a complicated protocol that requires multiple doses in a day (e.g. a rapid loading protocol for creatine) or a prolonged duration of intake (e.g. β-alanine loading). Sometimes the product is used in a dose that is sub-optimal; this can occur because of poor knowledge, inadequate finances to purchase the required amount or because early research failed to identify the therapeutic dose (e.g. beetroot juice; Hoon *et al.*, 2014b; Wylie *et al.*, 2013a). In other cases, the supplement may fail to achieve an ergogenic benefit because the use of an excessive dose causes harmful side effects or can impair performance. Excessive intakes may occur because early research failed to look for the smallest effective dose (e.g. caffeine use), or more often, because of consumer ignorance (failure to read product labels or to add up the total dose coming in from a range of supplements) or bravado in athletes (more is better). Athletes commonly share information about supplement protocols, and the 'word of mouth' testimonials frequently found on internet chat rooms and supplement discussion forums illustrate that real-life practices of supplement use can exceed the doses that are scientifically validated or even recommended by manufacturers.

In many situations, even in the case of products with a strong evidence base, successful supplementation strategies require practice and fine-tuning because the real-life world of sport means that the scenario in which they are to be used is different from anything that has been tested in a study. Occasionally, supplement research targets a specific event and simulates competition conditions and characteristics as closely as possible in the laboratory (e.g. Lane et al., 2014) or field (del Coso et al., 2013). In most situations, however, real-life practices occur in the face of variations of factors including environmental conditions, pre-competition nutrition status/strategies or pre-event training/ warm-up protocols; these characteristics are likely to affect the effectiveness of a supplement and may differ between individuals and events as well as from the researched conditions. A scenario that occurs frequently in real life is the multi-event competition where an athlete competes in heats and finals, or a series of games and stages, to determine the winner. Few studies have investigated whether supplement strategies that are effective in a single event can be repeated within hours (Hoon et al., 2014a) or days (Stadheim et al., 2014), and protocols may need to be tweaked in timing or amount to achieve the best outcome in terms of efficacy and absence of side effects.

Individual responses and characteristics

Real-life application of supplementation practices needs to consider the characteristics of the supplement consumer. The safety and efficacy of products require special attention when used by junior athletes, masters and veteran athletes, female athletes who are pregnant or breast-feeding, and athletes with disabilities or medical conditions. In many cases, safety is the issue of major priority, with factors of importance including altered physiology or nutritional requirements, differences in absolute or effective body size, interaction with medicines, and food intolerances and allergies. Some of these issues may also influence the efficacy of the protocol. The outcome may be a decision that the supplement or sports food isn't appropriate or suitable to use, or that a variation in the protocol or product source may be needed.

In real life as well as in studies, it is frequently observed that individuals respond differently to a supplement – again in terms of efficacy and side-effects. Many investigations now report the results of individual subjects as well as the group mean, and show that, even when the mean response suggests a

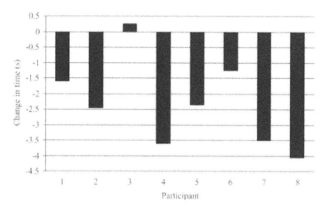

FIGURE 30   Individual responses to caffeine intake

Note: Eight well-trained cyclists consumed caffeine (5 mg/kg) prior to undertaking a laboratory simulation of the 1 km track cycling event. The mean outcome was an improvement of 2.3 s or ~ 3%; however, this ranged from a trivial performance impairment to a 4 s improvement. At the 2004 Olympic Games, the time difference between the first and 10th place getter was 2.39 s (Wiles *et al.*, 2006, with permission).

worthwhile improvement in performance, the individual experience can range from a negative effect through to a very large performance gain (see Figure 30).

Differences in the magnitude and direction of performance changes in individual subjects after consuming the same supplement in a randomized controlled trial are often interpreted as evidence of an innate responder vs. non-responder phenomenon. While this phenomenon undoubtedly occurs in the case of some products and individuals, some care should be taken in distinguishing it from the day-to-day variability in performance, which occurs even in the face of attempts to standardize or minimise extraneous variables within a scientific trial. Real differences in responsiveness to a supplement can arise due to a number of factors. These include differences in background nutritional status or body stores of the supplement substance; for example, creatine loading protocols achieve greater increases in muscle creatine stores in people such as vegetarians who have lower starting stores (Watt *et al.*, 2004). Genetic differences in metabolism may also account for a large fraction of the variability in responsiveness. For example, differences in the type, number and site of adenosine receptors around the body can explain differences in the responsiveness to caffeine which acts as an adenosine antagonist, while differences in liver metabolism of caffeine explain differences in the half-life of this chemical (Yang *et al.*, 2010).

Various sources of information can be used to explore or confirm the concept of individual responsiveness to a supplement. Techniques that have been used in scientific investigations include looking for a correlation between markers of altered biochemistry or physiology associated with a substance, and the change in performance (see Figure 31).

Undertaking repeated trials to confirm the robustness of a measured response to the supplement is also valuable (see Figure 32), while probing for genetic

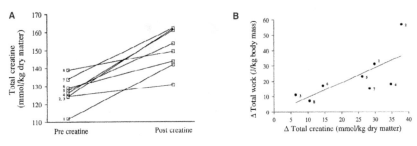

FIGURE 31 Individual responses to creatine loading

Note: Muscle creatine responses (panel A) to a rapid loading protocol in eight subjects. Only the five subjects who showed a substantial increase in muscle creatine content showed a meaningful increase in work done in a repeated sprint cycling test; furthermore there was a significant correlation between the increase in muscle creatine content due to the protocol (panel B) and the change in work achieved during the cycling test. The numerals in the figures identify the individual subjects (taken from Casey *et al.,* 1996, with permission). In this study, differences in response were confirmed by matching changes in physiology achieved by the supplement with changes in performance.

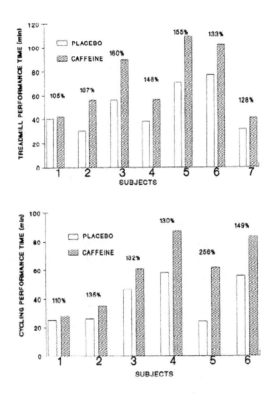

FIGURE 32 Individual response to caffeine supplementation

Note: Caffeine supplementation (9 mg/kg) was undertaken prior to exercise in two separate trials (cycling and running to exhaustion at 85% maximal aerobic capacity). Subject 1 showed a consistently smaller response to the treatment than other subjects (taken from Graham and Spriet, 1991, with permission). In this study, differences in response were confirmed by repeating the observation.

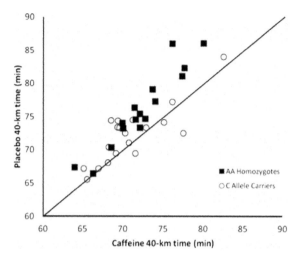

FIGURE 33   40 km time trial performance in 36 cyclists after caffeine intake (6 mg/kg)

Note: The group was subdivided according to the single nucleotide polymorphism of a gene associated with cytochrome P450 (CYP1A2), a family of proteins that metabolise drugs in the liver. The line of identity shows no difference in TT performance while plots above the line reflect improved 40 km time with caffeine. Overall, the 16 athletes who carry the AA version of the gene achieved a 5.9% improvement in 40 km time (P< 0.001) while the 19 athletes who carried the C allele achieved only a 1.8% improvement (p = 0.04). In this study, the tendency to be a responder was associated with a genetic marker.

polymorphisms in key proteins associated with the metabolism or response to a substance is becoming more common (see Figure 33).

Within real-life practice, high performance athletes who receive sports science support may have access to information about their signature responses to certain supplement protocols to enable them to identify successful strategies or tweak characteristics. For example, the athlete may be able to track blood pH and bicarbonate levels following bicarbonate loading strategies to optimize the right timing and dose to achieve an ergogenic benefit to a sustained high-intensity event. In the future, it may become possible to receive a genetic profiling report that could identify potential responsiveness to different kinds of supplement strategies. For the moment, the most pragmatic way for an athlete to identify if they are a non-responder or responder to various supplement strategies is via trial and error, aided by systematic reporting of the outcomes of their supplement activities.

Interaction between supplements

In most studies, experimental design focuses on a single intervention while standardizing all other variables, so that the effect of the intervention – in this case, the use of a supplement – can be clearly detected. In real life, however, many athletes use a number of supplements and sports foods that may have interactions ranging from negative to additive or synergistic. The deliberate

STACKING AND SUPPLEMENT INTERACTIONS

Louise M. Burke and Jeni Pearce

Supplement 'stacking' is the term originating from those undertaking anabolic steroid regimens (Antonio and Stout, 2001), to describe the consumption of two or more supplements at the same time in an attempt to increase the overall results of a supplement programme. 'Polypharmacy' is another term used to describe the simultaneous intake of several supplements although this is often used in the context of ad hoc and enthusiastic intake of many products without a unified programme. In other cases, athletes may use supplements in combinations on a few but deliberate occasions where they are aware that several different products may independently offer a performance advantage for the type of event or goal they are targeting. Finally, the athlete may unintentionally combine products because they purchase a multi-ingredient product in order to consume one of its substances, or inadvertently 'stack' their supplement use through failure to read from the labels of multiple products that a variety of ingredients is being thrown together or that different sources of the same ingredient are combining into an excessive dose. This can be a dangerous situation when a number of products containing caffeine or other stimulants are consumed over the day. Another scenario where multiple doses of single nutrients from a variety of supplements can lead to problematic intake involves minerals. For example, in the case of zinc, an athlete could combine dietary intake (15+mg) with one or more multivitamin mineral supplements (15+mg), protein shake (10 mg), recovery shake (10 mg), sports bar (15mg) and an immunity supplement (5+mg). Such an intake would be excessive, totalling over 70 mg/day (upper safe limits range from 40–45mg: FAO, 2014; NH&MRC and Ministry of Health, 2006) as well as interfering with the absorption of other minerals.

The interaction of different substances on sports performance may be negative, benign, additive or synergistic depending on the combination of products and the scenario of use. Figure 34 summarises examples of each outcome from the existing literature; as in the use of single supplements, the results are likely to be unique to the scenario and the protocols used. While stacking or combining some supplements may provide additional benefits, inadvertent stacking increases the risk of unintended negative consequences or adverse reactions including toxicity, loss of the performance effect of one supplement or interference with nutrient absorption. Athletes should be aware of combining supplements and possible adverse reactions, and should regularly review supplement use with a registered sport nutritionist or sports dietitian.

or inadvertent mixing and matching of supplements is covered in the article on 'Stacking' in this section, and constitutes a largely untouched area of sports science. It provides an obvious challenge for safety as well as efficacy.

Final thoughts on safety, efficacy and legality/ethics

A common thread throughout this book has been the requirement for each athlete to make his or her own informed choice about their use of supplements and sports foods. As much as resources, such as this text, try to support this goal by providing contemporary information about commonly available or topical substances, most athletes and their advisors still face challenges in staying sufficiently informed that good decisions can be made. The ability of the supplement industry to manufacture new products or product mixtures far outstrips the opportunity for researchers to undertake even the most cursory investigations of the claims that support them. Furthermore, products can be made with 'proprietary blends' which remain undisclosed, or can be reformulated so that old information about the product no longer applies. See 'Product reformulation' article below.

PRODUCT REFORMULATION

Ano Lobb

Rapid product reformulation appears to be a common practice among dietary supplement manufacturers, particularly as concerns about safety emerge. This appears to involve launching products into the lightly regulated dietary supplement market which contain often exotic-sounding ingredients that may have potent pharmacological effects, and whose safety and efficacy is commonly supported by very low quality research (Lobb, 2010, 2012). When safety concerns emerge, as is often the case when heavily marketed products reach tens of thousands of users, the formulation can change, though the name and marketing may remain essentially the same. Stimulants are often a consistent presence, with caffeine being the most common.

For example, Hydroxycut is a weight loss supplement whose original formulation contained hydroxycitric acid. After being linked to some two-dozen cases of liver damage and one death, the product was reformulated with a different botanical, Cissus quadrangularis, while retaining the same name, and making many of the same marketing claims (see respective sections in book). Numerous sub-formulations of Hydroxycut have been added to the product line, with various combinations of ingredients with little scientific evidence supporting their efficacy (see sections on these topics).

Scenario	Supplements	Study scenario	Underpinning theory	Outcome
Benign	Caffeine and nitrate (beetroot juice)	45 km cycling time trial in males (Lane et al., 2014) and female cyclists (Lane et al., 2014; Glaister et al., 2014)	Beetroot juice and caffeine believed to have independent effects on time trial performance; taken together the benefits may be additive	Only the caffeine enhanced performance; beetroot juice may have been sub-optimal dose or unable to enhance performance of this exercise protocol in competitive athletes. No apparent interaction between the supplements
Additive	Creatine and bicarbonate	Trained men undertaking 6 x 10 s cycling sprints with 60 sec recovery (Barber et al., 2013)	Creatine and bicarbonate believed to have independent effects on ability to undertake repeated sprints with short recovery interval; taken together the benefits may be additive	Relative peak power was significantly higher with creatine (4%) and creatine plus bicarbonate (7%). Combining creatine and bicarbonate supplementation increased peak and mean power and had the greatest attenuation of decline in relative peak power over the six repeated sprints
Adverse	Caffeine and bicarbonate	Well-trained rowers undertaking 2,000 m rowing ergometer time trial (Carr et al., 2011)	Bicarbonate and caffeine believed to have independent effects on sustained high-intensity events; taken together the benefits may be additive	Performance was enhanced by ~ 2% with caffeine but GI symptoms associated with bicarbonate counteracted this leading to unclear performance outcome
Synergistic	Bicarbonate and β-alanine	Well-trained male rowers undertaking 2,000 m rowing ergometer time trial (Hobson et al., 2013)	Chronic β-alanine loading increases intercellular buffering while acute bicarbonate loading enhances extra-cellular buffering; taken together they may provide optimal buffering of events involving sustained high-intensity exercise	β-alanine supplementation was very likely to be beneficial to 2,000-m rowing performance (6.4 ± 8.1 s effect compared with placebo), with the effect of sodium bicarbonate having a likely benefit (3.2 ± 8.8 s). There was a small (1.1 ± 5.6 s) but possibly beneficial additional effect of combining β-alanine with sodium bicarbonate compared with β-alanine supplementation alone

FIGURE 34 Examples of performance supplement protocols where different interactions between substances have been identified

Similarly, the supplement Jack3D (see section on Jack3D) removed the ingredient 1,3-dimethylamylamine, also known as DMAA, after the product was linked to haemorrhagic stroke (Young *et al.*, 2012), acute myocardial infarction (Smith *et al.*, 2014) and two deaths (Singer and Lattman, 2013). It remains on the market with different formulations making many of the same marketing claims, but we could find no published reports on the safety or efficacy of the current, DMAA-free formulation.

The presence of exotic and little-known substances, which may be frequently replaced during product reformulation, presents a marketing challenge. To maintain a market advantage, consumers must be educated about the merits of new and exotic substances. When health or fitness is at stake, consumers may want to see scientific evidence of safety and efficacy. To address this challenge, studies are frequently cited in marketing as evidence of effectiveness. In two reviews, Lobb (2010, 2012) suggested that such studies are typically:

1. of small size, short duration, and often un-blinded;
2. have authors associated with industry, and may not fully disclose conflicts of interest, or funding sources;
3. published in 'pay-to-publish' open access publications. Presumably this is due to the relative ease of publication in such journals, as well as ease of access by consumers. The peer-review process in such open access journals has been found to contain significant flaws by some investigators (Bohannon, 2013) although the papers published in open access journals have been found to be similar in impact and scientific quality as those in traditional journals in other reviews (Björk and Solomon, 2012).

In this environment characterized by dynamic information change, the internet is an optimal medium for the rapid updating of marketing messages. Internet commerce allows for round-the-clock sales to consumers in distant locations. Websites marketing supplements often appear as pseudo-news, research or science sites, generally enhanced with splashy multimedia content and links to published evidence of effectiveness. Further, websites provide one-stop for both marketing and easy product ordering (Lobb, 2012), and may in some territories lawfully circumvent state or national restrictions on the marketing (Rezaee *et al.*, 2012) or purchase of certain types of product. Even when a company's official material seems reasonably conservative or within regulations regarding marketing claims, the forums and chat-rooms associated with many websites typically host information of concern posted by users including incredible claims about the outcomes achieved with the use of the products, recommendations regarding high dose protocols, or the 'stacking' of numerous products (see p. 298).

As science evolves, the story about individual supplements may change – from finding evidence to support something that seemed too good to be true, to accumulating more evidence that suggests that the early promise or great theory doesn't quite pan out. Therefore research needs to be seen as a continuing activity, and evolving messages should be seen as a positive sign of a robust system that keeps adding new knowledge rather than a weak system that was wrong. Research and the education that emanates from it should endeavour to provide as much detail as possible about the known safety and efficacy issues for each product, allowing athletes and others in the sports system to make a cost:benefit analysis from their own perspective about supplement use. The issue of legality is often more black and white for competitive athletes since the rules about prohibited substances in Anti-Doping Codes are made clear. However, the ethics of supplement manufacture and use, which are perhaps more ephemeral, should be considered and provide the last piece of this chapter (See article on 'ethics and dietary supplements'.)

ETHICS AND DIETARY SUPPLEMENTS

Michael J. McNamee

One might reasonably question what ethical considerations could possibly arise when discussing the nature and role of dietary supplements. It would be impossible to survey particular products for the issues they give rise to and therefore this discussion is limited to a set of principles that occur very widely in medical ethics (Beauchamp and Childress, 2013). In summary some words are also aimed at the industry in terms of the promotion of products in terms of Truth and Trust.

If a person approaches a healthcare professional for advice, either for some disease, illness or disability, they reasonable expect – in the West at least – to receive a diagnosis and an explanation of the various possible paths to therapy or amelioration. Increasingly, individuals are seeking not simply to recover from various maladies but to enhance their well-being. Ingestion of dietary supplements is sought both as therapy and enhancement but the former has greater ethical urgency than the latter. If a person is healthy but wishes to feel better, no great loss is incurred if the product taken fails to deliver this, except in terms of cost, lost hope, or a developed distrust of the product or industry. A failure to assist in the recovery from a condition, where ingestion of dietary supplements is either an addition to, or surrogate for alternative therapies, leaves that individual in a deleterious state.

Where dietary supplements are taken as a health product, in relation to therapy rather than enhancement, their use ought to pass scrutiny under the principles of (i) Respect for autonomy; (ii) Non-maleficence; (iii) Beneficence;

and (v) Justice. This applies whether in terms of professional interactions with healthcare providers or in terms of the information that is used to market and sell products, and guide their use.

In terms of respect for autonomy, one should expect to make decisions based on reasonable information. This places a burden on producers to explain their products clearly and honestly. Mislabelling, or not clearly indicating substances/ dosages does not enable the individual to choose in an informed way. The failure to specify the high caffeine content in guarana-containing products may mean, for example, that parents choose this product inadvertently and potentially inappropriately for children (see Caffeine in this book). Indeed, mislabelling may be tantamount to misinformation. It is commonsensical that dietary substances should be non-maleficent (not harmful). Observing this principle, however, is not straightforward where dosage/usage maxima are not clearly stated. Moreover, it is not inconceivable that those taking dietary supplements also take a cornucopia of other substances. It is difficult to gain an appreciation of the effects of interactions between various compounds, but where particularly hazardous combinations exist these should be identified in a clear and comprehensible way. Moreover, it is clear that mislabelling of nutritional supplements has been the cause of many elite athletes falling foul of the World Anti-Doping Agency's Prohibited List (see Inadvertent Doping in this book). Given that strict liability operates there – where intention does not need to be proven – the failure to identify constituent chemical materials correctly can literally ruin an entire career and livelihood. Beneficence, that the intervention or substance should benefit the consumer of the product, is the third ethical principle. Here, serious issues have been raised concerning the efficacy of dietary supplements. This principle places limits on what claims can be made about the products. While not as serious as harm to the consumer, it is clearly unethical to make promises that generate reasonable expectations that the product cannot fulfil. Indeed, such claims may be considered fraudulent and not merely dishonest. The final principle, justice, demands that people are fair in their dealings with others. Where individuals or sports teams spend limited resources on dietary supplements or products there will be an opportunity cost; an inability to spend that money elsewhere. How to spend scarce resources for maximum benefit can raise issues of fairness. Contrast the choice of the following examples: iron supplements versus meat in a low-income household, or protein drinks versus flavoured milk in a high school athletics programme.

Finally, it is clear that these principles generate ethical duties for healthcare professionals who advise on the use of dietary supplements and the producers thereof. It is also clear that, where the growing nutrition industry fails to deal truthfully with consumers or indeed the healthcare professions, trust in them will diminish. In addition to governmental oversight of the industry, it is also clearly in the long-term interests of the producers and purveyors of dietary supplements to work towards the development of substantial and ethically justifiable codes of conduct and their robust application.

CONCLUSION

*Samantha J. Stear, Linda M. Castell and
Louise M. Burke*

Dietary/nutritional supplements, functional foods, nutraceuticals, sports/
performance-boosting supplements, ergogenic aids ...

Without doubt, there is widespread use of the products covered by the terms in
this list in the arenas of sport, exercise and health. Across the globe, it appears
that most athletes, from recreational to elite, use sports foods and supplements.
The rationale for this choice varies from the hope that they will compensate
for poor food choices, as well as making up for vital nutrients, to the belief that
there will be an ergogenic and/or health benefit which may translate into an
improvement in sports performance. Indeed, the popularity of certain types of
dietary supplements demonstrates that athletes may often be more motivated
by interests in health benefits and indirect performance enhancement rather
than the direct ergogenic effects. Furthermore, there seems to be a higher
dietary supplement usage with increasing age both in elite athletes and in the
general population. There is also increased use in athletes according to their
performance level.

Of course, the use of any product does not necessarily imply that it is used
correctly. In fact, surveys and professional experiences document that many
athletes fail to follow appropriate supplementation protocols (e.g. correct
source, dosage and timing of intake), even in the case of products that enjoy
good scientific proof of beneficial effects. The downside of flawed protocols
of supplement use includes the waste of resources and the failure to achieve a
potential benefit. However, the major concern is that all too often the mistake is
in exceeding the recommended product dose. This commonly occurs because
of the cultural belief among many athletes that, for example, taking twice the
dose will work twice as well. But more does not necessarily mean better: indeed,

in the case of some supplements, such as the fat-soluble vitamins (A, D, E and K) and iron, more can actually be toxic. Athletes and their support team are strongly recommended to take note of the tolerable 'upper intake levels' (UL) or 'safe upper levels' (SUL) that have been established for vitamins and minerals, as well as the evidence-based protocols that have been established for other nutrients and supplements (see relevant reviews in this book). In addition, medical concerns that may conflict with sports nutrition goals or advice should also be considered. For example: recommended protein requirements are reduced in diabetes; hypertension may have implications for sodium intake; use of caffeine may be contra-indicated in some medical conditions. Supplement dosages for special groups such as wheelchair athletes may also need to be altered because of decreased active muscle mass.

The decision to use a supplement should start with a cost: benefit analysis of whether it is safe, effective and legal/ethical to use. Sometimes specific information of this kind is not available. Studies examining the performance-enhancing effects of the vast array of supplements are relatively few, especially investigations which are relevant to sports events and elite athletes in the field. Subsequently, decisions regarding efficacy often have to be extrapolated from the best available research rather than from clear-cut evidence. Although athletes often wish for clear-cut answers, dietary supplements cannot simply be classified into two groups of 'useful' and 'not useful' or 'risky' versus 'beneficial'. Indeed, even when evidence for a product's benefits is reasonably well-established, the application to any particular athlete is questioned by specific circumstances and their individual response. Nevertheless, in this concluding chapter we have tried to provide a clarifying perspective on the complex world of sports foods and supplements. We embarked on this activity by taking all the current information provided in the supplement reviews throughout the book; then, with the help of our contributors, we attempted to standardise the level of efficacy in terms of sports and/or health performance into a framework summarised via a series of tables (Figures 35–48).

With regard to the safety of supplements, we considered the evidence of health risks from substances themselves as well as the potential for problems from undeclared ingredients or contaminants that have been linked to particular supplements or products in general. A further consideration, concerning legality/ethics, involved the risk of consuming substances that are banned by the anti-doping codes under which competitive sport is organised. Dietary supplements may contain some substances that are banned by WADA (WADA, 2014b) or other anti-doping agencies, either as listed ingredients, or more problematically as undeclared ingredients or contaminants. As highlighted in the expert commentaries on WADA and inadvertent doping (see Introduction chapter), competitive athletes remain solely responsible for their use of prohibited substances. These include the case of those who may be selected for urine or blood tests, the existence of prohibited substances in their system (strict liability). Therefore, the ethical/legal issues of sport can be contravened either by deliberate use of over-the-counter compounds that are prohibited by such codes (e.g. prohormones and stimulants) or by inadvertent intake of these products when they are hidden in supplements. Where this is a known issue for dietary supplements reviewed in this book, they have been assigned to the 'Caution' category in the summary tables that are presented in this chapter, with explanatory commentary provided.

Evaluation of supplements

There are numerous methods by which it is possible, albeit scientifically and practically difficult, to classify supplements on features of interest. When deciding on the efficacy of a supplement it is important to consider first the level of scientific evidence available to support the likelihood that it achieves the claimed outcomes. The traditional view of evidence is based on four levels, I–IV, as described in the introduction chapter (Figure 4) and represented here.

On assessing whether there is sufficient evidence to support the decision to use a supplement, the research should be at level III or IV. Caution should always be taken when considering a supplement if the research is only at levels I and II.

For this book's efficacy index, with the evidence level in mind, the strength of the direction of effect on sports performance and/or health is then considered. The direction of the effect is then ranked from 1–7 accordingly, ranging from: (1) strongly positive effect; (2) fairly positive effect; (3) mixed or no effect; (4) mostly no effect; (5) strong absence of effect and/or possible negative effect. The mid-way ranking (3) is given for those supplements where the evidence has produced mixed results, such that some research has shown positive results whereas others have found no effect or a negative result. Hence to be assigned category (3) there needs to be some evidence of positive effect, otherwise it is

Level I	Anecdotal evidence or expert opinion	These are common in the supplement marketplace, particularly when high-profile athletes promote the use of a particular supplement
Level II	Case series or observational studies	Less common in the supplement research literature
Level III	Randomised control trials (RCT)	The most common type of research undertaken in the supplement literature. However, it is key that the research is of suitable quality (Figure 5)
Level IV	Systematic reviews and meta-analysis	The highest level of evidence to show efficacy of a supplement. However, these are rare and may not always be available, especially for newer supplements which appear on the market

FIGURE 4 Levels of evidence

ranked to (4) 'mostly no effect'. In some instances, where there are known issues, for example, toxicity concerns, or being banned by WADA or FDA, we have assigned the supplement/product to a (6) 'Caution' category, with explanatory remarks provided in the comments column. As the majority of supplements have either supporting evidence for an effect on sports performance or for health, and not both, then the final ranking (7) is used for not applicable, where the evidence is neither clear nor focused.

Furthermore, it is also important to reflect on the discussion in the Introduction chapter regarding factors to consider when assessing research on supplements (see section on evaluation of supplements: Figures 5–9). This includes key factors to consider when assessing research on supplements (Figure 5) such as: study design; numbers and types of participants; type of performance test; study controls; and funding source. There are further factors that also need to be considered when measuring performance (Figure 7) such as the validity, reliability and sensitivity of the performance test, and indeed the type of performance test (e.g. 'Time to exhaustion' versus 'Time trials'), alongside environmental factors to control when measuring performance (Figure 8) including: climate; familiarisation; verbal encouragement; music; physiological measurements and feedback. In addition, an important aspect to consider in supplement research is the supplement's potential bioavailability and effectiveness (Figure 6). This must be coupled with other factors regarding supplement use (Figure 9) such as: financial cost; interaction with other nutrients/supplements; participants' habitual diet and overall nutritional status; adverse side effects in relation to health, adaption to training and performance; purity, contamination and inadvertent doping issues; and also the potential placebo effect.

For the purposes outlined above, regarding factors to consider when assessing research on supplements, a 'summary and comments' column is also provided as part of the efficacy index summary tables, where any key factors or issues with the research and/or supplement can be highlighted. For example, issues surrounding toxicology, safety, side-effects, nutrient-interactions, dosage and timing are highlighted in the comments column so that these are considered alongside the level of evidence and effect of sports performance and/or health. In addition, where there are known issues, for example the substance is considered problematical by WADA and/or the FDA, or there is evidence to suggest a potential risk of contamination with banned substances, then this is also highlighted in the comments column. We note that, in the case of safety issues, the level of evidence required to warrant a caution rating may not be as substantial as the evidence we required to rank the performance effects; this is important because the outcomes are more concerning. Conversely, some ingredients/supplements may be acceptable from a safety perspective but still have a negative impact on sports performance. All factors and aspects surrounding the supplement and the evidence need to be taken into consideration.

Efficacy Index summary

Based on the current evidence provided in the supplement reviews throughout this book, we have collated the following summary tables of our Efficacy Index of Supplements and Sports Foods.

Supplements with potential benefits

Sports performance

First, we consider those supplements with strong evidence (level IV) to suggest a 'strongly positive' effect on sports performance (Figure 35). Not surprising to those working in the field these are few and far between, and include carbohydrates, protein, electrolytes in terms of re-hydration, creatine and caffeine.

The next group is those supplements with good evidence (levels IV and III) to suggest a 'fairly positive' effect on sports performance (Figure 36). Here we find: β-alanine, nitrate, sodium in terms of specific roles (see comments) and as the buffer sodium bicarbonate, and guarana at evidence level IV. Leucine is placed here at the lower evidence level III.

It should be noted that there is some degree of subjectivity in the distinction between ratings of 'strongly positive' versus 'fairly positive' effects on sports performance at evidence levels III and IV, and generally all products in these categories should be regarded in a positive light for their potential to contribute to athletic goals. In undertaking this assessment, we noted that some products enjoy a long history and/or large literature of investigations on which decisions can be made. Furthermore, in many cases, the evidence of benefits to sports performance is relatively more clear cut because the mechanism is well-known, the range of scenarios in which benefits are seen is large and well-defined, and the successful protocol is clearly described and practical to achieve. Of course, we recognise that sometimes this is a feature of the available literature, rather than the product per se, in that some products have been fortunate to attract many well-conducted studies, with well-chosen design and protocols so that the potential to detect a performance benefit has been maximised. Where the literature still needs further development to isolate optimal protocols of use, specific scenarios of best use, or clear understanding of mechanisms of action, we erred on the side of providing a 'fairly positive' rating. We also provided this rating for products in which there may be a reasonable chance of side effects that could negate or reduce the positive performance effect. Finally, we had difficulty finding an appropriate rating for products which have received some evidence of beneficial effects in an isolated study, despite the confidence of the quality of the research, and the apparent robustness of the hypothetical mechanism of action. Some products may have been placed in the 'Mixed/no' effect rating, simply because of the principle that further corroborating evidence should be provided, preferably from other laboratories, before a more positive rating can be justified.

FIGURE 35 Supplements with a 'strongly positive' effect on sports performance at evidence level IV

Supplement/ ingredient	Level of evidence	Direction effect on sports performance	Direction effect on health	Summary and comments
Carbohydrate	Level IV: systematic reviews and meta-analysis	1. Strongly positive	2. Fairly positive	Carbohydrate provides an important fuel source for the muscle and central nervous system during exercise and, in many sports/exercise activities, strategies which maintain an adequate fuel source for muscle/CNS needs (= high carbohydrate availability) are associated with enhanced performance. By contrast, the depletion of these fuel sources is associated with fatigue and a reduction in performance. Carbohydrate supplements can play a useful role when consumed before, during and after exercise to achieve a desired goal of high carbohydrate availability, particularly when it is impractical to consume everyday foods. Some health concerns are noted in terms of oral health, and in the cases where athletes, like many sedentary people, consume carbohydrate in excess of needs.
Multiple Transportable Carbohydrates (MTC)	Level IV: systematic reviews and meta-analysis	1. Strongly positive	7. NOT APPLICABLE	During scenarios of prolonged exercise/sporting activities (> ~ 3 h), optimal performance requires high rates of provision of exogenous carbohydrate (up to ~ 90 g/h) to continue to meet high muscle fuel demands. Since intestinal absorption of glucose-based carbohydrates via the SGLT1 transporter is saturated at intakes of ~ 60 g/h, delivery of higher amounts to the muscle can only be achieved by the ingestion of multiple forms of carbohydrates with different intestinal absorption characteristics (= 'Multiple Transportable Carbohydrates'). Successful blends, including mixtures of glucose/fructose, maltodextrin/fructose and glucose/sucrose/fructose, have been used to achieve elevated rates of muscle carbohydrate oxidation, enhancing performance and reducing the gut discomfort often associated with such high rates of intake.
Sucrose	Level IV: systematic reviews and meta-analysis	1. Strongly positive	5. Strong absence of effect/possible negative effect	Sucrose has been used as a form of carbohydrate in various sports foods designed for intake during exercise (sports drinks, gels, confectionery), with some of these products also being designed to deliver the benefits of increased intestinal absorption of multiple transportable carbohydrates (MTC): glucose and fructose. When sucrose is used in this way, it can enhance sports performance [see also MTC and carbohydrates].

continued ...

Figure 35 continued

Supplement/ ingredient	Level of evidence	Direction effect on sports performance	Direction effect on health	Summary and comments
Electrolytes for rehydration	Level IV: systematic reviews and meta-analysis	1. Strongly positive	1. Strongly positive	The inclusion of electrolytes in rehydration beverages or drinking plans enhances the retention and distribution of water/fluid that is ingested to meet rehydration goals, which can indirectly assist in optimising performance. Although community health guidelines generally promote a reduction in dietary salt intake, the judicious use of electrolyte replacement products to replace sweat electrolytes losses may actually promote a more appropriate sodium replacement than other suggested strategies (intake of salty foods or salt added liberally to meals).
Protein	Level IV: systematic reviews and meta-analysis	1. Strongly positive	2. Fairly positive	The consumption of high quality sources of protein (~0.25-0.30 g/protein/ kg per Lean Body Mass) post-exercise and spread over the day at meals and snacks will maximize post –exercise muscle protein synthetic response. When dietary protein sources are impractical to consume, protein-rich powders and other sports foods can provide an alternative source of high quality protein. Animal-derived protein supplements (e.g. dairy, eggs) are considered high quality, providing all essential amino acids including the important leucine. Vegetable-derived protein sources (e.g. soy, hemp) may be less effective. Consuming in liquid form assists in the rapid digestion and absorption of the protein to increase blood amino acid levels quickly.
Whey protein	Level IV: systematic reviews and meta-analysis	1. Strongly positive	2. Fairly positive	Whey protein is a common form of rapidly digested high quality supplemental protein that can be used to achieve the desired protein serving of ~0.25-30 g/kg per LBM. It is particularly suited to the post-exercise situation where it may not be practical to prepare/consume everyday food sources of protein, and where the rapid digestion of a liquid form of protein quickly promotes muscle protein synthesis rates.

Supplement/ ingredient	Level of evidence	Direction effect on sports performance	Direction effect on health	Summary and comments
Caffeine	Level IV: systematic reviews and meta-analysis	1. Strongly positive	3. Mixed / no effect	There is clear evidence that caffeine is an ergogenic aid for a variety of sports, despite a lack of studies on elite athletes and in the field. Individual trialling is needed to define the range of protocols or sports activities benefiting from caffeine supplementation; in particular, optimal outcomes can be seen at small to moderate caffeine doses (2–3 mg/kg). Effects of caffeine on health and well-being are mixed; most say it adds to their quality of life. However, some individuals react negatively to caffeine or its withdrawal effects (headaches and fatigue); others use excessive doses (resulting in irritability, tremor, and heart rate increases) or mix it with other stimulants or alcohol. Caffeine consumption is safe at moderate intakes (400 mg/d or ~ 6 mg/kg/d); evidence shows that caffeine consumers have reduced health risks, rather than an increase in some diseases. This may be linked with other ingredients in the tea or coffee which is the vehicle for caffeine intake: it should not be extrapolated to intake via sugary energy drinks and colas.
Creatine	Level IV: systematic reviews and meta-analysis	1. Strongly positive	2. Fairly positive	Oral creatine supplementation can maximise muscle creatine levels by either: a 'rapid loading' dose of 20 g/ for ~5d followed by a 'maintenance' dose of 2–3 g/d; or by a 'slow loading dose' of 2–3 g/d for ~30d. Enhancement of muscle phosphocreatine content has been shown to increase capacity for exercise involving repeated high-intensity sprints including an enhancement of the outcomes of strength programmes. Other beneficial uses in sport may also be uncovered. Furthermore, there is also evidence to show creatine loading can improve both muscle and cognitive function in the elderly, as well as treating certain muscle diseases. It is recommended that individuals with pre-existing renal disease or those with a potential risk of renal dysfunction should not use creatine supplements. Vegetarians have lower dietary creatine intake and lower muscle creatine content.

FIGURE 36 Supplements with a 'fairly positive' effect on sports performance at evidence levels IV and III

Supplement/ ingredient	Level of evidence	Direction effect on sports performance	Direction effect on health	Summary and comments
β-alanine	Level IV: systematic reviews and meta-analysis	2. Fairly positive	7. NOT APPLICABLE	There is good evidence that muscle carnosine content can be increased by protocols of 4–8 weeks of supplementation with 3.2–6.4 g/d of β-alanine. Summaries of the literature of β-alanine supplementation show a moderate effect size for an enhancement of performance of high-intensity performance of 2–6 min. More research is needed to understand the mechanism of performance support better, with increased intracellular buffering capacity typically being identified but unlikely to be the sole explanation. Further research is needed to elucidate the potential of this product. β-alanine supplements can give rise to paraesthesia, i.e. a sensation of tingling, prickling or burning (e.g. >10mg/kg BW dose). But this is minimised/abolished by splitting the dose or using a sustained release formulation which mimics β-alanine appearance in blood after meat ingestion. Vegetarians have lower muscle carnosine content.
Nitrate	Level IV: systematic reviews and meta-analysis	2. Fairly positive	2. Fairly positive	Nitrate supplementation has promise as an ergogenic aid but the exact conditions under which it may be efficacious (e.g., subject population, duration and intensity of exercise, nitrate loading regimen) remain to be established, and are amongst the possible variables for the mixed results seen alongside a potential responder/non-responder effect. Nevertheless, there is evidence of an effect when an appropriate dose is used in sub-elite populations, and further studies are required to identify the scenarios of benefit for highly trained/elite competitors.
Sodium	Level IV: systematic reviews and meta-analysis	2. Fairly positive	3. Mixed / no effect	Sodium, the principle electrolyte in sweat, is involved in a number of roles in indirectly supporting sports performance. Supplemental intake of sodium is the most well-supported role as an aid to hydration/rehydration where its replacement is required for the restoration of a fluid deficit. Its intake as part of a pre-event hyperhydration strategy may help to increase body water stores, but how useful this is in assisting thermoregulation and performance in hot conditions is unclear and perhaps dependent on the situation of use. Sodium replacement during exercise that involves large sweat sodium losses (prolonged exercise, 'salty' sweaters etc.) has been purported to reduce the risk of hyponatraemia and to ameliorate exertional muscle cramping caused by a whole-body sodium deficit; again, the evidence for this depends on the

Supplement/ingredient	Level of evidence	Direction effect on sports performance	Direction effect on health	Summary and comments
Sodium bicarbonate	Level IV: systematic reviews and meta-analysis	2. Fairly positive	2. Fairly positive	Sodium bicarbonate loading protocols (e.g. 300mg/kg 90 min before) which increase extracellular buffering capacity are targeted to exercise protocols in which performance is limited due to excessive build up of H+ ions due to high rates of anaerobic glycolysis. They appear to be strongly positive in individual athletes who do not experience gastrointestinal (GI) upset. GI issues may be reduced by manipulating the loading protocol in various ways, using sodium citrate as an alternative (see Figure 37), and protocols may need to be highly individualised to the athlete and event. Resultant changes in pH level of urine may cause problems with standardised requirements for urine samples during Doping Control procedures. Sodium bicarbonate is also included in some urinary alkaliser preparations used to treat urinary tract infections.
Guarana	Level IV: systematic reviews and meta-analysis	2. Fairly positive	3. Mixed / no effect	Due to the popularity of this concentrated source of caffeine in supplements, particularly energy drinks, there have been a few recent reviews on its impact as an ergogenic aid in athletic performance and weight loss. The amounts of guarana found in popular supplements can be below the amounts expected to deliver therapeutic benefits, and/or be unstated, therefore making it a less practical form of caffeine. Emergency Room cases of caffeine overdoses after overindulging in guarana-based energy drinks have been reported.
Leucine	Level III: randomised controlled trials	2. Fairly positive	2. Fairly positive	The anabolic effects of leucine, in particular the stimulatory effect on protein synthesis, is well-documented (strongly positive). Adding extra leucine to a complete protein or EAA mixture has no effect, or only minor additional effect, on the rate of protein synthesis. The amount of leucine required to reach an optimal effect is 1.5–2.5 g in young individuals, and may need to be higher for the elderly.
L-carnitine consumed with carbohydrate	Level III: randomised controlled trials	2. Fairly positive	3. Mixed / no effect	Carnitine supplementation on its own has failed to result in an increased muscle carnitine content. However, breakthrough work from one laboratory has shown evidence that strenuous protocols can achieve this effect without apparent side effects: carnitine co-ingested with carbohydrate (3 g and 160 g per day, respectively, for up to 168 days). The elevation of muscle carnitine content mediates metabolic and genomic responses in skeletal muscle directly linked to muscle fuel metabolism. Further studies are needed to corroborate these findings and their implication.

FIGURE 37 Supplements with a 'strongly or fairly positive' effect on health/clinical situations only at evidence level IV

Supplement/ingredient	Level of evidence	Direction effect on sports performance	Direction effect on health	Summary and comments
Vitamin D for treating deficiency	Level IV: systematic reviews and meta-analysis`	3. Mixed / no effect	1. Strongly positive	The evidence for benefits of Vitamin D supplementation is strongly positive in individuals with Vitamin D deficiency, with athletes now recognised as a group that may develop deficiencies due to inadequate sunlight exposure. The current challenge is in understanding what levels are sufficient or optimal for an athlete. More research is needed in the area of Vitamin D supplementation and performance in athletes, particularly focused on altering Vitamin D levels that may be considered sub-optimal but not deficient.
Aspartame	Level IV: systematic reviews and meta-analysis	3. Mixed / no effect	2. Fairly positive	No current direct evidence of effects in relation to sports performance, but can be expected to have a positive effect via increasing acceptability of drinks for hydration and maintaining a healthy body weight, as per other intense sweeteners. Despite previous, ill-informed concerns, the weight of existing evidence is that aspartame is safe at current levels of consumption.
Calcium for addressing sub-optimal intake	Level IV: systematic reviews and meta-analysis	7. NOT APPLICABLE	2. Fairly positive	Calcium plays an important role in health and performance via its contributions to metabolism, muscle contraction, and skeletal health. Dietary intake should be able to meet requirements in a sound eating plan. However, supplements may be required in cases of increased requirements (growth, menopausal/amenorrhoeic females, high sweat losses) coupled with inadequate intake. If required, it is recommended to take calcium supplements in 400–500g maximum doses and in between meals to avoid adverse effects of extra calcium on absorption of other minerals, e.g. iron, zinc and magnesium.
Flavonoids	Level IV: systematic reviews and meta-analysis	3. Mixed / no effect	2. Fairly positive	Some flavonoid extracts ingested prior to an exercise challenge attenuate post-exercise oxidative stress, inflammation and DOMS. (See review on flavonoids for specific flavonoids and their sub-classes.)

Supplement/ ingredient	Level of evidence	Direction effect on sports performance	Direction effect on health	Summary and comments
Glutamine	Level IV: systematic reviews and meta-analysis	3. Mixed / no effect	2. Fairly positive	Although glutamine has been shown to be effective in decreasing the incidence of URTI (upper respiratory tract illness) in some populations, little evidence has been obtained of an effect on specific aspects of the immune system. More research is also needed to support the effects of glutamine on performance per se. Clinically, glutamine provision improves gut function, shortens recovery from surgery and helps maintains muscle protein mass.
Inositol	Level IV: systematic reviews and meta-analysis	7. NOT APPLICABLE	2. Fairly positive	Although research has been extensive to support its use in a range of clinical situations, very limited data has come from athlete-specific studies, in which it has been combined with other ergogenically active ingredients.
Iron for treating deficiency	Level IV: systematic reviews and meta-analysis	3. Mixed / no effect	2. Fairly positive	Appropriate supplementation of iron in athletes presenting with compromised iron stores is positive, but can have adverse side effects such as GI distress, constipation and/or black coloured stools (from oral preparations); and a degree of discomfort with the potential for anaphylactic shock (from parenteral administration, which should only be administered by trained medical personnel). Athletes should only take supplemental iron under medical guidance due to potential risk of iron overload, whereby excessive iron stores accumulate and cause organ dysfunction through the production of reactive oxygen species. There is some controversy over optimal iron levels for athletic performance, particularly in regard to response to altitude training.
Magnesium	Level IV: systematic reviews and meta-analysis	3. Mixed / no effect	2. Fairly positive	No significant effect of magnesium (Mg) supplementation on endurance or strength performance, at least in athletes with balanced Mg status, but Mg deficiency warrants correction both in terms of health and exercise capacity. For health effects of Mg a level of evidence III can be assumed with respect to insulin resistance/diabetes mellitus type 2.

continued …

Figure 37 continued

Supplement/ ingredient	Level of evidence	Direction effect on sports performance	Direction effect on health	Summary and comments
Probiotics (*Lactobacillus* and *Bifidobacterium* species)	Level IV: systematic reviews and meta-analysis	7. NOT APPLICABLE	2. Fairly positive	For probiotics. evidence is accumulating of a reduction in respiratory illness incidence in both general population and highly physically active people. Effects are dependent on strain and sufficient dose of live bacteria.
Sodium Citrate	Level IV: systematic reviews and meta-analysis	3. Mixed / no effect	2. Fairly positive	Sodium citrate provides an alternative buffer option to sodium bicarbonate (see Figure 36: sodium bicarbonate) with a slightly adapted loading protocol (e.g. 300–600mg/kg taken 1–2 h before exercise). This increases extracellular buffering capacity and is targeted to exercise protocols in which performance is limited by excessive build up of H+ ions due to high rates of anaerobic glycolysis. However, the evidence for a positive impact on exercise performance is not as conclusive as sodium bicarbonate, but has the advantage of reduced likelihood of GI distress. Similarly protocols may need to be highly individualised to the athlete and event. Resultant changes in pH level of urine may cause problems with standardised requirements for urine samples during Doping Control procedures. Sodium citrate is also included in some clinical preparations used to treat urinary tract infections.

FIGURE 38 Supplements with a 'strongly or fairly positive' effect on health/clinical situations only at evidence level III

Supplement/ ingredient	Level of evidence	Direction effect on sports performance	Direction effect on health	Summary and comments
Arginine	Level III: randomised controlled trials	3. Mixed / no effect	2. Fairly positive	Studies have shown varying results in terms of the effect of acute arginine supplementation on performance and chronic supplementation on muscle strength gains. They show potential health benefits and clinical use including wound healing.
Boron	Level III: randomised controlled trials	3. Mixed / no effect	2. Fairly positive	No conclusive evidence for an improved training effect but boron supplementation has been shown to improve bone health and osteoarthritis symptoms (6mg/d).
Copper for treating deficiency	Level III: randomised controlled trials	7. NOT APPLICABLE	2. Fairly positive	Copper deficiency will compromise physiological function. Copper is not ergogenic, but may have a beneficial role in bone health. Copper toxicity has been associated with water contamination over 1.6mg/L. Copper supplementation needs clinical justification due to toxicity issues.
Fish oils	Level III: randomised controlled trials	3. Mixed / no effect	2. Fairly positive	Mixed reports in athletes. Good evidence for positive physiological functions and for health benefits (cardiovascular disease, inflammation, possibly bone health, some cancers). Very high intakes of fish oil can cause nausea and GI upset. High dose (3.2g EPA plus 2g DHA daily) for 3 weeks improves lung function post-exercise in non-atopic elite athletes with exercise-induced bronchoconstriction and in asthmatic athletes.
Folate for treating deficiency	Level III: randomised controlled trials	7. NOT APPLICABLE	2. Fairly positive	Research has shown that low blood levels of key blood nutrients, including folate, impair exercise performance. In cases of diagnosed deficiency, a supplement may be needed. However, although folate supplementation improves blood folate levels, it does not affect performance.
Garlic	Level III: randomised controlled trials	3. Mixed / no effect	2. Fairly positive	More positive effect on health than on physical performance. Good evidence that regular and high intakes (6–10g fresh garlic daily) may improve the peripheral circulation.

continued …

Figure 38 continued

Supplement/ ingredient	Level of evidence	Direction effect on sports performance	Direction effect on health	Summary and comments
Glutathione precursors (Cysteine, Glycine, N-acetylcysteine)	Level III: randomised controlled trials	3. Mixed / no effect	2. Fairly positive	For sports and performance: Supplementation with glutathione (GSH) precursors may result in an increase in GSH in skeletal muscle, liver and erythrocytes; and may reduce oxidative stress and inflammation. However, it may delay exercise recovery and stress adaptation. For health: GSH deficiency was corrected by amino acid supplementation in diabetes, HIV-infected patients, older adults and those with Parkinson's disease. GSH is also a well-known antioxidant. (See comments for Vitamins A, C, E)
Histidine-containing-dipeptides (HCD)	Level III: randomised controlled trials	3. Mixed / no effect	2. Fairly positive	Carnosine is the only HCD (histidine-containing-dipeptide) found in human skeletal muscle, but is not stable in human blood and is rapidly degraded by serum carnosinase. HCD-rich supplements, such as chicken breast extract, are popular in Asia but warrant further research regarding performance improvements. Clinically, only a very few small-scale studies are available on Parkinson's disease, schizophrenia and autistic spectrum disorder.
Gamma linolenic acid	Level III: randomised controlled trials	5. Strong absence of effect / possible negative effect	2. Fairly positive	There is no scientific evidence to support improvements in sports performance with high doses thought to impair performance by having an adverse effect on mood, perhaps due to gamma linolenic acid (GLA) being a precursor of arachidonic acid. GLA has several beneficial clinical applications.
Melatonin	Level III: randomised controlled trials	3. Mixed / no effect	2. Fairly positive	An anti-oxidant, immunomodulator and anti-cancer agent associated with temperature regulation and sleep onset. Useful to modulate jet lag and, perhaps, thermal responses to exercise.
Methyl-sulfonyl-methane (MSM)	Level III: randomised controlled trials	7. NOT APPLICABLE	2. Fairly positive	Three small studies have shown slight but statistically significant improvement in osteoarthritic pain scores, pain and ankle hind foot scores in achilles tendinopathy, respectively. However, in some studies the supplement contained other active substances so MSM's contribution is unclear.

Supplement/ ingredient	Level of evidence	Direction effect on sports performance	Direction effect on health	Summary and comments
Plant sterols	Level III: randomised controlled trials	7. NOT APPLICABLE	2. Fairly positive	No direct ergogenic effects, but may improve lipid profiles or immune function.
Pycnogenol	Level III: randomised controlled trials	3. Mixed / no effect	2. Fairly positive	There are a limited number of sport performance-related studies using pycnogenol, with no convincing evidence of an ergogenic effect. Pycnogenol supplementation has been reported to have a wide array of health benefits including cardiovascular and anti-inflammatory effects.
Resveratrol	Level III: randomised controlled trials	3. Mixed / no effect	2. Fairly positive	Antioxidant properties. Evidence of sports performance effects are mainly in animal studies; human studies focus more on diseases like stroke, diabetes. Doses of 1600mg per day in a 70kg participant are regarded as safe, even long-term.
Selenium	Level III: randomised controlled trials	7. NOT APPLICABLE	2. Fairly positive	Selenium deficiency, although rare, will compromise physiological function. Selenium is not ergogenic, but has antioxidant properties.
Theobromine, theophylline	Level III: randomised controlled trials	3. Mixed / no effect	2. Fairly positive	Chemically similar to caffeine, and found in chocolate as well as the dietary sources of caffeine (tea, cola, coffee etc.). May also be found in some energy and sports foods although in amounts below the therapeutic dose of pure theophylline, which is a prescription drug used as an anti-asthmatic and under investigation as a treatment for other cardiorespiratory diseases. Theophylline has demonstrated immunomodulatory properties. Specific evidence regarding ergogenic properties for theophylline is sparse and provides mixed results; studies on theobromine are not available. WADA considered regulating these substances given their similarity to caffeine but, like caffeine, they are not included on the Prohibited List.

continued …

Figure 38 continued

Supplement/ ingredient	Level of evidence	Direction effect on sports performance	Direction effect on health	Summary and comments
Vanadyl Sulphate (Vanadium)	Level III: randomised controlled trials	4. Mostly no effect	2. Fairly positive	Five vanadyl sulphate supplementation studies failed to demonstrate a significant effect on body composition or muscle protein synthesis. Vanadium in various forms exert widespread biological effects and are currently the subject of research into antidiabetic therapeutics and anticancer agents. Vanadium in sulphate form has low toxicity or side effects.
Vitamin K for treating deficiency	Level III: randomised controlled trials	7. NOT APPLICABLE	2. Fairly positive	Given the mixed findings in the role of vitamin K in bone health generally, and the limited information available in athletic populations, further studies are required before it is routinely considered in the management of bone health in athletes.
Wheat Germ Oil	Level III: randomised controlled trials	7. NOT APPLICABLE	2. Fairly positive	There is a lack of supporting evidence regarding a role for wheat germ oil (WGO) in sports performance. There is some evidence for a positive role in cholesterol metabolism. WGO, however, contains significant quantities of bioactive compounds, and in particular is the richest plant origin source of tocopherols (vitamin E).
Zinc for treating deficiency	Level III: randomised controlled trials	3. Mixed / no effect	2. Fairly positive	The scientific evidence for any performance benefit is weak in the absence of a Zn deficiency. Tolerable Upper Intake Level of Zn for adults is 40 mg/d, with >100 mg/d causing adverse health effects e.g. headache, abdominal cramps and nausea, together with copper deficiency, which can cause anaemia, leucopaenia and neutropaenia.

Health

Finally, the third group is those supplements with good evidence (levels IV and III) to suggest a 'strongly or fairly positive' effect on health and/or clinical situations at level IV (Figure 37) and level III (Figure 38).

In Figure 37 with strong evidence (level IV) we find: vitamin D in terms of treating deficiency to be 'strongly positive' whereas 'fairly positive' are: aspartame; calcium in terms of addressing sub-optimal intake; flavonoids; glutamine, inositol, iron in terms of treating deficiency; magnesium; probiotics (*Lactobacillus* and *Bifidobacterium* species); and sodium citrate.

Also from the previous two figures (Figures 35 and 36) we find a strong level of evidence (level IV) to suggest a 'strongly positive' effect on health for electrolytes in terms of re-hydration (Figure 35); and 'fairly positive' for health for: carbohydrates, protein and creatine (Figure 35); and nitrate and sodium bicarbonate (Figure 36).

In Figure 38, with good evidence (level III) to suggest a 'fairly positive' effect on health and/or clinical situations we have twenty products: copper, folate, vitamin K and zinc in terms of treating deficiencies; arginine; boron; fish oils; garlic; glutathione precursors; histidine-containing peptides (HCD); gamma-linoleic acid; melatonin; methyl-sulphonyl-methane (MSM); plant sterols; pycnogenol; resveratrol; selenium; theobromine and theophylline; vanadyl sulphate (vanadium); and wheat germ oil; plus leucine from Figure 36.

Supplements with mixed results or no effect

The next group is the huge list of supplements ($n=33$) with albeit good evidence (levels IV and III) but with only a mixed or no significant effect on sports performance and/or health. It is worth noting that to be assigned to this category there needs to be some evidence of positive results, but the culmination of results, due to some research showing no or negative effects, is mixed or no effect. In Figure 39, with strong evidence (level IV) to suggest a 'mixed or no' effect on both sports performance and health are: antioxidants; vitamins A, C and E; chromium picolinate; conjugated linoleic acid (CLA); ginseng; green tea; alpha-liopic acid (ALA); and rhodiola rosea.

Also from Figure 37 with strong evidence (level IV) to suggest a 'mixed or no' effect on sports performance we have: iron and vitamin D in terms of treating deficiencies; aspartame; flavonoids; glutamine; magnesium; and sodium citrate.

In Figure 40, still with strong evidence (level IV) to suggest a 'mixed or no' effect on health only are: chondroitin and glucosamine; chlorogenic acids; and echinacea. From previous figures, also with strong evidence (Level IV) to

FIGURE 39 Supplements with a 'mixed or no' effect on sports performance and health at evidence level IV

Supplement/ ingredient	Level of evidence	Direction effect on sports performance	Direction effect on health	Summary and comments
Vitamins A, C, E	Level IV: systematic reviews and meta-analysis	3. Mixed / no effect	3. Mixed / no effect	These vitamins undertake many roles in the body including functioning as antioxidants. The need for supplemental forms of these vitamins should be minimal if the athlete can follow a nutrient-dense eating plan. There is some evidence that supplementation with large amounts of Vitamins C and E can cause an imbalance to the body's complex anti-oxidant system and may actually impair performance by blunting the adaptive responses to exercise that are mediated by oxidative signalling.
Antioxidants	Level IV: systematic reviews and meta-analysis	3. Mixed / no effect	3. Mixed / no effect	Consumption of supplemental dietary antioxidants attenuate exercise-induced oxidative stress, but also mitigate the benefits of ROS-induced adaptations to exercise training. (See comments for Vitamins A, C, E)
Chromium picolinate	Level IV: systematic reviews and meta-analysis	3. Mixed / no effect	3. Mixed / no effect	Although the data on the effects of chromium picolinate on muscle gain, fat loss, and management of diabetes strongly suggest little or no effect, there are far fewer data available on long -erm safety. Clinically, more work needs to be done to understand fully any potential value of chromium picolinate in the management of diabetes.
Conjugated lin-oleic acid (CLA)	Level IV: systematic reviews and meta-analysis	3. Mixed / no effect	3. Mixed / no effect	Mixed effects reported in both athletes and non-athletes probably due to isomer mix, and doses used. Inconclusive evidence of CLA producing any clinically relevant effects on body composition in the long term.
Ginseng	Level IV: systematic reviews and meta-analysis	3. Mixed / no effect	3. Mixed / no effect	Ergogenic properties of ginseng have not been substantiated scientifically. Often used in energy drinks. Great heterogeneity in supplements based on pre-consumer factors. Side effects are often related to over-consumption.

Supplement/ ingredient	Level of evidence	Direction effect on sports performance	Direction effect on health	Summary and comments
Green tea	Level IV: systematic reviews and meta-analysis	3. Mixed / no effect	3. Mixed / no effect	EGCG (epigallocatechin-3-gallate), a catechin (subclass of flavonoids), is a widely-studied biologically active component abundant in green tea. Side effects are often related to over-consumption. Caffeine component is more likely to affect performance with health concerns being raised over catechins (see review on Yerba maté).
Alpha-lipoic acid (ALA)	Level IV: systematic reviews and meta-analysis	3. Mixed / no effect	3. Mixed / no effect	Supportive evidence is specific to diabetic neuropathy. Although often added to combination sport supplements, this is based on equivocal research findings and applications.
Rhodiola rosea	Level IV: systematic reviews and meta-analysis	3. Mixed / no effect	3. Mixed / no effect	Evidence is inconclusive as to whether Rhodiola supplementation, in doses of 100–600 mg/day, can enhance either mental and/or exercise performance. May possess antioxidant properties.

FIGURE 40 Supplements with a 'mixed or no' effect on health only at evidence level IV

Supplement/ ingredient	Level of evidence	Direction effect on sports performance	Direction effect on health	Summary and comments
Chondroitin	Level IV: systematic reviews and meta-analysis	7. NOT APPLICABLE	3. Mixed / no effect	No ergogenic effect; mixed results for treatment of osteoarthritis regarding symptom treatment – appears safe with minimal side effect profile.
Chlorogenic acids (CGA)	Level IV: systematic reviews and meta-analysis	7. NOT APPLICABLE	3. Mixed / no effect	The evidence to support the isolated application and use of CGA as a supplement, at least in humans, on type 2 diabetes or on weight loss is unclear, largely limited to animal research, with the reduction seen in body weight being generally clinically insignificant. It is also unlikely that CGA will alter the ergogenic effects of caffeine when consumed as coffee.
Echinacea	Level IV: systematic reviews and meta-analysis	7. NOT APPLICABLE	3. Mixed / no effect	Great heterogeneity in supplements based on pre-consumer factors. Limited studies on health effects in athletes, with effects seemingly stronger than in non-athletes. No effect on sports performance.
Glucosamine	Level IV: systematic reviews and meta-analysis	7. NOT APPLICABLE	3. Mixed / no effect	No ergogenic effect; mixed results for the treatment of osteoarthritis regarding symptom treatment – appears safe with minimal side effect profile

FIGURE 41 Supplements with a 'mixed or no' effect on sports performance and health at evidence level III

Supplement/ ingredient	Level of evidence	Direction effect on sports performance	Direction effect on health	Summary and comments
Citrulline	Level III: randomised controlled trials	3. Mixed / no effect	3. Mixed / no effect	Evidence to support the use of L-citrulline as an ergogenic aid, although promising, is lacking and further research with this relatively new supplement in sports performance is required.
Co-Enzyme Q10	Level III: randomised controlled trials	3. Mixed / no effect	3. Mixed / no effect	Mixed results from supplementation studies. Note the general caution about antioxidant supplementation in terms of blunting the adaptive response to exercise (See comments for vitamins A, C, E)
Cordyceps (Ophiocordyceps)	Level III: randomised controlled trials	3. Mixed / no effect	3. Mixed / no effect	May affect oxygen metabolism. Often given in combination with other herbal preparations.
Glycine	Level III: randomised controlled trials	3. Mixed / no effect	3. Mixed / no effect	At present there is insufficient evidence for glycine supplementation in sports performance. However, further research on the ergogenic effectiveness of GPLC (Glycine-Propionyl-L-Carnitine) is warranted. In addition glycine's anti-inflammatory role is being investigated.
HMB	Level III: randomised controlled trials	3. Mixed / no effect	3. Mixed / no effect	3g daily dose is well tolerated but effects are small, if any, amongst trained individuals, especially if dietary protein intake is optimised. Application amongst clinical populations, including disuse atrophy following injury, warrants further investigation.
N-acetylcysteine (NAC)	Level III: randomised controlled trials	3. Mixed / no effect	3. Mixed / no effect	Performance data limited to small studies under laboratory conditions; only cycling and specific muscle group endurance evaluated (no competitive sports); side effects, nausea and vomiting, may limit use at doses that increase performance. The potential for blunting adaptive response to training should also be considered. (See comments for vitamins A, C, E)

continued …

Figure 41 continued

Supplement/ ingredient	Level of evidence	Direction effect on sports performance	Direction effect on health	Summary and comments
Tyrosine	Level III: randomised controlled trials	3. Mixed / no effect	3. Mixed / no effect	More research is necessary to demonstrate any potential exercise and cognitive performance enhancing effects of tyrosine. There is individual responsiveness to tyrosine supplementation. Acute or short-term administration appears to be safe, not inducing side effects, but there is no information on long-term use.
Tryptophan	Level III: randomised controlled trials	3. Mixed / no effect	3. Mixed / no effect	Currently, there is no credible evidence that tryptophan supplementation has any beneficial effects on athletes. In fact an increase in the plasma concentration of tryptophan might actually be detrimental and lead to premature fatigue, e.g. in endurance events. Clinically, tryptophan is prescribed to alleviate depression.
Yerba maté	Level III: randomised controlled trials	3. Mixed / no effect	3. Mixed / no effect	Another plant source of caffeine. There have only been a couple of RCT studies, both using a commercial product. Therefore specific evidence for an effect on athletic performance is limited and cannot be attributed to yerba maté per se. There remains an increased risk of adverse effects using herbal supplements particularly those containing multiple ingredients.

FIGURE 42 Supplements with a 'mixed or no' effect on sports performance only at evidence level III

Supplement/ ingredient	Level of evidence	Direction effect on sports performance	Direction effect on health	Summary and comments
Branched chain amino acids	Level III: randomised controlled trials	3. Mixed / no effect	7. NOT APPLICABLE	There is some evidence to suggest that BCAA supplementation during sustained physical activity can exert positive effects on cognitive and physical performance. Amount of BCAA recommended is 0.03–0.05g/kg BW/h or 2–4g/h ingested repeatedly during recovery. Large doses of BCAA (~30g/d) are well tolerated; however, they may be detrimental to performance due to increased production of ammonia by the exercising muscle.
Cysteine & cystine	Level III: randomised controlled trials	3. Mixed / no effect	7. NOT APPLICABLE	Very little evidence to support its use. Most research has studied the N-acetylcysteine form (see comments for NAC). Further research needed, particularly looking at oral cysteine ingestion and exercise performance and the effect of cystine supplementation on the immune response to training.
Electrolytes for hyperhydration	Level III: randomised controlled trials	3. Mixed / no effect	7. NOT APPLICABLE	Limited evidence. Specific to efficacy of sodium supplementation in hyperhydration protocols to enhance thermoregulation capacity and performance by increasing body fluid stores prior to exercise in hot conditions. Used as alternative to glycerol; few studies currently available.
HICA	Level III: randomised controlled trials	3. Mixed / no effect	7. NOT APPLICABLE	There is currently limited evidence to support the use of HICA in athletes. However, it is promising and warrants further research.
AKG (α-ketoglutarate)	Level III: randomised controlled trials	3. Mixed / no effect	4. Mostly no effect	Currently, there is insufficient evidence to support the use of AKG supplements enhancing athletic performance. No negative side effects reported for doses up to 2g/d.
KIC (α-ketoisocaproate)	Level III: randomised controlled trials	3. Mixed / no effect	7. NOT APPLICABLE	At present there is insufficient evidence to support the use of KIC supplementation in enhancing exercise performance or reducing muscle damage. No negative side effects reported for doses up to 10g per day. Has been investigated in conjunction with glycine and L-arginine and HMB with mixed results.

continued …

Figure 42 continued

Supplement/ ingredient	Level of evidence	Direction effect on sports performance	Direction effect on health	Summary and comments
Medium Chain Triglycerides (MCT)	Level III: randomised con- trolled trials	3. Mixed / no effect	7. NOT APPLICABLE	Despite some support for MCT use during prolonged exercise, MCT ap- pear to have limited application to most sporting situations. In addition, the theoretical metabolic benefits are likely to be outweighed by the associated gastrointestinal distress.
Ornithine	Level III: randomised con- trolled trials	3. Mixed / no effect	7. NOT APPLICABLE	There is some evidence that L-ornithine hydrochloride supplementation prior to high-intensity exercise may improve sports performance, but further research is needed using valid measures of performance. In the clinical setting, ornithine-α-ketoglutarate has been shown to improve recovery of individuals from burns, trauma and in the post-operative state.
Phenylalanine	Level III: randomised con- trolled trials	3. Mixed / no effect	7. NOT APPLICABLE	No studies supplementing directly with phenylalanine (level of evidence from tyrosine supplementation studies); excess phenylalanine converted to tyrosine by liver; no effect of tyrosine supplementation on exercise performance.
Phosphate	Level III: randomised con- trolled trials	3. Mixed / no effect	7. NOT APPLICABLE	Although there is some evidence of an ergogenic benefit of phosphate supple- mentation it has only correlated well with increases in 2,3 DPG levels in some instances. Supplementation may also be necessary to correct deficiencies but can have adverse side effects. Furthermore, excessive phosphate loading may place unnecessary strain on the kidneys: consequently, athletes with known kidney disorders should refrain from using phosphate.
Taurine	Level III: randomised con- trolled trials	3. Mixed / no effect	7. NOT APPLICABLE	There is no scientific evidence to support an ergogenic effect of supplemental taurine in human subjects. Despite large increases in plasma taurine following acute ingestion of a large dose of taurine, it does not enhance endurance per- formance in well-trained athletes and does not accumulate in skeletal muscles when consumed chronically (5g/d for 7d).

FIGURE 43 Supplements with a 'mixed or no' effect on health only at evidence level III

Supplement/ ingredient	Level of evidence	Direction effect on sports performance	Direction effect on health	Summary and comments
D-Aspartic acid (D-AA)	Level III: randomised controlled trials	4. Mostly no effect	3. Mixed / no effect	At this stage there is limited evidence with regard to the efficacy of this supplement for athletes. 2–3g/day is the range of standard doses. There have been no reported side effects within the dosing ranges and time course (approximately 1 month maximum), and further study is required.
Bee pollen	Level III: randomised controlled trials	4. Mostly no effect	3. Mixed / no effect	Little evidence from well–controlled trials to support the broad range of health claims or ergogenic properties; no clinical trials to assess appropriate dosages or health risks properly; some case study reports of allergic/anaphylactic reactions stemming from supplementation.
Cissus quadrangularis	Level III: randomised controlled trials	7. NOT APPLICABLE	3. Mixed / no effect	Animal and *in vitro* research is promising for both its potential bone influencing properties and use for weight loss. However, well-controlled research data in humans, particularly in the athletic population, is scarce. Currently there is no evidence that CQ poses a safety issue in humans but data is limited.
Ginger	Level III: randomised controlled trials	7. NOT APPLICABLE	3. Mixed / no effect	May exhibit analgesic or anti-inflammatory properties in certain contexts, but ergogenic properties are unproven.
Ginkgo	Level III: randomised controlled trials	7. NOT APPLICABLE	3. Mixed / no effect	Often discussed in the context of altitude sickness. May have haemorrheological effects, but effects are likely to be inconsistent due to variations in manufacturing processes.
Nootkatone	Level III: randomised controlled trials	7. NOT APPLICABLE	3. Mixed / no effect	There are no reports on the effects of grapefruit, including nootkatone, on physical performance in humans and scant evidence for its role in weight loss. Further studies are required to clarify the efficacy of nootkatone as an ergogenic and anti-obesity compound.

continued …

Figure 43 continued

Supplement/ ingredient	Level of evidence	Direction effect on sports performance	Direction effect on health	Summary and comments
Octacosanol and Policosanol	Level III: randomised controlled trials	4. Mostly no effect	3. Mixed / no effect	Although supplementing with octacosanol and policosanol has been shown to have favourable effects on hypercholesterolaemia and hyperlipidaemia, more recent studies have found no positive effects. Research on athletic performance is lacking and remains unclear. No negative side effects reported for doses up to 12 mg per day.
Papain	Level III: randomised controlled trials	7. NOT APPLICABLE	3. Mixed / no effect	In most research, papain was tested in conjunction with other proteases, or other supplements, making it difficult to isolate effectiveness, as well as producing some equivocal results.
Potassium	Level III: randomised controlled trials	4. Mostly no effect	3. Mixed / no effect	Potassium (K) is a minor electrolyte in sweat and does not appear to require specific replacement during and/or after exercise. The consumption of very high levels of supplemental forms of K might result in hyperkalaemia which could lead to cardiac arrhythmias and even cardiac arrest. Individuals with kidney failure or compromised kidney function or other chronic clinical conditions should seek clinical advice before taking any K supplement or consuming potassium-rich foods.
Spirulina	Level III: randomised controlled trials	4. Mostly no effect	3. Mixed / no effect	The current literature on spirulina supplementation in athletes is extremely sparse and does not address the many claims made for this product. There are some concerns over the safety of spirulina supplements due to contamination with heavy metals or toxins with excessive dosage leaving the recommended maximum dose at 15g/day; nutrient interactions unknown.
Phlogenzym and Wobenzyme	Level III: randomised controlled trials	7. NOT APPLICABLE	3. Mixed / no effect	Studies in the athletic population are lacking. Other findings have been mixed, but suggest that phlogenzym and wobenzyme could be used as an effective anti-inflammatory and analgesic, but further research is needed to elucidate the potential mechanisms of action. No toxic or side effects reported in doses of 540 mg bromelain, 288 mg trypsin, 600 mg rutin.

Supplement/ ingredient	Level of evidence	Direction effect on sports performance	Direction effect on health	Summary and comments
D-pinitol	Level III: randomised controlled trials	7. NOT APPLICABLE	3. Mixed / no effect	Although pinitol may have some benefit in disease-related outcomes, there has been no evidence to support its use in athletes.
Prebiotics	Level III: randomised controlled trials	7. NOT APPLICABLE	3. Mixed / no effect	There is no specific investigation of whether prebiotics directly affect sports performance. Trials have provided mixed evidence of health effects but there is no indication of a negative health effect.
Probiotics (species and combinations of different species or strains other than *Lactobacillus* and *Bifidobacterium*)	Level III: randomised controlled trials	7. NOT APPLICABLE	3. Mixed / no effect	Limited evidence of reduction in respiratory illness incidence in both general population and highly physically active people. Effects are dependent on species, strain and sufficient dose of live bacteria.
Wolfberry (Goji berry)	Level III: randomised controlled trials	7. NOT APPLICABLE	3. Mixed / no effect	Some peer-reviewed publications suggest some specific health benefits via: prevention of diabetic retinopathy and inhibition of prostate cancer progression. No evidence for benefits for sports performance.

suggest a 'mixed or no' effect on health are: caffeine (Figure 35); plus sodium and guarana (Figure 36).

In Figure 41, with good evidence (level III) to suggest a 'mixed or no' effect on both sports performance and health are: L-carnitine consumed with carbohydrate; citrulline; co-enzyme Q10; cordyceps (ophiocordyceps); glycine; HMB; N-acetylcysteine (NAC); tyrosine; tryptophan; and yerba maté.

Next, in Figure 42, with good evidence (level III) to suggest a 'mixed or no' effect on sports performance only are: branched chain amino acids (BCAA); cysteine and cystine; electrolytes with regard to hyperhydration; HICA; α-ketoglutarate (AKG); α-ketoisocaproate (KIC); medium chain triglycerides (MCTs); ornithine; phenylalanine; phosphate; and taurine.

Also from Figure 38, with good evidence (level III) to suggest a 'mixed or no' effect on sports performance we have: arginine; boron; fish oils; garlic; glutathione precursors; histidine-containing peptides (HCD); melatonin; pycnogenol; resveratrol; theobromine and theophylline; and zinc in terms of treating deficiency.

Finally, in Figure 43 with good evidence (level III) to suggest a 'mixed or no' effect on health only are: D-Aspartic acid (D-AA); bee pollen; cissus quadrangularis; ginger; ginkgo; nootkatone; octacosanol and policosanol; papain; potassium; spirulina; phlogenzym and wobenzyme; D-pinitol; prebiotics; probiotics (species and combinations of different species or strains other than *Lactobacillus* and *Bifidobacterium*); and wolfberry (goji berry).

Supplements with mostly no effect

In Figure 44 are those supplements which suggest good evidence (levels IV and III), but have 'mostly no effect' on sports performance and/or health.

With strong evidence (level IV) but 'mostly no' effect on sports performance is aspartate.

With good evidence (level III) but 'mostly no' effect on sports performance are: choline bitartrate plus acetylcholine; cytochrome C; dihydroxyacetone phosphate (DHAP) and pyruvate; dimethyglycine; ferulic acid and gamma-oryzanol; lecithin; phosphatidlyserine (plant-derived); ribose; succinate; valine; water (oxygenated); B vitamins; and ZMA; plus vanadyl sulphate (vanadium) from Figure 38.

With good evidence (level III) but 'mostly no' effect on health are: choline bitartrate plus acetylcholine; phosphatidylserine (plant-derived); and the B vitamins; plus α-ketoglutarate (AKG) from Figure 42.

FIGURE 44 Supplements with a 'mostly no' effect on sports performance and/or health at evidence levels IV and III

Supplement/ingredient	Level of evidence	Direction effect on sports performance	Direction effect on health	Summary and comments
Aspartate	Level IV: systematic reviews and meta-analysis	4. Mostly no effect	7. NOT APPLICABLE	Various forms of aspartate including L-aspartate, D-aspartate and N-methyl-D-aspartate. Lack of evidence to support an ergogenic effect. No toxicity or side effects yet reported.
Choline bitartrate plus acetylcholine	Level III: randomised controlled trials	4. Mostly no effect	4. Mostly no effect	Despite several studies showing choline supplementation elevating plasma choline concentrations there is no evidence this has translated into benefits in athletic performance or reductions in fatigue. Small supplemental doses are currently not considered harmful and the upper safe limit is set at 3–3.5 g for adults, although some forms of choline supplements may cause gastrointestinal side effects leading to fishy body odours; individuals with gout are advised to avoid them altogether.
Cytochrome C	Level III: randomised controlled trials	4. Mostly no effect	7. NOT APPLICABLE	Commonly studied as part of antioxidant formulations. No effect on sports performance.
Dihydroxyacetone phosphate (DHAP) & pyruvate	Level III: randomised controlled trials	4. Mostly no effect	7. NOT APPLICABLE	There is currently no scientific basis for the use of DHAP/pyruvate as an ergogenic aid. Furthermore, it is unlikely that the ingested compounds could even reach skeletal muscle and have a direct effect on metabolism.
Dimethylglycine	Level III: randomised controlled trials	4. Mostly no effect	7. NOT APPLICABLE	Lack of evidence to support an ergogenic effect. Elevated plasma dimethylglycine is associated with higher cardiovascular mortality, though study was not based on supplementation.
Ferulic Acid and gamma-oryzanol	Level III: randomised controlled trials	4. Mostly no effect	7. NOT APPLICABLE	Only one full peer-reviewed study. No evidence to support their use in athletic populations.

continued …

Figure 44 continued

Supplement/ingredient	Level of evidence	Direction effect on sports performance	Direction effect on health	Summary and comments
Lecithin	Level III: randomised controlled trials	4. Mostly no effect	7. NOT APPLICABLE	Lecithin supplementation appears to prevent the decrease in choline levels after exercise, but there is no clear evidence to indicate any performance benefits.
Phosphatidlyserine – plant derived	Level III: randomised controlled trials	4. Mostly no effect	4. Mostly no effect	Typical dose range 100–500 mg/d; no effect on cognitive function or performance.
Ribose	Level III: randomised controlled trials	4. Mostly no effect	7. NOT APPLICABLE	Although ribose supplementation appears to improve the rate of de novo synthesis of ATP in muscle, existing scientific evidence does not support the use of ribose as an ergogenic aid in young healthy individuals.
Succinate	Level III: randomised controlled trials	4. Mostly no effect	7. NOT APPLICABLE	No performance benefit based on very limited research; underlying theoretical rationale is questionable.
Water (oxygenated)	Level III: randomised controlled trials	4. Mostly no effect	7. NOT APPLICABLE	There is no scientific evidence for the ergogenic claims for oxygenated water.
Valine	Level III: randomised controlled trials	4. Mostly no effect	7. NOT APPLICABLE	Valine is an important essential amino acid but, in isolation from other BCAA, it has no significant effect on exercise performance or muscle protein synthesis.
Vitamin B	Level III: randomised controlled trials	4. Mostly no effect	4. Mostly no effect	According to current evidence, when adequate intakes and status of B vitamins are present, further supplementation does not enhance exercise performance.
ZMA	Level III: randomised controlled trials	4. Mostly no effect	7. NOT APPLICABLE	At present, there is little evidence to support the use of ZMA as an anabolic nutritional intervention.

FIGURE 45 Supplements with a 'strong absence of effect/possible negative effect' on sports performance and/or health at evidence levels IV and III

Supplement/ ingredient	Level of evidence	Direction effect on sports performance	Direction effect on health	Summary and comments
Arnica	Level IV: systematic reviews and meta-analysis	5. Strong absence of effect/possible negative effect	5. Strong absence of effect/possible negative effect	There is little compelling evidence that herbal or homeopathic arnica preparations have a role in sports medicine or health apart from potentially reducing bruising when applied topically. Herbal arnica is administered topically, because arnica can be neurotoxic when given orally. Consequently oral homeopathic arnica preparations are typically highly diluted (pillule form).
GABA (γ-aminobutyric acid)	Level III: randomised controlled trials	5. Strong absence of effect/possible negative effect	7. NOT APPLICABLE	Some effects of GABAergic manipulation and response to resistance training, but more research is needed to elucidate the role of GABA. An overdose might result in cognitive impairments, hallucinations, loss of consciousness. Alcohol reinforces the effects of benzodiazepines.
Inosine	Level III: randomised controlled trials	5. Strong absence of effect/possible negative effect	7. NOT APPLICABLE	Despite its physiological role, little has been shown to support the use of inosine as an ergogenic aid. Some work suggests that high dose inosine, a uric acid precursor, combined with elevated urinary excretion, could be detrimental and result in kidney stones or acute renal failure.
Royal jelly	Level III: randomised controlled trials	7. NOT APPLICABLE	5. Strong absence of effect/possible negative effect	Little benefits in exercise have been observed. Case reports of anaphylaxis, haemorrhagic colitis and asthma.
Smilax (Sarsaparilla)	Level III: randomised controlled trials	5. Strong absence of effect/possible negative effect	5. Strong absence of effect/possible negative effect	There is presently no evidence of ergogenic benefits from Smilax supplementation and its use is discouraged. May produce kidney and stomach problems. May interact with other drugs.

FIGURE 46 Supplements with only the lowest level of evidence at levels II and I

Supplement/ingredient	Level of evidence	Direction effect on sports performance	Direction effect on health	Summary and comments
Electrolytes & hyponatraemia	Level II: case series or observational studies	7. NOT APPLICABLE	2. Fairly positive	Specifically related to efficacy of consumption of higher-sodium-content fluids to mitigate risk of developing hyponatraemia. Although prevention of hyponatraemia is primarily related to avoidance of overhydration or excessive fluid intake, it is theoretically possible for mild hyponatraemia to occur when salty sweat losses are replaced by low-sodium fluid. Therefore, addition of sodium to fluids consumed during exercise helps to mitigate this effect.
Linoleic acid	Level II: case series or observational studies	7. NOT APPLICABLE	3. Mixed / no effect	No role as a supplement: dietary intake is high. Increased dietary intake lowers cholesterol, so reducing risk of cardiovascular disease, but there are (mainly theoretical) concerns about increasing inflammation and cancer risk.
Electrolytes for exertional (heat) cramps	Level I: anecdotal evidence or expert opinion	2. Fairly positive	7. NOT APPLICABLE	Specifically related to the efficacy of sodium supplementation to prevent or resolve exertional muscle cramping related to extensive sweating and a whole-body sodium deficit – not muscle cramping due to overload and fatigue.
Ketone bodies	Level I: anecdotal evidence or expert opinion	2. Fairly positive	7. NOT APPLICABLE	Interesting concept and some anecdotal reports from athletes of successful outcomes from use of ketone body product. Data from some studies are unpublished, thus too soon to make conclusive statements regarding the novel role of supplemental forms of ketone bodies as a fuel in exercise, or their impact on performance. Some safety data published but tests of efficacy and commercial production will also be needed before ketones can be considered as useful for athletic performance.
Yucca	Level I: anecdotal evidence or expert opinion	7. NOT APPLICABLE	2. Fairly positive	Widely used in folk medicine in South America for several purported indications. Yucca extract used as animal feed additive to increase growth rate and ease joint pains in animals. No evidence of an ergogenic benefit in sports performance in humans, only shown in animals.

Supplements with strong absence of effect or possible negative effect

Figure 45 contains those supplements where there is good evidence (levels IV and III), but a 'strong absence of effect or possible negative effect' on sports performance and/or health.

Here with a 'strong absence of effect or possible negative effect' on both sports performance and health is arnica (level IV) and smilax (level III). With good evidence (level III) but a 'strong absence of effect or possible negative effect' on sports performance are: GABA (γ-aminobutyric acid) and inosine (Figure 45); and gamma-linolenic acid (Figure 38). With a 'strong absence of effect or possible negative effect' on health are: sucrose at level IV (Figure 35); and royal jelly at level III (Figure 45).

Supplements with lack of evidence

The next group of supplements (Figure 46) is where the evidence to date is only at levels II and I and therefore restraint is advised when considering these supplements, despite their seemingly positive effects, due to the lack of scientific evidence.

Here, with the evidence only at level II are: electrolytes with regard to hyponatraemia; and linoleic acid. At level I are: electrolytes with regard to exertional heat cramps, ketone bodies and yucca, only having evidence at the lowest level I. Noteworthy in this group is ketone bodies which, although a potentially promising concept as a supplement, was, at the time of going to press, unable to be supported by published data.

Supplements with lack of application to sports performance or health

This next group of supplements are those where there are no studies or credible evidence for sports performance and/or health, regardless of the level of evidence (IV, III, II or I). In Figure 47 are those supplements where the evidence to date does not provide an obvious application in either sports performance or health: serine (level IV); leptin (level III); and glandulars, methionine; proline; and threonine at level I.

From previous figures the following supplements also have no studies or credible evidence of a direct benefit to sports performance: calcium, inositol and the *Lactobacillus* and *Bifidobacterium* species of probiotics (Figure 37). Copper, folate, MSM, plant sterols, selenium, vitamin K and wheat germ oil (Figure 38). Chondroitin and glucosamine, chlorogenic acids, and echinacea (Figure 40). Cissus quadrangularis; ginger; ginkgo; nootkatone; papain; phlogenzym and wobenzyme; D-pinitol; prebiotics; probiotics (species and combinations of different species or strains other than *Lactobacillus* and *Bifidobacterium*); and

FIGURE 47 Supplements with no studies or credible evidence for sports performance or health at evidence levels IV–I

Supplement/ ingredient	Level of evidence	Direction effect on sports performance	Direction effect on health	Summary and comments
Serine	Level IV: systematic reviews and meta-analysis	7. NOT APPLICABLE	7. NOT APPLICABLE	There is no evidence to suggest the exogenous consumption of serine has any health or sports performance benefits or risks.
Leptin	Level III: randomised controlled trials	7. NOT APPLICABLE	7. NOT APPLICABLE	Leptin is a hormone which could be abused, but so far there is no record of it being misused. There is no evidence of leptin ergogenic effects. Chronic leptin administration may be associated with unknown side effects.
Glandulars	Level I: anecdotal evidence or expert opinion	7. NOT APPLICABLE	7. NOT APPLICABLE	There is no scientific evidence that glandular tissue concentrates enhance organ and gland activities, nor work ergogenically, other than through their vitamin, mineral and protein content.
Methionine	Level I: anecdotal evidence or expert opinion	7. NOT APPLICABLE	7. NOT APPLICABLE	No ergogenic effect if consuming daily requirement (13–15 mg/kg/d).
Proline	Level I: anecdotal evidence or expert opinion	7. NOT APPLICABLE	7. NOT APPLICABLE	It is not possible to make any claims about the safety or even effectiveness of proline supplements due to an almost complete lack of data.
Threonine	Level I: anecdotal evidence or expert opinion	7. NOT APPLICABLE	7. NOT APPLICABLE	No ergogenic effect if consuming daily requirement (15 mg/kg/d).

wolfberry (goji berry) (Figure 43). Royal jelly (Figure 45) and electrolytes with regard to hyponatraemia; linoleic acid and yucca (Figure 46). Of course, some of these have been reviewed as having evidence of providing a positive effect on an athlete's health, which may in turn lead to better preparation for competition. However, in other cases, there is no evidence of any benefit.

In addition, from previous figures the following supplements also have no studies or credible evidence for health: multiple transportable carbohydrates (Figure 35) and β-alanine (Figure 36). From Figure 42: branched chain amino acids (BCAA); cysteine and cystine; electrolytes with regard to hyperhydration; HICA; α-ketoisocaproate (KIC); medium chain triglycerides (MCTs); ornithine; phenylalanine; phosphate; and taurine. Figure 44: aspartate; cytochrome C; dihydroxyacetone phosphate (DHAP) and pyruvate; dimethyglycine; ferulic acid and gamma-oryzanol; lecithin; ribose; succinate; water (oxygenated); and ZMA. Electrolytes with regard to exertional heat cramps and ketone bodies (Figure 46) also belong here.

Supplements assigned to the 'Caution' category

The final group of supplements are those which in our opinion could be assigned to a 'Caution' category, where there are known issues or a high risk of problems, as well as an uncertain risk where a substance was present but has been removed, related to sporting outcomes (particularly an anti-doping rule violation) or health. Definite issues include scenarios where the actual product is subject to bans by WADA and/or the FDA, while high risk typically involves evidence of potential contamination with banned or harmful substances. Please see figure summary and comments alongside more detailed explanation within the individual reviews in the book. This is not an extensive list, for example it does not comprise the full WADA banned substances list (WADA, 2014), but is merely a list of the supplements reviewed within this book that we believe warrant being assigned to the 'Caution' category.

In Figure 48, the supplements reviewed in this book that we have assigned to the 'Caution' category are: androstenediol (prohormone); androstenedione (DIONE); DHEA (Didehydroepiandrosterone); prohormones (19-nor steroid group); DMAA; Jack3D; OxyElite Pro; colostrum-bovine; ephedra; γ-hydroxybutyrate and γ-butyrolactone (GHB and GBL); glucuronolactone; glycerol; Hydroxycut; melamine; pangamic acid; peptides-synthetic; tribulus; weight loss supplements: herbal; and yohimbine. The rationale for the rating of caution for each product is explained in the summary and comments section of the table.

In conclusion, it is important to note that, in consideration of current scientific research and increasing innovation and development in the sports nutrition arena, all supplement frameworks, including this book's own efficacy index, are working documents that are only accurate to the date of the most recent publication.

FIGURE 48 Supplements assigned to the 'Caution' category

Supplement/ ingredient	Level of evidence	Direction effect on sports performance	Direction effect on health	Summary and comments
Androstenediol (prohormone)	Level III: randomised controlled trials	6. CAUTION	6. CAUTION	Reasonably strong evidence of lack of anabolic or ergogenic effects in supplement form at supraphysiological doses. Strong evidence of dose and time-related widespread adverse effects resulting in several negative health consequences (see review). Classified as an androgenic/anabolic steroid and included on the WADA Prohibited List (WADA, 2014).
Androstenedione (DIONE)	Level III: randomised controlled trials	6. CAUTION	6. CAUTION	Reasonably strong evidence of lack of anabolic or ergogenic effects in supplement form at supraphysiological doses. Strong evidence of dose and time-related widespread adverse effects resulting in several negative health consequences (see review). Classified as an androgenic/anabolic steroid and included on the WADA Prohibited List (WADA, 2014).
DHEA (Didehydroepiandrosterone)	Level III: randomised controlled trials	6. CAUTION	6. CAUTION	Reasonably strong evidence of lack of anabolic or ergogenic effects in supplement form at supraphysiological doses. Strong evidence of dose and time-related widespread adverse effects resulting in several negative health consequences (see review). Classified as an androgenic/anabolic steroid and included on the WADA Prohibited List (WADA, 2014).
Prohormones: 19-nor steroid group	Level III: randomised controlled trials	6. CAUTION	6. CAUTION	Reasonably strong evidence of lack of anabolic or ergogenic effects in supplement form at supraphysiological doses. Strong evidence of dose and time-related widespread adverse effects resulting in several negative health consequences (see review). Classified as an androgenic/anabolic steroid and included on the WADA Prohibited List (WADA, 2014). UK law legislates prohormones under Schedule 4 of the Misuse of Drugs Act 1971, and the current list of 54 'class C' substances includes both prohormones and anabolic steroids in recognition of their biochemical similarity, thus closing a previous loophole. Similar restrictions apply under the Anabolic and Steroid Control Act (2004) in US law.

Supplement/ingredient	Level of evidence	Direction effect on sports performance	Direction effect on health	Summary and comments
DMAA (methyl-hexanamine/di-methylamylamine)	Level II: case series or observational studies	6. CAUTION	6. CAUTION	DMAA is included on the WADA Prohibited List as a stimulant (WADA, 2014). DMAA-containing supplements are also banned in several countries, including the US where they were linked to 86 adverse events, including hypertension, stroke, heart attack, seizure, psychiatric disorders and death.
Jack3D	Level I: anecdotal evidence or expert opinion	6. CAUTION	6. CAUTION	Jack3D originally contained DMAA (see DMAA), which is included on the WADA Prohibited List (WADA, 2014). Although it no longer contains DMAA, there are no published reports on the safety or efficacy of the current, DMAA-free formulation of Jack3D and for this reason we believe it should be treated with caution until such evidence has been established.
OxyElite Pro	Level I: anecdotal evidence or expert opinion	6. CAUTION	6. CAUTION	OxyElite Pro contains DMAA (see reviews OxyElite Pro and DMAA), which is included on the WADA Prohibited List (WADA, 2014).
Colostrum-bovine (non-hyperium-mue)	Level III: randomised con-trolled trials	6. CAUTION	2. Fairly positive	Limited evidence to support consistent improvements in acute exercise performance after bovine colostrum supplementation, but appears to reduce upper respiratory tract illness symptoms, and may prove beneficial to improve recovery/maintain exercise performance during periods of intensified exercise training or competition with longer term dosing at 10–60g for 8–12 weeks. Some colostrum preparations may contain lactose. WADA does not recom-mend the ingestion of this product (see review).
Ephedra	Level IV: system-atic reviews and meta-analysis	6. CAUTION	6. CAUTION	Carries serious adverse effects. Included on the WADA Prohibited List (WADA, 2014).
γ-hydroxybutyrate and γ-butyrolact-one (GHB and GBL)	Level II: case series or observational studies	6. CAUTION	6. CAUTION	Currently, there is no available evidence to support the use of GHB & GBL in the athletic population. Side effects include drowsiness, alcohol-like inebria-tion, dizziness, and induction of sleep. In overdose it can potentially cause coma, respiratory depression and death.

continued …

Figure 48 continued

Supplement/ ingredient	Level of evidence	Direction effect on sports performance	Direction effect on health	Summary and comments
Glucuronolactone	Level I: anecdotal evidence or expert opinion	7. NOT APPLICABLE	6. CAUTION	No available study testing the potential ergogenic effect of this molecule alone. Safety concerns raised over the level of glucuronolactone present in beverages with potential toxicity issues.
Glycerol	Level IV: systematic reviews and meta-analysis	6. CAUTION	7. NOT APPLICABLE	A metabolite of fat utilisation and an ingredient in many foods and cosmetics, glycerol acts as an osmolite which can be used to increase plasma osmolality and thus enhance retention of ingested fluids. Glycerol hyperhydration prior to exercise in hot environments has been shown to enhance fluid balance and endurance performance, while it may also be used to enhance the effectiveness of rehydration strategies. Occasional side effects of glycerol hyperhydration strategies include nausea, gut discomfort and headaches from increased intracranial pressure. Despite controversy over the real effect on plasma volume and alteration of physiological changes indicative of doping, the specific use of glycerol to aid/enhance hydration has been banned by WADA under S5: Diuretics and other masking agents as a plasma expander (WADA, 2014). Urinary thresholds for glycerol can distinguish between this deliberate use of glycerol versus its normal intake from foodstuffs or appearance via metabolism.
Hydroxycut	Level I: anecdotal evidence or expert opinion	6. CAUTION	6. CAUTION	A previous formulation of Hydroxycut was withdrawn from the market after being associated with 23 cases of hepatotoxicity and one death, but the suspected hepatotoxic ingredients (e.g. HCA) have been removed from the current formulation (see review). However, there are no published reports on the safety or efficacy of the current formula and for this reason we believe it should be treated with caution until such evidence has been established.
Melamine	Level II: case series or observational studies	6. CAUTION	6. CAUTION	Adulterant found in protein supplements. No documented ergogenic capacity. Melamine and derivatives (e.g. cyanuric acid) are toxic to humans even at low quantities, with strong effects on the kidneys (see review). Tolerable daily intake amounts are ~0.5 mg/kg/d for adults.

Supplement/ ingredient	Level of evidence	Direction effect on sports performance	Direction effect on health	Summary and comments
Pangamic acid	Level II: case series or observational studies	6. CAUTION	6. CAUTION	The USA FDA considers pangamic acid products to be unsafe and recommends they be seized, with injunctions against manufacturers (see review).
Peptides – synthetic	Level II: case series or observational studies	6. CAUTION	6. CAUTION	Included in various sections of the WADA Prohibited List (WADA, 2014). Research is limited but provides no evidence of performance-enhancing effects. Unknown side effects (see review).
Tribulus	Level III: randomised controlled trials	6. CAUTION	7. NOT APPLICABLE	Has been found contaminated with WADA-prohibited substances (see review).
Weight Loss supplements: herbal	Level III: randomised controlled trials	6. CAUTION	3. Mixed / no effect	Most have tenuous claims. Most found in combination therapies, with contaminants (some of which are prohibited by WADA). Bitter melon, ginger, and green tea have the strongest support as candidate therapies for weight loss, but most sources recommend making diet, exercise and lifestyle adjustments before considering supplements (see review).
Yohimbine	Level III: randomised controlled trials	6. CAUTION	6. CAUTION	Research findings do not support any ergogenic effect for yohimbine and there are acute negative nervous system effects with the severity of these effects increasing with dose (see review).

Finally, each athlete should always make his or her own decisions regarding the use of any supplement based on an assessment of the pros and cons of use, including considerations such as expense and the issues of efficacy, safety and legality/ethics. Unfortunately, all too frequently, the specific information needed to complete such an analysis is limited. Furthermore, due to poor manufacturing practice, some supplements do not contain (a) an adequate dose of the labelled ingredients but do contain (b) impurities such as glass, lead or animal faeces. Moreover, the FDA regularly reports on products found to contain effective amounts of prescription drugs, which could lead to detrimental side effects. As also discussed in the Introduction chapter, another potential health risk is from contamination or fake supplements which can cause a positive doping test for those athletes competing under the WADA code. Athletes, particularly those competing under the WADA code, need to be extremely cautious about using supplements and are advised always to work with a qualified professional to minimise the risks of supplement use.

The authors, editors and publishers cannot be held responsible for advice given on the purity of the supplement or failure to improve health or performance of any specific dose discussed.

REFERENCES

Abbasi, B., Kimiagar, M., Sadeghniiat, K., *et al.* (2012). The effect of magnesium supplementation on primary insomnia in elderly: a double-blind placebo-controlled clinical trial. *J Res Med Sci* 17(12): 1161–9.

Abdelmalki, A., Merino, D., Bonneau, D., *et al.* (1997). Administration of a GABAB agonist baclofen before running to exhaustion in the rat: effects on performance and on some indicators of fatigue. *Int J Sport Med* 18: 75–8.

Abidov, M., Crendal, F., Grachev, S., *et al.* (2003). Effects of extracts from Rhodiola rosea and Rosea crenulata (Crassulaceae) roots on ATP content in mitochondria of skeletal muscles. *Bull Exp Biol Med* 136: 585–7.

Acosta, P.B., Elsas, L.J. (1999). Nutritional management of phenylketonuria. In: Sadler, M.J., Strain, J.J., Caballero, A.(eds). *Encyclopedia of Human Nutrition*. San Diego: Academic Press: 1088–96.

ACSM (2009). American Dietetic Association, Dietitians of Canada, American College of Sports Medicine, *et al.* American College of Sports Medicine position stand. Nutrition and athletic performance. *Med Sci Sports Exerc* 41: 709–31.

ACSM, Sawka, M.N., Burke, L.M., Eichner, E.R., Maughan, R.J., Montain, S.J., Stachenfeld, N.S. (2007). American College of Sports Medicine (ACSM) position stand. Exercise and fluid replacement. *Med Sci Sports Exerc* 39: 377–90.

Adkison, J.D., Bauer, D.W., Chang, T. (2010). The effect of topical arnica on muscle pain. *Ann Pharmacother* 44: 1579–84.

AFSSA (2004). Avis relatif à la publicité portant sur des substances de développement musculaire et de mise en forme contenue dans un magazine spécialisé. Available at https://www.anses.fr/fr/content/avis-relatif-%C3%A0-une-demande-d%C3%A9valuation-relative-%C3%A0-la-publicit%C3%A9-portant-sur-des-substances--0. Accessed 28 January 2015.

Ahlborg, B., Ekelund, L.G., Nilsson, C.G. (1965). Effect of potassium-magnesium-aspartate on the capacity for prolonged exercise in man. *Acta Physiol Scand* 74: 238–45.

Akasaka, Y., Tsunoda, M., Ogata, T., Ide, T., Murakami, K. (2010). Direct evidence for leptin-induced lipid oxidation independent of long-form leptin receptor. *Biochim Biophys Acta* 1801: 1115–22.

Alessandri, C., Pignatelli, P., Loffredo, L., *et al.* (2006). Alpha-linolenic acid-rich wheat germ oil decreases oxidative stress and CD40 ligand in patients with mild hypercholesterolemia. *Arterioscler Thromb Vasc Biol* 26: 2577–8.

Aloia, J.F., Li-Ng, M. (2007). Correspondence: Epidemic influenza and vitamin D. *Epidemiol Infect* 135: 1095–8.

Andersen, T., Fogh, J. (2001). Weight loss and delayed gastric emptying following a South American herbal preparation in overweight patients. *J Hum Nutr Diet* 14: 243–50.

Andersson, A., Sjödin, A., Hedman, A., Olsson, R., Vessby, B. (2000). Fatty acid profile of skeletal muscle phospholipids in trained and untrained young men. *Am J Physiol Endocrinol Metab* 279: E744–51.

Andrade-Cetto, A., Wiedenfeld, H. (2001). Hypoglycemic effect of Cecropia obtusifolia on streptozotocin diabetic rats. *J Ethnopharmacol* 78: 145–9.

Andreini, C., Bertini, I., Cavallaro, G. (2011). Minimal functional sites allow a classification of zinc sites in proteins. *PloS One* 6: e26325.

Angus, D.J., Hargreaves, M., Dancey, J., Febbraio, M.A. (2000). Effect of carbohydrate or carbohydrate plus medium-chain triglyceride ingestion on cycling time trial performance. *J Appl Physiol* 88: 113–19.

Antonio, J., Sanders, M.S., Van Gammeren, D. (2001). The effects of bovine colostrum supplementation on body composition and exercise performance in active men and women. *Nutrition* 17: 243–7.

Antonio, J., Stout, J. (2001). *Sports Supplements*. Philadelphia: Lippincott Williams & Wilkins, p. 16.

Arena, B., Mafulli, N., Maffulli, F., Morleo, M.A. (1995). Reproductive hormones and menstrual changes with exercise in female athletes. *Sports Med* 19: 278–87.

Arendt, J. (1998). Melatonin and the pineal gland: influence on mammalian seasonal and circadian physiology. *Rev. Reprod* 3: 13–22.

Areta, J.L., Burke, L.M., Ross, M.L., Camera, D.M., West, D.W., Broad, E.M., Jeacocke, N.A., Moore, D.R., Stellingwerff, T., Phillips, S.M., Hawley, J.A., Coffey, V.G. (2013). Timing and distribution of protein ingestion during prolonged recovery from resistance exercise alters myofibrillar protein synthesis. *J Physiol* 591: 2319–31.

Armstrong, L.E. (2002). Caffeine, body fluid-electrolyte balance, and exercise performance. *Int J Sport Nutr Exerc Metab* 12: 189–206.

Arnaud, M.J. (2011). Pharmacokinetics and metabolism of natural methylxanthines in animal and man. *Handb Exp Pharmacol* 200: 33–91.

ASADA (2014a). Australian Sports Anti-Doping Authority. Supplements Warning. Available at www.asada.gov.au/substances/supplements.html. Accessed 21 August 2014.

ASADA (2014b). Important Athlete Advisory: prohibited stimulants found in supplement, 2014. Available at http://asada.govspace.gov.au/2014/06/26/important-athlete-advisory-prohibited-stimulants-found-in-supplements. Accessed 26 June 2014.

Aschenbach, W., Ocel, J., Craft, L., Ward, C., Spangenburg, E., Williams, J. (2000). Effect of oral sodium loading on high-intensity arm ergometry in college wrestlers. *Med Sci Sports Exerc* 32: 669–75.

Ashton, K., Hooper, L., Harvey, L.J., Hurst, R., Casgrain, A., Fairwather-Tait, S.J. (2009). Methods of assessment of selenium status in humans: a systematic review. *Am J Clin Nutr* 89s: 2025S–39S.

Atanasovska, T., Petersen, A.C., Rouffet, D.M., *et al.* (2014). Plasma K^+ dynamics and implications during and following intense rowing exercise. *J Appl Physiol* 117: 60–8.

Athayde, M.L., Coelho, G.C., Schenkel, E.P. (2000). Caffeine and theobromine in epicuticular wax of Ilex paraguariensis A. St.-Hil. *Phytochemistry* 55: 853–7.

Atherton, P.J., *et al.* (2010a). Distinct anabolic signalling responses to amino acids in C2C12 skeletal muscle cells. *Amino Acids* 38: 1533–9.

Atherton, P.J., Etheridge, T., Watt, P.W., *et al.* (2010b). Muscle full effect after oral protein: time-dependent concordance and discordance between human muscle protein synthesis and mTORC1 signaling. *Am J Clin Nutr* 92: 1080–8.

Atkinson, G., Buckley, P., Edwards, B., *et al.* (2001). Are there hangover effects on physical performance when melatonin is ingested by athletes before nocturnal sleep? *Int J Sport Med* 22: 231–4.

Atkinson, G., Drust, B., Reilly, T., Waterhouse, J. (2003).The relevance of melatonin to sports medicine and science. *Sports Med* 33: 809–11.

Atkinson, G., Jones, H., Edwards, B.J., Waterhouse, J.M. (2005). Effects of daytime ingestion of melatonin on short-term athletic performance. *Ergonomics* 48: 1512–22.

Auersperger, I., Knap, B., Jerin, A., *et al.* (2012). The effects of 8 weeks of endurance running on hepcidin concentrations, inflammatory parameters, and iron status in female runners. *Int J Sport Nutr Exer Metab* 22: 55–63.

Austin, K.G., Travis, J., Pace, G., *et al.* (2014). Analysis of 1.3 dimethylamylamine concentrations in Geraniaceae, geranium oil and dietary supplements. *Drug Test Anal* 6: 797–804.

Australian Government (2006). Department of Health and Aging, National Health and Medical Research Council. *Nutrient Reference Values for Australia and New Zealand.* Canberra.

Australian National Health and Medical Research Council, Health NZMo. (2006). Nutrient Reference Values for Australia and New Zealand Including Recommended Dietary Intakes. In: *Department of Health and Aging*, editor: Commonwealth of Australia, pp. 147–51.

Avery, N.G., Kaiser, J.L., Sharman, M.J., Scheett, T.P., Barnes, D.M., Gomez, A.L., Kraemer, W.J., Volek, J.S. (2003). Effects of Vitamin E supplementation on recovery from repeated bouts of resistance exercise. *J Str Cond Re*s 17: 801–9.

Avois, L., Robinson, N., Saudan, C., *et al.* (2006). Central nervous system stimulants and sport practice. *Br J Sports Med* 40: i16–20.

Baer, D.J., Rumpler, W.V., Miles, C.W., Fahey, G.C. (1997). Dietary fiber decreases the metabolizable energy content and nutrient digestibility of mixed diets fed to humans. *J Nutr* 127: 579–86.

Bagheri, H., Schmitt, L., Berlan, M., Montastruc, J.L. (1997). A comparative study of the effects of yohimbine and anetholtrithione on salivary secretion in depressed patients treated with psychotropic drugs. *Eur J Clin Pharmacol* 52: 339–42.

Baguet, A., Everaert, I., Yard, B., Peters, V., Zschocke, J., Zutinic, A., de Heer, E., Podgorski, T., Domaszewska, K., Derave, W. (2014). Does low serum carnosinase activity favor high-intensity exercise capacity? *J Appl Physiol* 116: 553–9.

Baguet, A., Koppo, K., Pottier, A., Derave, W. (2010). Beta-Alanine supplementation reduces acidosis but not oxygen uptake response during high-intensity cycling exercise. *Eur J Appl Physiol* 108: 495–503.

Baguet, A., Reyngoudt, H., Pottier, A., Everaert, I., Callens, S., Achten, E., Derave, W. (2009). Carnosine loading and washout in human skeletal muscles. *J Appl Physiol* 106: 837–42.

Bahrke, M.S., Morgan, W.P., Stegner, A. (2009). Is ginseng an ergogenic aid? *Int J Sport Nutr Exerc Metab* 19: 298–322.

Bailey, D.M., Davies, B. (2001). Acute mountain sickness: prophylactic benefits of antioxidant vitamin supplementation at high altitude. *High Alt Med Biol* 2: 21–9.

Bailey, S.J., Fulford, J., Vanhatalo, A., Winyard, P.G., Blackwell, J.R., DiMenna, F.J., Wilkerson, D.P., Benjamin, N., Jones, A.M. (2010). Dietary nitrate supplementation enhances muscle contractile efficiency during knee-extensor exercise in humans. *J Appl Physiol* 109: 135–48.

Bailey, S.J., Winyard, P., Vanhatalo, A., Blackwell, J.R., Dimenna, F.J., Wilkerson, D.P., Tarr, J., Benjamin, N., Jones, A.M. (2009). Dietary nitrate supplementation reduces the O_2 cost of low-intensity exercise and enhances tolerance to high-intensity exercise in humans. *J Appl Physiol* 107: 1144–55.

Baillie, J.K., Thompson, A.A., Irving, J.B., Bates, M.G., Sutherland, A.I., Macnee, W., Maxwell, S.R., Webb, D.J. (2009). Oral antioxidant supplementation does not prevent acute mountain sickness: double-blind, randomized placebo-controlled trial. *QJM* 102: 341–8.

Bakker, G.C., van Erk, M.J., Pellis, L., et al. (2010). An antiinflammatory dietary mix modulates inflammation and oxidative and metabolic stress in overweight men: a nutrigenomics approach. *Am J Clin Nutr* 91: 1044–59.

Balage, M., Dardevet, D. (2010). Long-term effects of leucine supplementation on body composition. *Curr Opin Clin Nutr Metab Care* 13: 265–70.

Ballard, S.L., Wellborn-Kim, J.J., Clauson, K.A. (2010). Effects of commercial energy drink consumption on athletic performance and body composition. *Phys Sportsmed* 38: 107–17.

Bannert, N., Starke, I., Mohnike, K., Frohner, G. (1991). Parameters of mineral metabolism in children and adolescents in athletic training. *Kinderarztl Prax* 59: 153–6.

Banu, J., Varela, E., Bahadur, A.N., Soomro, R., Kazi, N., Fernandes, G. (2012). Inhibition of bone loss by cissus quadrangularis in mice: a preliminary report. *J Osteoporosis* 2012: 101206. [EPub]

Banuelos, C., Beas, B.S., McQuail, J.A., et al. (2014). Prefrontal cortical GABAergic dysfunction contributes to age-related working memory impairment. *J Neurosci* 34: 3457–66.

Barber, J.J., McDermott, A.Y., McGaughey, K.J., Olmstead, J.D., Hagobian, T.A. (2013). Effects of combined creatine and sodium bicarbonate supplementation on repeated sprint performance in trained men. *J Strength Cond Res* 27: 252–8.

Barbul, A. (2008). Proline precursors to sustain mammalian collagen synthesis. *J Nutr* 138: 2021S–2024S.

Barceloux, D.G.J. (1999). Vanadium. *Toxicol Clin Toxicol* 37: 265–78.

Barger-Lux, M.J., Heaney, R.P. (1995). Caffeine and the calcium economy revisited. *Osteoporosis Int* 5: 97–102.

Barile, D., Rastall, R.A. (2013). Human milk and related oligosaccharides as prebiotics. *Curr Opin Biotechnol* 24: 214–19.

Barker, T., Martins, T.B., Hill, H.R., Kjeldsberg, C.R., Trawick, R.H., Weaver, L.K., et al. (2011). Low vitamin D impairs strength recovery after anterior cruciate ligament surgery. *J Evid Based Complement Altern Med* 16: 201–9.

Basile-Filho, A., El-Khoury, A.E., Beaumier, L., Wang, S.Y., Young, V.R. (1997). Continuous 24-h L-[1-13C]phenylalanine and L-[3,3-2H2]tyrosine oral-tracer studies at an intermediate phenylalanine intake to estimate requirements in adults. *Am J Clin Nutr* 65: 473–88.

Bassarello, C., Bifulco, G., Montoro, P., Skhirtladze, A., Benidze, M., Kemertelidze, E., Pizza, C., Piacente, S. (2007). Yucca gloriosa: a source of phenolic derivatives with strong antioxidant activity. *J Agric Food Chem* 55: 6636–42.

Bassini-Cameron, A., Monteiro, A., Gomes, A., Werneck-de-Castro, J.P., Cameron, L. (2008). Glutamine protects against increases in blood ammonia in football players in an exercise intensity-dependent way. *Br J Sports Med* 42: 260–6.

Bassit, R.A., Sawada, L.A., Bacurau, R.F., Navarro, F., Costa Rosa, L.F. (2000). The effect of BCAA supplementation upon the immune response of triathletes. *Med Sci Sports Exerc* 32: 1214–19.

Basu, T.K., Donaldson, D. (2003). Intestinal absorption in health and disease: micronutrients. *Best Pract Res Clin Gastroenterol* 17: 957–79.

Batterham, A.M., Hopkins, W.G. (2006). Making meaningful inferences about magnitudes. *Int J Sport Physiol Perform* 1: 50–7.

Baur, J.A., Sinclair, D.A. (2006). Therapeutic potential of resveratrol: the in vivo evidence. *Nature* 5: 493–506.

Baylis, A., Cameron-Smith, D., Burke, L.M. (2001). Inadvertent doping through supplement use by athletes: assessment and management of the risk in Australia. *Int J Sport Nutr Exerc Metab* 11: 365–83.

Beals, K.A., Manore, M.M. (1998). Nutritional status of female athletes with subclinical eating disorders. *J Am Diet Assoc* 98: 419–25.

Beard, J., Tobin, B. (2000). Iron status and exercise. *Am J Clin Nutr* 72: 594S–597S.

Beauchamp, T., Childress, J. (2013). *The Principles of Biomedical Ethics*. Oxford: Oxford University Press.

Beaudoin, M.S., Graham, T.E. (2011). Methylxanthines and human health: epidemiological and experimental evidence. *Handb Exp Pharmacol* 200: 509–48.

Beavers, K.M., Serra, M.C., Beavers, D.P., et al. (2010). Soy and the exercise-induced inflammatory response in postmenopausal women. *Appl Physiol Nutr Metab* 35: 261–9.

Beck, T.W., Housh, T.J., Johnson, G.O., Schmid, R.J., Housh, D.J., Coburn, J.W., et al. (2007). Effects of a protease supplement on eccentric exercise-induced markers of delayed-onset muscle soreness and muscle damage. *J Strength Cond Res* 21: 661–7.

Beedie, C.J., Coleman, D.A., Foad, A.J. (2007). Positive and negative placebo effects resulting from the deceptive administration of an ergogenic aid. *Int J Sport Nutr Exerc Metab* 17: 259–69.

Beedie, C.J., Foad, A.J. (2009). The placebo effect in sports performance. *Sports Med* 39: 313–29.

Behne, D., Alber, D., Kyriakopoulos, A. (2010). Long-term selenium supplementation of humans: selenium status and relationships between selenium concentrations in skeletal muscle and indicator materials. *J Trace Elements Med Biol* 24: 99–105.

Beis, L., Mohammad, Y., Easton, C., Pitsiladis, Y.P. (2011). Failure of glycine-arginine-α-ketoisocaproic acid to improve high-intensity exercise performance in trained cyclists. *Int J Sport Nutr Exerc Metab* 21: 33–9.

Bell, D.G., McLellan, T.M. (2003). Effect of repeated caffeine ingestion on repeated exhaustive exercise endurance. *Med Sci Sports Exerc* 35: 1348–54.

Bellar, D., Moody, K.M., Richard, N.S., et al. (2014). Efficacy of a botanical supplement with concentrated echinacea purpurea for increasing aerobic capacity. *ISRN Nutr* 2014: 1–5.

Bendahan, D., Mattei, J.P., Ghattas, B., et al. (2002). Citrulline/malate promotes aerobic energy production in human exercising muscle. *Br J Sports Med* 36: 282–9.

Bendtsen, L.Q., Lorenzen, J.K., Bendsen, N.T., Rasmussen, C., Astrup, A. (2013). Effect of dairy proteins on appetite, energy expenditure, body weight, and composition: a review of the evidence from controlled clinical trials. *Adv Nutr* 4: 418–38.

Benesch, R., Benesch, R.E. (1969). Intracellular organic phosphates as regulators of oxygen release by haemoglobin. *Nature* 221: 618–22.

Bentley, D.J., Dank, S., Coupland, R., *et al.* (2012). Acute antioxidant supplementation improves endurance performance in trained athletes. *Research in Sports Med* 20: 1–12.

Benzie, I.F.F., Chung, W.Y., Wang, J., *et al.* (2006). Enhanced bioavailability of zeaxanthin in a milk-based formulation of wolfberry (Gou Qi Zi; Fructus barbarum L.). *Br J Nutr* 96: 154–60.

Berardi, J.M., Ziegenfuss, T.N. (2003). Effects of ribose supplementation on repeated sprint performance in men. *J Strength Cond Res* 17: 47–52.

Bergeron, M.F. (2003). Heat cramps: fluid and electrolyte challenges during tennis in the heat. *J Sci Med Sport* 6: 19–27.

Bergeron, M.F. (2008). Muscle cramps during exercise: is it fatigue or electrolyte deficit? *Curr Sports Med Rep* 7: S50–S55.

Bergeron, M.F. (2014). Hydration and thermal strain during tennis in the heat. *Br J Sports Med* 48: i 12–17.

Bergeron, M.F., Senchina, D.S., Burke, L.M., Stear, S.J., Castell, L.M. (2010). BJSM reviews: A–Z of nutritional supplements: dietary supplements, sports nutrition foods and ergogenic aids for health and performance Part 13: Electrolytes, Ephedra, Echinacea. *Br J Sports Med* 44: 985–6.

Berggren, A., Lazou Ahrén, I., Larsson, N., Önning, G. (2011). Randomised, double-blind and placebo-controlled study using new probiotic lactobacilli for strengthening the body immune defence against viral infections. *Eur J Nutr* 50: 203–10.

Bergström, J., Hermansen, L., Hultman, E., Saltin, B. (1967). Diet, muscle glycogen and physical performance. *Acta Physiol Scand* 71: 140–50.

Berthold, H.K., Unverdorben, S., Degenhardt, R., Bulitta, M., Gouni-Berthold, I. (2006). Effect of policosanol on lipid levels among patients with hypercholesterolemia or combined hyperlipidemia: a randomized control trial. *JAMA* 295: 2262–9.

Bérubé-Parent, S., Pelletier, C., Doré, J., Tremblay, A. (2005). Effects of encapsulated green tea and guarana extracts containing a mixture of epigallocatechin-3-gallate and caffeine on 24h energy expenditure and fat oxidation in men. *Br J Nutr* 94: 432–6.

Beulens, J.W., Booth, S.L., van den Heuvel, E.G., Stoecklin, E., Baka, A., Vermeer, C. (2013). The role of menaquinones (vitamin K(2)) in human health. *Br J Nutr* 110: 1357–68.

Bex, T., Chung, W., Baguet, A., Stegen, S., Stautemas, J., Achten, E., Derave, W. (2014). Muscle carnosine loading by beta-alanine supplementation is more pronounced in trained vs. untrained muscles. *J Appl Physiol* 116: 204–9.

Bhattacharya, A., Banu, J., Rahman, M., Causey, J., Fernandes, G. (2006). Biological effects of conjugated linoleic acids in health and disease. *J Nutr Biochem* 17: 789–810.

Bhujade, A.M., Talmale, S., Kumar, N., Gupta, G., Reddanna, P., Das, S.K., *et al.* (2012). Evaluation of Cissus quadrangularis extracts as an inhibitor of COX, 5-LOX, and proinflammatory mediators. *J Ethnopharmacology* 141: 989–96.

Biolo, G., Maggi, S.P., Williams, B.D., Tipton, K.D., Wolfe, R.R. (1995). Increased rates of muscle protein turnover and amino acid transport after resistance exercise in humans. *Am J Physiol* 268: E514–20.

Biolo, G., Tipton, K.D., Klein, S., Wolfe, R.R. (1997). An abundant supply of amino acids enhances the metabolic effect of exercise on muscle protein. *Am J Physiol* 273: E122–9.

Bishop, D., Edge, J., Davis, C., Goodman, C. (2004). Induced metabolic alkalosis affects muscle metabolism and repeated-sprint ability. *Med Sci Sports Exerc* 36: 807–13.

Bishop, P.A., Smith, J.F., Young, B. (1987). Effects of N' N'-dimethylglycine on physiological response and performance in trained runners. *J Sports Med Phys Fitness* 27: 53–7.

Bjelakovic, G., Nikolova, D., Gluud, L.L., Simonetti, R.G., Gluud, C. (2007). Mortality in randomized trials of antioxidant supplements for primary and secondary prevention: systematic review and meta-analysis. *JAMA* 297: 842–57.

Björk, B.C., Solomon, D. (2012). Open access versus subscription journals: a comparison of scientific impact. *BMC Med* 10: 73.

Black, C.D., Herring, M.P., Hurley, D.J., *et al.* (2010). Ginger (Zingiber officinale) reduces muscle pain caused by eccentric exercise. *J Pain* 11: 894–903.

Blasbalg, T.L., Hibbeln, J.R., Ramsden, C.E., Majchrzak, S.F., Rawlings, R.R. (2011). Changes in consumption of omega-3 and omega-6 fatty acids in the United States during the 20th century. *Am J Clin Nutr* 93: 950–62.

Blau, N., van Spronsen, F.J., Levy, H.L. (2010). Phenylketonuria. *Lancet* 376: 1417–27.

Blomstrand, E., Hassmén, P., Ek, S., Ekblom, B., Newsholme, E.A. (1997). Influence of ingesting a solution of branched-chain amino acids on perceived exertion during exercise. *Acta Physiol Scand* 159: 41–9.

Blomstrand, E., Saltin, B. (2001). BCAA intake affects protein metabolism in muscle after but not during exercise in humans. *Am J Physiol Endocrinol Metab* 281: E365–74.

Bloomer, R.J. (2007). The role of nutritional supplements in the prevention and treatment of resistance exercise-induced skeletal muscle injury. *Sports Med Auckl NZ* 37: 519–32.

Bloomer, R.J., Goldfarb, A.H., McKenzie, M.J. (2006). Oxidative stress response to aerobic exercise: comparison of antioxidant supplements. *Med Sci Sports Exerc* 38: 1098–105.

Bloomer, R.J., Smith, W.A. (2009). Oxidative stress in response to aerobic and anaerobic power testing: influence of exercise training and carnitine supplementation. *Res Sports Med* 17: 1–16.

Bohannon, J. (2013). Who's afraid of peer review? *Science* 342: 60–5.

Bohe, J., Low, A., Wolfe, R.R., Rennie, M.J. (2003). Human muscle protein synthesis is modulated by extracellular, not intramuscular amino acid availability: a dose-response study. *J Physiol* 552: 315–24.

Boldyrev, A.A., Aldini, G., Derave, W. (2013). Physiology and pathophysiology of carnosine. *Physiol Rev* 93: 1803–45.

Bond, H., Morton, L., Braakhuis, A.J. (2012). Dietary nitrate supplementation improves rowing performance in well-trained rowers. *Int J Sport Nutr Exerc Metab* 22: 251–6.

Bonner, B., Warren, B., Bucci, L. (1990). Influence of ferulate supplementation on postexercise stress hormone levels after repeated exercise stress. *J Appl Sports Sci Res* 4: 110.

Boorsma, R.K., Whitfield, J., Spriet, L.L. (2014). Beetroot juice supplementation does not improve performance in elite 1500-m runners. *Med Sci Sports Exerc* 46: 2326–34.

Booth, S.L., Tucker, K.L., Chen, H., *et al.* (2000). Dietary vitamin K intakes are associated with hip fracture but not with bone mineral density in elderly men and women. *Am J Clin Nutr* 71: 1201–8.

Borchers, A.T., Selmi, C., Meyer, F.J., *et al.* (2009). Probiotics and immunity. *J Gastroenterol* 44: 26–46.

Bordia, A., Verma, S.K., Srivastava, K.C. (1998). Effect of garlic (Allium sativum) on blood lipids, blood sugar, fibrinogen and fibrinolytic activity in patients with coronary artery disease. *Prostaglandins Leukot Essent Fatty Acids* 58: 257–63.

Borgenvik, M., Apró, W., Blomstrand, E. (2012). Intake of branched-chain amino acids influences the levels of MAFbx mRNA and MuRF-1 total protein in resting and exercising human muscle. *Am J Physiol Endocrinol Metab* 302: E510–21.

Borsheim, E., Tipton, K.D., Wolf, S.E., Wolfe, R.R. (2002). Essential amino acids and muscle protein recovery from resistance exercise. *Am J Physiol Endocrinol Metab* 283: E648–57.

Bos, C., Metges, C.C., Gaudichon, C., *et al.* (2003). Postprandial kinetics of dietary amino acids are the main determinant of their metabolism after soy or milk protein ingestion in humans. *J Nutr* 133: 1308–15.

Bouic, P.J., Clark, A., Lamprecht, J., *et al.* (1999). The effects of B-sitosterol (BSS) and B-sitosterol glucoside (BSSG) mixture on selected immune parameters of marathon runners: inhibition of post marathon immune suppression and inflammation. *Int J Sport Med* 20: 258–62.

Bowery, N.G. (1993). GABA$_B$ receptor pharmacology. *Annu Rev Pharmacol Toxicol* 33: 109–47.

Bowtell, J.L., Marwood, S., Bruce, M., *et al.* (2007). Tricarboxylic acid cycle intermediate pool size: functional importance for oxidative metabolism in exercising human skeletal muscle. *Sports Med* 37: 1071–88.

Braakhuis, A.J. (2012). Effect of vitamin C supplements on physical performance. *Curr Sports Med Rep* 11: 180–4.

Braam, L.A., Knapen, M.H., Geusens, P., Brouns, F., Vermeer, C. (2003). Factors affecting bone loss in female endurance athletes: a two-year follow-up study. *Am J Sports Med* 31: 889–95.

Branch, J.D. (2003). Effect of creatine supplementation on body composition and performance: a meta-analysis. *Int J Sport Nutr Exerc Metab* 13: 198–226.

Brandolini, A., Hidalgo, A. (2012). Wheat germ: not only a by-product. *Int J Food Sci Nutr* 63: 71–4.

Brass, E.P. (2000). Supplemental carnitine and exercise. *Am J Clin Nutr* 72: 618S–623S.

Braun, B., Clarkson, P.M., Freedson, P.S., *et al.* (1991). Effects of coenzyme Q10 supplementation on exercise performance, VO$_{2max}$, and lipid peroxidation in trained cyclists. *Int J Sport Nutr* 2: 353–65.

Braun, H., Koehler, K., Geyer, H., *et al.* (2009a). Dietary supplement use among elite young German athletes. *Int J Sport Nutr Exer Metab* 19: 97–109.

Braun, H., Koehler, K., Geyer, H., Thevis, M., Schaenzer, W. (2009b). Dietary supplement use of elite German athletes and knowledge about the contamination problem. In: Loland, S., Bø, K., Fasting, K., Hallén, J., Ommundsen, Y., Roberts, G., Tsolakidis, E. (eds). *14th Annual Congress of the European College of Sport Sciences, Book of Abstracts.* Oslo, Norway: 378.

Bredle, D.L., Stager, J.M., Brechue, W.F., *et al.* (1988). Phosphate supplementation, cardiovascular function, and exercise performance in humans. *J Appl Physiol* 65: 1821–6.

Breen, L., Philp, A., Witard, O.C., *et al.* (2011). The influence of carbohydrate-protein co-ingestion following endurance exercise on myofibrillar and mitochondrial protein synthesis. *J Physiol* 589: 4011–25.

Breen, L., Phillips, S.M., Watford, M., Burke, L.M., Stear, S.J., Castell, L.M. (2012). BJSM reviews: A–Z of nutritional supplements: dietary supplements, sports nutrition foods and ergogenic aids for health and performance Part 32: Protein and Proline. *Br J Sports Med* 46: 454–6.

Bremner, K., Bubb, W.A., Kemp, G.J., *et al.* (2002). The effect of phosphate loading on erythrocyte 2,3-bisphosphoglycerate levels. *Clin Chim Acta* 323: 111–14.

Brenneisen, R., Elsohly, M.A., Murphy, T.P., *et al.* (2004). Pharmacokinetics and excretion of gamma-hydroxybutyrate (GHB) in healthy subjects. *J Anal Toxicol* 28: 625–30.

Brien, S., Prescott, P., Lewith, G. (2011). Meta-analysis of the related nutritional supplements dimethyl sulfoxide and methylsulfonylmethane in the treatment of osteoarthritis of the knee. *J Evid Based Complement Alternat Med* 2011: 528403.

Brilla, L.R., Conte, V. (2000). Effects of a novel zinc-magnesium formulation on hormones and strength. *J Exerc Physiol* (Online) 3: 26–36.

Brinkhaus, B., Wilkens, J.M., Lüdtke, R., Hunger, J., Witt, C.M., Willich, S.N. (2006). Homeopathic arnica therapy in patients receiving knee surgery: results of three randomised double-blind trials. *Complement Ther Med* 14: 237–46.

Brinkworth, G.D., Buckley, J.D., Slavotinek, J.P., Kurmis, A.P. (2004). Effect of bovine colostrum supplementation on the composition of resistance trained and untrained limbs in healthy young men. *Eur J Appl Physiol* 91: 53–60.

Broad, E.M., Maughan, R.J., Galloway, S.D.R. (2005). Effects of L-Carnitine L-Tartrate ingestion on substrate utilisation during prolonged exercise. *Int J Sport Nutr Exerc Metab* 15: 665–79.

Broeder, C.E., Quindry, J., Brittingham, L., Panton, J., Thomson, S., Appakondu, K., Breuel, R., Byrd, J., Douglas, C., Earnest, C., Mitchell, M., Olson, T., Roy, C., Yarlagadda, C. (2000). The Andro Project: physiological and hormonal influences of androstenedione supplementation in men 35 to 65 years old participating in a high-intensity resistance training program. *Arch Intern Med* 160: 3093–104.

Broome, C., McArdle, F., Kyle, J., Andrews, F., Lowe, N.M., Hart, C.A., Arthur, J.R., Jackson, M.J. (2004). An increase in selenium intake improves immune function and poliovirus handling in adults with marginal selenium status. *Am J Clin Nutr* 80: 154–62.

Brown, A.C., Macrae, H.S., Turner, N.S. (2004). Tricarboxylic-acid-cycle intermediates and cycle endurance capacity. *Int J Sport Nutr Exerc Metab* 14: 720–9.

Brown, G.A., Vukovich, M., King, D.S. (2006). Testosterone prohormone supplements. *Med Sci Sports Exerc* 38: 1451–61.

Brown, G.A., Vukovich, M.D., King, D.S., Wolfe, R.R., Newsholme, E.A., Trudeau, F., Curi, R., Burke, L.M., Stear, S.J., Castell, L.M. (2009). BJSM reviews: A–Z of supplements: dietary supplements, sports nutrition foods and ergogenic aids for health and performance Part 2: Amino acids, Androstenedione, Arginine, Asparagine and Aspartate. *Br J Sports Med* 43: 807–10.

Brown, G.A., Vukovich, M.D., Sharp, R.L., Reifenrath, T.A., Parsons, K.A., King, D.S. (1999). Effect of oral DHEA on serum testosterone and adaptations to resistance training in young men. *J Appl Physiol* 87: 2274–83.

Brown, R.P., Gerberg, P.L., Ramazanov, Z. (2002). Rhodiolo rosea: a phytomedicinal overview. *Herbal Gram* 56: 40–52.

Bruce, M., Constantin-Teodosiu, D., Greenhaff, P.L., *et al.* (2001). Glutamine supplementation promotes anaplerosis but not oxidative energy delivery in human skeletal muscle. *Am J Physiol Endocrinol Metab* 280: E669–75.

Brukner, P. (2013). Challenging beliefs in sports nutrition: are two 'core principles' proving to be myths ripe for busting? *Br J Sports Med* 47: 663.

Bucci, L.R. (2000). Selected herbals and human exercise performance. *Am J Clin Nutr* 72: 624S–36S.

Bucci, L.R., Blackman, G., Defoyd, W., Kaufman, R., Mandel-Tayes, C., Sparks, W.S., Stiles, J.C., Hickson, J.F. (1990a). Effect of ferrulate on strength and body composition of weightlifters. *J Appl Sports Sci Res* 4: 110. Abstract.

Bucci, L., Hickson Jr, J.F., Pivarnik, J.M., Wolinsky, I., McMahon, J.C., Turner, S.D. (1990b). Ornithine ingestion and growth hormone release in bodybuilders. *Nutr Res* 10: 239–45.

Buchman, A.L., Awal, M., Jenden, D., *et al.* (2000). The effect of lecithin supplementation on plasma choline concentrations during a marathon. *J Am Coll Nutr* 19: 768–70.

Buchman, A.L., Jenden, D., Roch, M. (1999). Plasma free, phospholipid-bound and urinary free choline all decrease during a marathon run and may be associated with impaired performance. *J Am Coll Nutr* 18: 598–601.

Buck, C.L., Wallman, K.E., Dawson, B., Guelfi, K.J. (2013). Sodium phosphate as an ergogenic aid. *Sports Med* 43: 425–35.

Buford, T.W., Cooke, M.B., Redd, L.L., Hudson, G.M., Shelmadine, B.D., Willoughby, D.S. (2009). Protease supplementation improves muscle function after eccentric exercise. *Med Sci Sports Exerc* 41: 1908–14.

Buono, M.J., Ball, K.D., Kolkhorst, F.W. (2007). Sodium ion concentration vs. sweat rate relationship in humans. *J Appl Physiol* 103: 990–4.

Burd, N.A., Hamer, H.M., Pennings, B., *et al.* (2013). Substantial differences between organ and muscle specific tracer incorporation rates in a lactating dairy cow. *PloS One* 8: e68109.

Burd, N.A., Jeukendrup, A., Reid, M.B., Burke, L.M., Stear, S.J., Castell, L.M. (2011a). BJSM reviews: A–Z of nutritional supplements: dietary supplements, sports nutrition foods and ergogenic aids for health and performance Part 26: Methionine, Multiple Transportable Carbohydrates and N-acetylcysteine. *Br J Sports Med* 45: 1163–4.

Burd, N.A., Stear, S.J., Burke, L.M., Castell, L.M. (2013). BJSM reviews: A–Z of nutritional supplements: dietary supplements, sports nutrition foods and ergogenic aids for health and performance Part 47: Peptides. *Br J Sports Med* 47: 933–4.

Burd, N.A., West, D.W., Moore, D.R., *et al.* (2011b). Enhanced amino acid sensitivity of myofibrillar protein synthesis persists for up to 24 h after resistance exercise in young men. *J Nutr* 141: 568–73.

Burke, D.G., Chilibeck, P.D., Parise, G., Tarnopolsky, M.A., Candow, D.G. (2003). Effect of alpha-lipoic acid combined with creatine monohydrate on human skeletal muscle creatine and phosphagen concentration. *Int J Sport Nutr Exerc Metab* 13: 294–302.

Burke, L.M. (2007). *Practical Sports Nutrition*. Champaign, IL: Human Kinetics Publishers.

Burke, L.M. (2008). Caffeine and sports performance. *Appl Physiol Nutr Metab* 33: 1319–34.

Burke, L.M. (2010). Fueling strategies to optimize performance: training high or training low? *Scand J Med Sci Sports* 20: 48–58.

Burke, L.M. (2013). Practical considerations for bicarbonate loading and sports performance. *Nestlé Nutr Inst Workshop Ser* 75: 15–26.

Burke, L.M., Desbrow, B., Spriet, L. (2013). *Caffeine for Sports Performance*. Champaign, Ill: Human Kinetics Publishers.

Burke, L.M., Hawley, J.A., Wong, S.H.H., Jeukendrup, A.E. (2011). Carbohydrates for training and competition. *J Sports Sci* 29: S17–S27.

Burke, L.M., Kiens, B. (2006). 'Fat adaptation' for athletic performance: the nail in the coffin? *J Appl Physiol* 100: 7–8.

Cade, R., Conte, M., Zauner, C., *et al.* (1984). Effects of phosphate loading on 2,3-diphosphoglycerate and maximal oxygen uptake. *Med Sci Sports Exerc* 16: 263–8.

Cahill Jr., G.F. (1970). Starvation in man. *N Engl J Med* 282: 668–75.

Cahill Jr., G.F., Owen, O.E. (1968). Starvation and survival. *Trans Am Clin Climatol Assoc* 79: 13.

Calbet, J.A., Mooren, F.C, Burke, L.M., Stear, S.J., Castell, L.M. (2011). BJSM reviews: A–Z of nutritional supplements: dietary supplements, sports nutrition foods and ergogenic aids for health and performance Part 24: Leptin, Magnesium and Medium Chain Triglycerides. *Br J Sports Med* 45: 1005–7.

Calder, P.C. (2012). Mechanisms of action of (n-3) fatty acids. *J Nutr* 142: 592S–9S.

Calder, P.C., Burdge, G.C. (2004). Fatty Acids. In: Nicolaou, A., Kafatos, G. (eds), *Bioactive Lipids*, The Oily Press: Bridgewater, pp. 1–36.

Calder, P.C., Lindley, M.R., Burke, L.M., Stear, S.J., Castell, L.M. (2010). BJSM reviews: A–Z of nutritional supplements: dietary supplements, sports nutrition foods and ergogenic aids for health and performance Part 14: Fatty acids and Fish oils. *Br J Sports Med* 44: 1065–7.

Calder, P.C., Yaqoob, P. (2009). Understanding omega-3 polyunsaturated fatty acids. *Postgrad Med* 121: 148–57.

Campbell, B., Roberts, M., Kerksick, C., *et al.* (2006). Pharmokinetics, safety, and effects on exercise performance of L-arginine a-ketoglutarate in trained adult men. *Nutr* 22: 872–81.

Campbell, B., Wilborn, C., La Bounty, P., *et al.* (2013). International society of sports nutrition position stand: energy drinks. *J Int Soc Sports Nutr* 10: 1.

Cannell, J.J., Hollis, B.W. (2008). Use of vitamin D in clinical practice. *Altern Med Rev* 13: 6–20.

Cannell, J.J., Hollis, B.W., Sorenson, M.B., Taft, T.N., Anderson, J.J. (2009). Athletic performance and vitamin D. *Med Sci Sports Exerc* 41: 1102–10.

Carlomagno, G., Unfer, V., Buffo, S., D'Ambrosio, F. (2011). Myo-inositol in the treatment of premenstrual dysphoric disorder. *Human Psychopharmacol Clin Exp* 26: 526–30.

Carmeli, E., Moa, M., Reznick, A.Z., *et al.* (2004). Matrix metalloproteinases and skeletal muscle: a brief review. *Muscle Nerve* 29: 191–7.

Carnés, J., de Larramendi, C.H., Ferrer, A., *et al.* (2013). Recently introduced foods as new allergenic sources: sensitisation to Goji berries (Lycium barbarum). *Food Chem* 137: 130–5.

Carol, A., Witkamp, R.F., Wichers, H.J., Mensink, M. (2011). Bovine colostrum supplementation's lack of effect on immune variables during short-term intense exercise in well-trained athletes. *Int J Sport Nutr Exerc Metab* 21: 135–45.

Carr, A.J., Gore, C.J., Dawson, B. (2011). Induced alkalosis and caffeine supplementation: effects on 2,000-m rowing performance. *Int J Sport Nutr Exerc Metab* 21: 357–64.

Carr, A.J., Hopkins, W.G., Gore, C.J. (2011a). Effects of acute alkalosis and acidosis on performance: a meta-analysis. *Sports Medicine* 41: 801–14.

Carr, A.J., Slater, G.J., Gore, C.J., *et al.* (2011b). Effect of sodium bicarbonate on [HCO3-], pH, and gastrointestinal symptoms. *Int J Sport Nutr Exerc Metab* 21: 189–94.

Carter, J.M., Jeukendrup, A.E., Jones, D.A. (2004). The effect of carbohydrate mouth rinse on 1-h cycle time trial performance. *Med Sci Sports Exerc* 36: 2107–11.

Casey, A., Constantin-Teodosiu, D., Howell, S., Hultman, E., Greenhaff, P.L. (1996). Creatine ingestion favorably affects performance and muscle metabolism during maximal exercise in humans. *Am J Physiol* 271: E31–7.

Castell, L.M. (2003). Glutamine supplementation in vitro and in vivo, in exercise and in immunodepression. *Sports Med.* 33: 323–45.

Castell, L.M., Poortmans, J.R., Newsholme, E.A. (1996). Does glutamine have a role in reducing infections in athletes? *Eur J Appl Physiol* 73: 488–90.

Castell, L.M., Stear, S.J., Burke, L.M. (2009). BJSM reviews: A–Z of supplements: dietary supplements, sports nutrition foods and ergogenic aids for health and performance Part 1. *Br J Sports Med* 43: 728–9.

Castell, L.M., Vance, C., Abbott, R., Marquez, J., Eggleton, P. (2004). Granule localization of glutaminase in human neutrophils and the consequence of glutamine utilization for neutrophil activity. *J Biol. Chem* 279: 13305–10.

Catlin, D.H., Fitch, K.D., Ljungqvist, A. (2008) Medicine and science in the fight against doping in sport. *J Intern Med* 264: 99–114.

CDC (2013). Acute hepatitis and liver failure following the use of a dietary supplement intended for weight loss or muscle building. *MMWR* 62: 817–18.

Cellini, M., Attipoe, S., Seales, P., *et al.* (2013). Dietary supplements: physician knowledge and adverse event reporting. *Med Sci Sports Exerc* 45: 23–8.

Cermak, N.M., Gibala, M.J., van Loon, L.J. (2012a). Nitrate supplementation's improvement of 10-km time-trial performance in trained cyclists. *Int J Sport Nutr Exerc Metab* 22: 64–71.

Cermak, N.M., Res, P.T., de Groot, L.C., Saris, W.H., van Loon, L.J. (2012b). Protein supplementation augments the adaptive response of skeletal muscle to resistance-type exercise training: a meta-analysis. *Am J Clin Nutr* 96: 1454–64.

Cermak, N.M., van Loon, L.J. (2013). The use of carbohydrates during exercise as an ergogenic aid. *Sports Med* 43: 1139–55.

Cermak, N., Yamamoto, T., Meeusen, R., Burke, L.M., Stear, S.J., Castell, L.M. (2012c). BJSM reviews: A–Z of nutritional supplements: dietary supplements, sports nutrition foods and ergogenic aids for health and performance Part 38: Threonine, Tryptophan and Tyrosine. *Br J Sports Med* 46: 1027–8.

Chandra, S., De Mejia, G.E. (2004). Polyphenolic compounds, antioxidant capacity, and quinone reductase activity of an aqueous extract of Ardisia compressa in comparison to mate (Ilex paraguariensis) and green (Camellia sinensis) teas. *J Agric Food Chem* 52: 3583–9.

Chasapis, C.T., Loutsidou, A.C., Spiliopoulou, C.A., *et al.* (2012). Zinc and human health: an update. *Arch Toxicol* 86: 521–34.

Cheeke, P.R., Piacente, S., Olezek, W. (2006). Anti-inflammatory and anti-arthritic effects of yucca schidigera: a review. *J Inflamm* 3: 6.

Chen, C.Y., Bakheit, R.M., Hart, V., *et al.* (2005a). Isoflavones improve plasma homocysteine status and antioxidant defense system in healthy young men at rest but do not ameliorate oxidative stress induced by 80% VO2pk exercise. *Ann Nutr Metab* 49: 33–41.

Chen, J.T., Wesley, R., Shamburek, R.D., *et al.* (2005b). Meta-analysis of natural therapies for hyperlipidemia: plant sterols and stanols versus policosanol. *Pharmocotherapy* 25: 171–83.

Cheng, S.M., Yang, L.L., Chen, S.H., Hsu, M.H., Chen, I.J., Cheng, F.C. (2010). Magnesium sulfate enhances exercise performance and manipulates dynamic changes in peripheral glucose utilization. *Eur J Appl Physiol* 108: 363–9.

Chesley, A., Howlett, R.A., Heigenhauser, G.J.F., Hultman, E., Spriet, L.L. (1998). Regulation of muscle glycogenolytic flux during intense aerobic exercise after caffeine ingestion. *Am J Physiol* 275: R596–R603.

Cheung, A.M., Tile, L., Lee, Y., *et al.* (2008). Vitamin K supplementation in postmenopausal women with osteopenia (ECKO trial): a randomized controlled trial. *PLoS Med* 5: e196.

Chinevere, T.D., Sawyer, R.D., Creer, A.R., Conlee, R.K., Parcell, A.C. (2002). Effects of L-tyrosine and carbohydrate ingestion on endurance exercise performance. *J Appl Physiol* 93: 1590–7.

Cho, A.S., *et al.* (2010). Chlorogenic acid exhibits anti-obesity property and improves lipid metabolism in high-fat diet-induced obese mice. *Food Chem Toxicol* 48: 937–43.

Choi, S., Disilvio, B., Fernstrom, M.H., Fernstrom, J.D. (2013). Oral branched-chain amino acid supplements that reduce brain serotonin during exercise in rats also lower brain catecholamines. *Amino Acids* 45: 1133–42.

Chopra, S.S., Patel, M.R., Awadhiya, R.P. (1976). Studies of Cissus quadrangularis in experimental fracture repair: a histopathological study. *Indian J Med Res* 64: 1365–8.

Chowdhury, I., Sengupta, A., Maitra, S.K. (2008). Melatonin: fifty years of scientific journey from the discovery in bovine pineal gland to delineation of functions in human. *Indian J Biochem Biophys* 45: 289–304.

Christensen, P.M., Nyberg, M., Bangsbo, J. (2013). Influence of nitrate supplementation on VO_2 kinetics and endurance of elite cyclists. *Scand J Med Sci Sports* 23: e21–31.

Christie, Á., *et al.* (1968). Observations on the performance of a standard exercise test by claudicants taking gamma-linolenic acid. *J Atherosclerosis Res* 8: 83–90.

Chun, O.K., Floegel, A., Chung, S.J., *et al.* (2010). Estimation of antioxidant intakes from diet and supplements in U.S. adults. *J Nutr* 140: 317–24.

Chung, K.W., Kim, S.Y., Chan, W.Y., *et al.* (1986). Androgen receptors in ventral prostate glands of zinc deficient rats. *Life Sciences* 38: 351–6.

Cimolai, N., Cimolai, T. (2011). Yohimbine use for physical enhancement and its potential toxicity. *J Diet Suppl* 8: 346–54.

Clancy, R.L., Gleeson, M., Cox, A., *et al.* (2006). Reversal in fatigued athletes of a defect in interferon gamma secretion after administration of Lactobacillus acidophilus. *Br J Sports Med* 40: 351–4.

Clancy, S.P., Clarkson, P.M., DeCheke, M.E., *et al.* (1994). Effects of chromium picolinate supplementation on body composition, strength, and urinary chromium loss in football players. *Int J Sport Nutr* 4: 142–53.

Clark, M., Reed, D.B., Crouse, S.F., Armstrong, R.B. (2003). Pre- and post-season dietary intake, body composition, and performance indices of NCAA Division I female soccer players. *Int J Sport Nutr Exerc Metab* 13: 303–19.

Clarke, K., Tchabenenko, K., Pawlosky, R., Carter, E., *et al.* (2012). Kinetics, safety and tolerability of (R)-3-hydroxybutyl (R)-3-hydroxybutyrate in healthy adult subjects. *Regul Toxicol Pharmacol* 63: 401–8.

Clarke, R., Halsey, J., Bennett, D., Lewington, S. (2011). Homocysteine and vascular disease: review of published results of the homocysteine-lowering trials. *J Inherited Metabolic Dis* 34: 83–91.

Clarke, R., Halsey, J., Lewington, S., Lonn, E., Armitage, J., et al (2010). Effects of lowering homocysteine levels with B vitamins on cardiovascular disease, cancer, and cause-specific mortality: meta-analysis of 8 randomized trials involving 37,485 individuals. *Arch Intern Med* 170: 1622–31.

Clegg, D.O., Reda, D.J., Harris, C.L., Klein, M.A., O'Dell, J.R., Hooper, M.M., *et al.* (2006). Glucosamine, chondroitin sulfate, and the two in combination for painful knee osteoarthritis. *N Engl J Med* 354: 795–808.

Close, G., Ashton, T., Cable, T., *et al.* (2006). Ascorbic acid supplementation does not attenuate post-exercise soreness following muscle-damaging exercise but may delay the recovery process. *Br J Nutr* 95: 976–81.

Close, G.L., Leckey, J., Patterson, M., Bradley, W., Owens, D.J., Fraser, W.D., *et al.* (2013b). The effects of vitamin D3 supplementation on serum total 25[OH]D concentration and physical performance: a randomised dose-response study. *Br J Sports Med* 47: 692–6.

Close, G.L., Russell, J., Cobley, J.N., Owens, D.J., Wilson, G., Gregson, W., *et al.* (2013a). Assessment of vitamin D concentration in non-supplemented professional athletes and healthy adults during the winter months in the UK: implications for skeletal muscle function. *J Sports Sci* 31: 344–53.

Cockayne, S., Adamson, J., Lanham-New, S., Shearer, M.J., Gilbody, S., Torgerson, D.J. (2006). Vitamin K and the prevention of fractures: systematic review and meta-analysis of randomized controlled trials. *Arch Intern Med* 166: 1256–61.

Cohen, P.A. (2012). DMAA as a dietary supplement ingredient. *Arch Int Med* 172: 1038–9.

Colakoglu, S., Colakoglu, M., Taneli, F., Cetinoz, F., Turkmen, M. (2006). Cumulative effects of conjugated linoleic acid and exercise on endurance development, body composition, serum leptin and insulin levels. *J Sports Med Phys Fitness* 46: 570–7.

Collins, J.K., Wu, G., Perkins-Veazie, P., *et al.* (2007). Watermelon consumption increases plasma arginine concentrations in adults. *Nutrition* 23: 261–6.

Collomp, K., Fortier, M., Cooper, S., *et al.* (1985). Performance and metabolic effects of benzodiazepine during submaximal exercise. *J Appl Physiol* 77: 828–33.

Colson, S.N., Wyatt, F.B., Johnston, D.L., *et al.* (2005). Cordyceps sinensis- and Rhodiola rosea-based supplementation in male cyclists and its effect on muscle tissue oxygen saturation. *J Strength Cond Res* 19: 358–63.

Colzato, L.S., Jongkees, B.J., Sellaro, R., Hommel, B. (2013). Working memory reloaded: tyrosine repletes updating in the *N*-back task. *Front Behav Neurosci* 7: 200.

Conlay, L.A., Sabounjian, L.A., Wurtman, R.J. (1992). Exercise and neuromodulators: choline and acetylcholine in marathon runners. *Int J Sport Med* 13: S141–2.

Conlay, L., Wurtman, R., Blusztajn, K., *et al.* (1986). Decreased plasma choline concentrations in marathon runners. *New Engl J Med* 315: 892.

Connolly, D.A., McHugh, M.P., PadillA–Zakour, O.I., *et al.* (2006). Efficacy of a tart cherry juice blend in preventing the symptoms of muscle damage. *Br J Sports Med* 40: 679–83.

Consumer Reports Magazine. (2010a). *Protein drinks.* Available at: www.consumerreports. org/cro/magazine-archive/2010a/july/food/protein-drinks/overview/index.htm. Accessed 15 September 2014.

Consumer Reports Magazine. (2010b). *Athletes complain.* Available at: www. consumerreports.org/cro/magazine-archive/2010/july/food/protein-drinks/athletes-complain/index.htm. Accessed 15 September 2014.

Coppola, A., Wenner, B.R., Ilkayeva, O., *et al.* (2013). Branched-chain amino acids alter neurobehavioral function in rats. *Am J Physiol Endocrinol Metab* 304: E405–13.

Cornelis, M.C., El-Sohemy, A., Campos, H. (2007). Genetic polymorphism of the adenosine A2A receptor is associated with habitual caffeine consumption. *Am J Clin Nutr* 86: 240–4.

Cornish, S.M., Candow, D.G., Jantz, N.T., Chilibeck, P.D., Little, J.P., Forbes, S., Abeysekara, S., Zello, G.A. (2009). Conjugated linoleic acid combined with creatine monohydrate and whey protein supplementation during strength training. *Int J Sport Nutr Exerc Metab* 19: 79–96.

Couzy, F., Kastenmayer, P., Vigo, M., Clough, J., Munoz-Box, R., Barclay, D.V. (1995). Calcium bioavailability from a calcium- and sulphur-rich mineral water, compared with milk, in young adult women. *Am J Clin Nutr* 62: 1239–44.

Cox, A.J., Pyne, D.B., Saunders, P.U., Fricker, P.A. (2010). Oral administration of the probiotic Lactobacillus fermentum VRI-003 and mucosal immunity in endurance athletes. *Br J Sports Med* 44: 222–6.

Cox, G.R., Desbrow, B., Montgomery, P.G., Anderson, M.E., Bruce, C.R., *et al.* (2002). Effect of different protocols of caffeine intake on metabolism and endurance performance. *J Appl Physiol* 93: 990–9.

Cox, P. (2012). The effects of a novel substrate on exercise energetics in elite athletes. *DPhil thesis.* University of Oxford: Oxford.

Cox, P.J., Clarke, K. (2014) Acute nutritional ketosis: implications for exercise performance and metabolism. *Extrem Physiol Med* 3: 17.

Coyle, E.F. (2004). Fluid and fuel intake during exercise. *J Sports Sci* 22: 39–55.

Craciun, A.M., Wolf, J., Knapen, M.H., Brouns, F., Vermeer, C. (1998). Improved bone metabolism in female elite athletes after vitamin K supplementation. *Int J Sport Med* 19: 479–84.

Craig, W.J. (1994). Iron status of vegetarians. *Am J Clin Nutr* 59: 1233S–1237S.

Cronin, J. (1999). The biochemistry of alternative therapies. Methylsulfonylmethane – Nutraceutical of the next century? *Alternative and Complementary Therapies* 5: 386–9.

Crooks, C., Wall, C., Cross, M., Rutherfurd-Markwick, K. (2006). The effect of bovine colostrum supplementation on salivary IgA in distance runners. *Int J Sport Nutr Exerc Metab* 16: 47–64.

Croze, M.L., Soulage, C.O. (2013). Potential role and therapeutic interests of myo-inositol in metabolic diseases. *Biochimie* 95: 1811–27.

Crozier, R.L., Robinson, D.K., Naughten, R.E., *et al.* (1991). Hyperhomocysteinemia: an independent risk factor for vascular disease. *N Engl J Med* 324: 1149–55.

Crozier, S.J., Kimball, S.R., Emmert, S.W., Anthony, J.C., Jefferson, L.S. (2005). Oral leucine administration stimulates protein synthesis in rat skeletal muscle. *J Nutr* 135: 376–82.

Crozier, T.W., *et al.* (2012). Espresso coffees, caffeine and chlorogenic acid intake: potential health implications. *Food Funct* 3: 30–3.

Cruzat, V.F., Tirapegui, J. (2009). Effects of oral supplementation with glutamine and alanyl-glutamine on glutamine, glutamate, and glutathione status in trained rats and subjected to long-duration exercise. *Nutr* 25: 428–35.

Cryan, J.F., Kaupmann, K. (2005). Don't worry 'B' happy!: a role for GABA(B) receptors in anxiety and depression. *Trends Pharmacol Sci* 26: 26–43.

Cui, J., Garle, M., Eneroth, P., *et al.* (1994). What do commercial ginseng preparations contain? *Lancet* 344: 134.

Cureton, K.J., Tomporowski, P.D., Singhal, A., *et al.* (2009). Dietary quercetin supplementation is not ergogenic in untrained men. *J Appl Physiol* 107: 1095–104.

Currell, K., Derave, W., Everaert, I., McNaughton, L., Slater, G., Burke, L.M., Stear, S.J., Castell, L.M. (2011). BJSM reviews: A–Z of nutritional supplements: dietary supplements, sports nutrition foods and ergogenic aids for health and performance Part 20: Glycine, Histidine-containing peptides, HMB and Inosine. *Br J Sport Med* 45: 530–2.

Currell, K., Jeukendrup, A. (2008a). Superior performance with ingestion of multiple transportable carbohydrates. *Med Sci Sports Exerc* 40: 275–81.

Currell, K., Jeukendrup, A.E. (2008b). Validity, reliability and sensitivity of performance tests. *Sports Med* 38: 297–316.

Currell, K., Moore, D.R., Peeling, P., Burke, L.M., Stear, S.J., Castell, L.M. (2012). BJSM reviews: A–Z of nutritional supplements: dietary supplements, sports nutrition foods and ergogenic aids for health and performance Part 28: Ornithine, Phenylalanine, Phosphate and Pangamic Acid. *Br J Sport Med* 46: 75–6.

Currell, K., Syed, A., Dziedzic, C.E., King, D.S., Spriet, L.L., Collins, J., Castell, L.M., Stear, S.J., Burke, L.M. (2010). BJSM reviews: A–Z of nutritional supplements: dietary supplements, sports nutrition foods and ergogenic aids for health and performance Part 12: Cysteine, Cystine, Cytochrome C, Dehydroepiandrosterone, Dihydroxyacetone Phosphate, Pyruvate, Dimethylglycine. *Br J Sport Med* 44: 905–7.

Currell, K., Urch, J., Cerri, E., *et al.* (2008). Plasma deuterium oxide accumulation following ingestion of different carbohydrate beverages. *Applied Physiol Nutr Metab* 33: 1067–72.

Cynober, L. (2004). Ornithine α-ketoglutarate as a potent precursor of arginine and nitric oxide: a new job for an old friend. *J Nutr* 134: 2858S–62S.

D'Aniello, A. (2007). D-Aspartic acid: an endogenous amino acid with an important neuroendocrine role. *Brain Res Rev* 53: 215–34.

D'Aniello, A., di Cosmo, A., Di Cristo, C., Annunziato, L., Petrucelli, L., Fisher, G. (1996). Involvement of D-aspartic acid in the synthesis of testosterone in rat testes. *Life Sciences* 59: 97–104.

D'Aniello, A., di Fiore, M.M., Fisher, G.H., Milone, A., Seleni, A., D'Aniello. S., *et al.* (2000). Occurrence of D-aspartic acid and N-methyl-D-aspartic acid in rat neuroendocrine tissues and their role in the modulation of luteinizing hormone and growth hormone release. *FASEB J* 14: 699–714.

Dang, R., Chow, T.-J. (2010). Hypolipidemic, antioxidant, and anti-inflammatory activities of microalgae spirulina. *Cardiovasc Ther* 28: e33–45.

Daniels, M.C., Popkin, B.M. (2010). Impact of water intake on energy intake and weight status: a systematic review. *Nutr Rev* 68: 505–21.

Dara, L., Hewett, J., Lim, J.K. (2008). Hydroxycut hepatotoxicity: a case series and review of liver toxicity from herbal weight loss supplements. *World J Gastroenterol* 14: 6999–7004.

Darbinyan, V., Kteyan, A., Panossian, A., *et al.* (2000). Rhodiola rosea in stress induced fatigue – a double blind cross-over study of a standardized extract SHR-5 with a repeated low-dose regimen on the mental performance of healthy physicians during night duty. *Phytomedicine* 7: 365–71.

Darra, E., Ebner, F.H., Shoji, K., Suzuki, H., Mariotto, S. (2009). Dual cross-talk between nitric oxide and D-serine in astrocytes and neurons in the brain. *Cent Nerv Syst Agents Med Chem* 9: 289–94.

Davis, A., Christiansen, M., Horowitz, J.F., Klein, S., Hellerstein, M.K., Ostlund, R.E. (2000). Effect of pinitol treatment on insulin action in subjects with insulin resistance. Diabetes Care. *Am Diabetes Assoc* 23: 1000–5.

Davis, J.M., Murphy, A., Carmichael, M.D., Davis, B. (2008). Quercetin increases brain and muscle mitochondrial biogenesis and exercise tolerance. *Am J Physiol Regul Integr Comp Physiol* 296: 1071–7.

Davison, G., Diment, B.C. (2010). Bovine colostrum supplementation attenuates the decrease of salivary lysozyme and enhances the recovery of neutrophil function after prolonged exercise. *Br J Nutr* 103: 1425–32.

Dawson, B., Goodman, C., Blee, T., *et al.* (2006). Iron supplementation: oral tablets versus intramuscular injection. *Int J Sport Nutr Exerc* 16: 180–6.

Dawson, K.D., Howarth, K.R., Tarnopolsky, M.A., *et al.* (2003). Short-term training attenuates muscle TCA cycle expansion during exercise in women. *J Appl Physiol* 95: 999–1004.

de Bock, K., Eijinde, B.O., Ramaekers, M., *et al.* (2004). Acute Rhodiola rosea intake can improve endurance exercise performance. *Int J Sport Nutr Exerc Metab* 14: 298–307.

de Hon, O., Coumans, B. (2007). The continuing story of nutritional supplements and doping infractions. *Br J Sport Med* 41: 800–5.

de la Hunty, A., Gibson, S., Ashwell, M. (2006). A review of the effectiveness of aspartame in helping with weight control. *Br Nutri Foundation Nutri Bull* 31: 115–28.

de Paulis, T., *et al.* (2002). Dicinnamoylquinides in roasted coffee inhibit the human adenosine transporter. *Eur J Pharmacol* 442: 215–23.

de Salles Painelli, V., Saunders, B., Sale, C., Harris, R.C., Solis, M.Y., Roschel, H., Gualano, B., Artioli, G.G., Lancha Jr, A.H. (2014). Influence of training status on high-intensity intermittent performance in response to β-alanine supplementation. *Amino Acids* 46: 1207–15.

de Sanctis, R., De Bellis, R., Scesa, C., *et al.* (2004). In vitro protective effect of Rhodiola rosea extract against hypochlorous acid-induced oxidative damage in human erythrocytes. *Biofactors* 20: 147–59.

de Vrese, M., Winkler, P., Rautenberg, P., *et al.* (2005). Effect of Lactobacillus gasseri PA 16/8, Bifidobacterium longum SP 07/3, B. bifidum MF 20/5 on common cold episodes: a double blind, randomized, controlled trial. *Clin Nutr* 24: 481–91.

Dean, S., Braakhuis, A., Paton, C. (2009). The effects of EGCG on fat oxidation and endurance performance in male cyclists. *Int J Sport Nutr Exerc Metab* 19: 624–44.

Defa, L., Changting, X., Shiyan, Q., Jinhui, Z., Johnson, E.W., Thacker, P.A. (1999). Effects of dietary threonine on performance, plasma parameters and immune function of growing pigs. *Animal Feed Sci Technol* 78: 179–88.

del Coso, J., Portillo, J., Muñoz, G., Abián-Vicén, J., Gonzalez-Millán, C., Muñoz-Guerra, J. (2013). Caffeine-containing energy drink improves sprint performance during an international rugby sevens competition. *Amino Acids* 44: 1511–9.

del Favero, S., Roschel, H., Solis, M.Y., *et al.* (2012). Beta-alanine (Carnosyn) supplementation in elderly subjects (60–80 years): effects on muscle carnosine content and physical capacity. *Amino Acids* 43: 49–56.

Delbeke, F.T., de Backer, P. (1996). Threshold level for theophylline in doping analysis. *J Chromatogr B Biomed Appl* 687: 247–52.

Demura, A.C., Morishita, K., Yamada, T., *et al.* (2011). Effect of L-ornithine hydrochloride ingestion on intermittent maximal anaerobic cycle ergometer performance and fatigue recovery after exercise. *Eur J Appl Physiol* 111: 2837–43.

Department of Health (1991). Report 41: *Dietary Reference Values for Food and Energy and Nutrients for the United Kingdom*. London: HMSO.

Deuster, P.A., Day, B.A., Singh, A., *et al.* (1989). Zinc status of highly trained women runners and untrained women. *Am J Clin Nutr* 49: 1295–1301.

Deuster, P.A., Hodgson, A.B., Stear, S.J., Burke, L.M., Castell, L.M. (2013). BJSM reviews: A–Z of nutritional supplements: dietary supplements, sports nutrition foods and ergogenic aids for health and performance Part 46: Zinc and ZMA. *Br J Sports Med* 47: 809–10.

Deuster, P.A., Kyle, S.B., Moser, P.B., *et al.* (1986). Nutritional survey of highly trained women runners. *Am J Clin Nutr* 44: 954–62.

Deuster, P., Maier, S., Moore, V., *et al.* (2004). *Dietary Supplements and Military Divers: a Synopsis for Undersea Medical Officers*. Bethesda, MD: Uniformed Services University of the Health Sciences, Department of Military and Emergency Medicine.

Deutz, N.E., Wolfe, R.R. (2013). Is there a maximal anabolic response to protein intake with a meal? *Clin Nutr* 32: 309–13.

di Donato, D.M., West, D.W., Churchward-Venne, T.A., Breen, L., Baker, S.K., Phillips, S.M. (2014). Influence of aerobic exercise intensity on myofibrillar and mitochondrial protein synthesis in young men during early and late postexercise recovery. *Am J Physiol Endocrinol Metab* 306: E1025–32.

di Giacomo, C., Acquaviva, R., Sorrenti, V., *et al.* (2009). Oxidative and antioxidant status in plasma of runners: effect of oral supplementation with natural antioxidants. *J Med Food* 12: 145–50.

di Santolo, M., Banfi, G., Stel, G., Cauci, S. (2009). Association of recreational physical activity with homocysteine, folate and lipid markers in young women. *Eur J Appl Physiol* 105: 111–8.

Diaz-Castro, J., Guisado, R., Kajarabille, N., *et al.* (2012). Coenzyme Q (10) supplementation ameliorates inflammatory signaling and oxidative stress associated with strenuous exercise. *Eur J Nutr* 51: 791–9.

DiMarco, N.M., West, N.P., Burke, L.M., Stear, S.J., Castell, L.M. (2012). BJSM reviews: A–Z of nutritional supplements: dietary supplements, sports nutrition foods and ergogenic aids for health and performance Part 30: Potassium and Prebiotics. *Br J Sports Med* 46: 299–300.

Ding, X., Ma, N., Nagahama, M., Yamada, K., Semba, R. (2011). Localization of D-serine and serine racemase in neurons and neuroglias in mouse brain. *Neurol Sci* 32: 263–7.

Doessing, S., Heinemeier, K.M., Holm, L., *et al.* (2010). Growth hormone stimulates the collagen synthesis in human tendon and skeletal muscle without affecting myofibrillar protein synthesis. *J Appl Physiol* 588: 341–51.

Dominguez, L.J., Barbagallo, M., Lauretani, F., Bandinelli, S., Bos, A., Corsi, A.M., Simonsick, E.M., Ferrucci, L. (2006). Magnesium and muscle performance in older persons: the InCHIANTI study. *Am J Clin Nutr* 84: 419–26.

Drakoularakou, A., Tzortzis, G., Rastall, R.A., Gibson, G.R. (2010). A double-blind, placebo-controlled, randomized human study assessing the capacity of a novel galacto-oligosaccharide mixture in reducing travellers' diarrhoea. *Eur J Clin Nutr* 64: 146–52.

Dreschfeld, J. (1886). The Bradshawe Lecture on Diabetic Coma. *Br J Med* 2: 358–63.

Drincic, A.T., Armas, L.A., Van Diest, E.E., Heaney, R.P. (2012). Volumetric dilution, rather than sequestration best explains the low vitamin D status of obesity. *Obesity* 20: 1444–8.

Droge, W., Schulze-Osthoff, K., Mihm, S., Galter, D., Schenk, H., Eck, H.-P., Roth, S., Gmunder, H. (1994). Functions of glutathione and glutathione disulfide in immunology and immunopathology. *FASEB J* 8: 1131–8.

Dubnov-Raz, G., Livne, N., Raz, R., Rogel, D., Cohen, A., Constantini, N. (2013). Vitamin D concentrations and physical performance in competitive adolescent swimmers. *Pediatr Exerc Sci* 26: 64–70.

Duff, W.R., Chilibeck, P.D., Rooke, J.J., Kaviani, M., Krentz, J.R., Haines, D.M. (2014). The effect of bovine colostrum supplementation in older adults during resistance training. *Int J Sport Nutr Exerc Metabol* 24: 276–85.

Duffield, A.J., Thomson, C.D., Hill, K.E., Williams, S. (1999). An estimation of selenium requirements for New Zealanders. *Am J Clin Nutr* 70: 896–903.

Dulin, M.F., Hatcher, L.F., Sasser, H.C., Barringer, T.A. (2006). Policosanol is ineffective in the treatment of hypercholesterolemia: a randomized control trial. *Am J Clin Nutr* 84: 1543–8.

Duncan, C., Dougall, H., Johnston, P., Green, S., Brogan, R., Smith, L., Golden, M., Benjamin, N. (1995). Chemical generation of nitric oxide in the mouth from the enterosalivary circulation of dietary nitrate. *Nat Med* 1: 546–51.

Dunne, L., Worley, S., Macknin, M. (2006). Ribose versus dextrose supplementation, association with rowing performance: a double-blind study. *Clin J Sport Med* 16: 68–71.

Dutka, T.L., Lamboley, C.R., McKenna, M.J., Murphy, R.M., Lamb, G.D. (2012). Effects of carnosine on contractile apparatus Ca2+-sensitivity and sarcoplasmic reticulum Ca2+ release in human skeletal muscle fibers. *J Appl Physiol* 112: 728–36.

Dutka, T.L., Lamboley, C.R., Murphy, R.M., *et al.* (2014). Acute effects of taurine on sarcoplasmic reticulum Ca^{2+} accumulation and contractility in human type I and type II skeletal muscle fibres. *J Appl Physiol* 117: 797–805.

Dyck, D.J. (2004). Pyruvate and dihydroxyacetone. In: Wolinsky, I., Driskell, J.A. (eds), *Nutritional Ergogenic Aids*. Boca Raton, FL: CRC Press: pp. 445–54.

Earnest, C.P., Morss, G.M., Wyatt, F., *et al.* (2004). Effects of a commercial herbal-based formula on exercise performance in cyclists. *Med Sci Sports Exerc* 36: 504–9.

Eaton-Evans, J., McIlrath, E.M., Jackson, W.E., McCartney, H. and Strain, J.J. (1998) Copper supplementation and the maintenance of bone mineral density in middle aged women. *The Journal of Trace Elements in Experimental Medicine.* 9 (3):87–94.

Edge, J., Bishop, D., Goodman, C. (2006). Effects of chronic NaHCO3 ingestion during interval training on changes to muscle buffer capacity, metabolism and short-term endurance performance. *J Appl Physiol* 101: 918–25.

EFSA (2005). EFSA Scientific Panel on Dietetic Products, Nutrition and Allergies. Opinion of the scientific panel on dietetic products, nutrition and allergies on a request from the commission related to the tolerable upper intake level of sodium. *EFSA J* 209: 1–26.

EFSA (2006). Tolerable upper intake levels for vitamins and minerals. Available at: www.efsa.europa.eu/EFSA/Scientific_Document/upper_level_opinions_full-part33.pdf. Accessed 20 June 2014.

Eichenberger, P., Mettler, S., Arnold, M., *et al.* (2010). No effects of three-week consumption of a green tea extract on time trial performance in endurance-trained men. *Int J Vitam Nutr Res* 80: 54–64.

Eijnde, B.O., van Leemputte, M., Brouns, F., van der Vusse, G.J., Labarque, V., *et al.* (2001). No effects of oral ribose supplementation on repeated maximal exercise and de novo ATP resynthesis. *J Appl Physiol* 91: 2275–81.

Eliason, M.J., Eichner, A., Cancio, A., *et al.* (2012). Case reports: death of active duty soldiers following ingestion of dietary supplements containing 1,3-dimethylamylamine (DMAA). *Mil Med* 177: 1455–9.

Elsohly, M.A., Gul, W., Elsohly, K.M., *et al.* (2012). Pelargonium oil and methyl hexaneamine (MHA): analytical approaches supporting the absence of MHA in authenticated Pelargonium graveolens plant material and oil. *J Anal Toxicol* 36: 457–71.

Erdtman, H., Hirose, Y. (1962). The chemistry of the natural order *Cupressales. Acta Chem Scand* 16: 1311–14.

Ernst, E., Pittler, M.H. (1998). Efficacy of homeopathic arnica. A systematic review of placebo-controlled clinical trials. *Arch Surg* 133: 1187–90.

Escames, G., Ozturk, G., Baño-Otálora, B., Pozo, M.J., Madrid, J.A., Reiter, R.J., Serrano, E.,Concepción, M., Acuña-Castroviejo, D. (2012). Exercise and melatonin in humans: reciprocal benefits. *J. Pineal Res* 52: 1–11.

Everaert, I., Mooyaart, A., Baguet, A., Zutinic, A., Baelde, H., Achten, E., Taes, Y., de Heer, E., Derave, W. (2011). Vegetarianism, female gender and increasing age, but not CNDP1 genotype, are associated with reduced muscle carnosine levels in humans. *Amino Acids* 40: 1221–9.

Everaert, I., Stegen, S., Vanheel, B., Taes, Y., Derave, W. (2013). Effect of beta-alanine and carnosine supplementation on muscle contractility in mice. *Med Sci Sports Exerc* 45: 43–51.

EVM (2003). Safe upper levels for vitamins and minerals. Available at: http://cot.food.gov.uk/pdfs/vitmin2003.pdf. Accessed 20 June 2014.

Fang, Y., Hu, C., Tao, X., Wan, Y., Tao, F. (2012). Effect of vitamin K on bone mineral density: a meta-analysis of randomized controlled trials. *J Bone Miner Metab* 30: 60–8.

FAO (2014). Chapter 16. Available at: www.fao.org/docrep/004/y2809e/y2809e0m.htm. Accessed 29 January 2015.

Faria, I.E., Faria, E.W., Parker, D.L. (2002). Effect of cytochrome C supplementation on aerobic running performance. *J Exerc Physiol* 5: 35–40.

Farney, T.M., Mccarthy, C.G., Canale, R.E., *et al.* (2012). Hemodynamic and hematologic profile of healthy adults ingesting dietary supplements containing 1,3-dimethylamylamine and caffeine. *Nutr Metabolic Insights* 5: 1–12.

Favier, A.E. (1992). The role of zinc in reproduction. Hormonal mechanisms. *Biol Trace Elem Res* 32: 363–82.

Fawcett, J.P., Farquhar, S.J., Thou, T., Shand, B.I. (1997). Oral vanadyl sulphate does not affect blood cells, viscosity or biochemistry in humans. *Pharmacol Toxicol* 80: 202–6.

FDA (1995). Inspections, compliance, enforcement, and criminal investigations. www.fda.gov/ICECI/ComplianceManuals/CompliancePolicyGuidanceManual/ucm074396.htm. Accessed 29 January 2015.

Fehrenbach, E., Neiss, A. (1999). Role of heat shock proteins in the exercise response. *Exerc Immunol Rev* 5: 57–77.

Felig, P., Owen, O.E., Wahren, J., Cahill, G.F.Jr. (1969). Amino acid metabolism during prolonged starvation. *J Clin Invest.* 48: 584–94.

Fernstrom, J.D., Fernstrom, M.H. (2007). Tyrosine, phenylalanine, and catecholamine synthesis and function in the brain. *J Nutr* 137: 539S–47S.

Fernstrom, J.D., Wurtman, R.J. (1972). Brain serotonin content: physiological regulation by plasma neutral amino acids. *Sci* 178: 414–16.

Ferrando, A.A., Green, N.R. (1993). The effect or boron supplementation on lean body mass, plasma testosterone levels, and strength in male bodybuilders. *Int J Sport Nutr* 3: 140–9.

Ferreira, L.F., Behnke, B.J. (2011). A toast to health and performance! Beetroot juice lowers blood pressure and the O_2 cost of exercise. *J Appl Physiol* 110: 585–6.

Ferreira, L.F., Campbell, K.S., Reid, M.B. (2011). N-acetylcysteine in handgrip exercise: plasma thiols and adverse reactions. *Int J Sport Nutr Exerc Metab* 21: 146–54.

Fery, F., Balasse, E.O. (1983). Ketone-body turnover during and after exercise in overnight-fasted and starved humans. *Am J Physiol* 245: E318–E325.

Finaud, J., Lac, G., Filaire, E. (2006). Oxidative stress: relationship with exercise and training. *Sports Med Auckl NZ* 36: 327–58.

Fitschen, P.J., Wilson, G.J., Wilson, J.M., *et al.* (2013). Efficacy of beta-hydroxy-beta-methylbutyrate supplementation in elderly and clinical populations. *Nutr* 29: 29–36.

Flanagan, J., *et al.* (2014). Lipolytic activity of svetol(R), a decaffeinated green coffee bean extract. *Phytother Res* 28: 946–8.

Flaring, U.B., Rooyackers, O.E., Wernerman, J., Hammarqvist, F. (2003). Glutamine attenuates post-traumatic glutathione depletion in human muscle. *Clin Sci* (Lond) 104: 275–82.

Fleischauer, A.T., Poole, C., Arab, L. (2000). Garlic consumption and cancer prevention: meta-analyses of colorectal and stomach cancers. *Am J Clin Nutr* 72: 1047–52.

Fleming, H.L., Ranaivo, P.L., Simone, P.S. (2012). Analysis and confirmation of 1,3-DMAA and 1,4-DMAA in geranium plants using high performance liquid chromatography with tandem mass spectrometry at ng/g concentrations. *Anal Chem Insights* 7: 59–78.

FNB (2000). Dietary reference intakes: a risk assessment model for establishing upper intake levels for nutrients. Available at: www.nap.edu/openbook.php?isbn=0309063485.

Foad, A.J., Beedie, C.J., Coleman, D.A. (2008). Pharmacological and psychological effects of caffeine ingestion in 40 km cycling performance. *Med Sci Sports Exerc* 40: 158–65.

Fogarty, M.C., Devito, G., Hughes, C.M., Burke, G., Brown, J.C., McEneny, J., Brown, D., McClean, C., Davison, G.W. (2013). Effects of α-lipoic acid on mtDNA damage after isolated muscle contractions. *Med Sci Sports Exerc* 45(8): 1469–77.

Fogelholm, G.M. (1992). Micronutrient status in females during a 24-week fitness-type exercise program. *Ann Nutr Metab* 36: 209–18.

Fogelholm, G.M., Näveri, H.K., Kiilavuori, K.T., Härkönen, M.H. (1993a). Low-dose amino acid supplementation: no effects on serum human growth hormone and insulin in male weightlifters. *Int J Sport Nutr Exerc Metab* 3: 290–7.

Fogelholm, G.M., Ruokonen, I., Laakso, J.T., *et al.* (1993b). Lack of association between indicies of vitamin B-1, B-2 and B-6 status and exercise-induced blood lactate in young adults. *Int J Sport Nutr* 3: 165–76.

Fogelholm, M., Laakso, J., Lehto, J., *et al.* (1991). Dietary-intake and indicators of magnesium and zinc status in male athletes. *Nutr Res* 11: 1111–18.

Folland, J.P., Stern, R., Brickley, G. (2008). Sodium phosphate loading improves laboratory cycling time-trial performance in trained cyclists. *J Sci Med Sport* 11: 464–8.

Fontani, G., Lodi, L., Migliorini, S., Corradeschi, F. (2009). Effect of omega-3 and policosanol supplementation on attention and reactivity in athletes. *J Am Coll Nutr* 28 Suppl: 473S–81S.

Forrester, M.B. (2013). Exposures to 1,3-dimethylamylamine-containing products reported to Texas poison centers. *Hum Exp Toxicol* 32: 18–23.

Forsythe, P. (2014). Probiotics and lung immune responses. *Ann Am Thorac Soc* 11 Suppl 1: S33–7.

Fransen, M., Agaliotis, M., Narin, L., Votrubec, M., Bridgett, L., Su, S., *et al.* (2014). Glucosamine and chondroitin for knee osteoarthritis: a double-blind randomised placebo-controlled clinical trial evaluating single and combination regimens. *Ann Rheum Dis*. doi: 10.1136/annrheumdis-2013-203954. [Epub ahead of print]

Frayn, K.N. (2010). *Metabolic Regulation – A Human Perspective* (Third Edition). Wiley-Blackwell: Chichester.

Friedman, J.M., Halaas, J.L. (1998). Leptin and the regulation of body weight in mammals. *Nature* 395: 763–70.

Friedmann, B., Weller, E., Mairbaeurl, H., *et al.* (2001). Effects of iron repletion on blood volume and performance capacity in young athletes. *Med Sci Sport Ex*erc 33: 741–6.

Fry, A.C., Bronner, E., Lewis, D.L., Johnson, R.L., Stone, M.H., Kraemer, W.J. (1997). The effects of gamma-oryzanol supplementation during resistance exercise training. *Int J Sport Nutr* 7: 318–29.

Fu, L., Yun, F., Oczak, M., Wong, B.Y., Vieth, R., Cole, D.E. (2009). Common genetic variants of the vitamin D binding protein (DBP) predict differences in response of serum 25-hydroxyvitamin D [25(OH)D] to vitamin D supplementation. *Clin Biochem* 42: 1174–7.

Fuentes, T., Ara, I., Guadalupe-Grau, A., Larsen, S., Stallknecht, B., Olmedillas, H., Santana, A., Helge, J.W., Calbet, J.A., Guerra, B. (2010). Leptin receptor 170 kda (ob-r170) protein expression is reduced in obese human skeletal muscle: a potential mechanism of leptin resistance. *Exp Physiol* 95: 160–71.

Fujioka, K., Greenway, F., Sheard, J., *et al.* (2006). The effects of grapefruit on weight and insulin resistance: relationship to the metabolic syndrome. *J Med Food* 9: 49–54.

Fuller Jr., J.C., Sharp, R.L., Angus, H.F., *et al.* (2011). Free acid gel form of beta-hydroxy-beta-methylbutyrate (HMB) improves HMB clearance from plasma in human subjects compared with the calcium HMB salt. *Br J Nutr* 105: 367–72.

Furuchi, T., Homma, H. (2005). Free D-aspartate in mammals. *Biol Pharma Bull* 28: 1566–70.

Galloway, S.D.R., Talanian, J.L., Shoveler, A.K., *et al.* (2008). Seven days of oral taurine supplementation does not increase muscle taurine content or alter substrate metabolism during prolonged exercise in humans. *J Appl Physiol* 105: 643–51.

Ganio, M.S., Klau, J.F., Casa, D.J., Armstrong, L.E., Maresh, C.M. (2009). Effect of caffeine on sport-specific endurance performance: a systematic review. *J Strength Cond Res* 23: 315–24.

Gannon, M.C., Nuttall, J.A., Nuttall, F.Q. (2002). The metabolic response to glycine. *Am J Clin Nutr* 76: 1302–7.

Garlick, P.J. (2004). The nature of human hazards associated with excessive intake of amino acids. *J Nutr* 134: 1633S–1639S.

Garlick, P.J. (2006). Toxicity of methionine in humans. *J Nutr* 136: 1722S–1725S.

Garvican, L.A., Lobigs, L., Telford, R., *et al.* (2011). Haemoglobin mass in an anaemic female endurance runner before and after iron supplementation. *Int J Sport Physiol Perform* 6: 137–40.

Garvican, L.A., Saunders, P.U., Cardoso, T., *et al.* (2014). Intravenous iron supplementation in distance runners with low or suboptimal ferritin. *Med Sci Sports Exerc* 46: 376–85.

Gauthier, T.D. (2013). Evidence for the presence of 1,3-dimethylamylamine (1,3-DMAA) in geranium plant materials. *Anal Chem Insights* 8: 29–40.

Gee, P., Tallon, C., Long, N., *et al.* (2012). Use of a recreational drug 1,3-dimethylethylamine (DMAA) associated with cerebral hemorrhage. *Ann Emer Med* 60: 431–4.

Geiss, K.R., Jester, I., Falke, W., *et al.* (1994). The effect of taurine-containing drink on performance in 10 endurance-athletes. *Amino Acids* 7: 45–56.

Geyer, H., Braun, H., Burke, L.M., Stear, S.J., Castell, L.M. (2011). BJSM reviews: A–Z of nutritional supplements: dietary supplements, sports nutrition foods and ergogenic aids for health and performance Part 22: Inadvertent Doping. *Br J Sports Med* 45: 752–4.

Geyer, H., Gülker, A., Mareck, U., *et al.* (2004a). Some good news from the field of nutritional supplements. *In Recent Advances in Doping Analysis* (12), Schänzer, W., Geyer, H., Gotzmann, A., Mareck, U. (eds). Sportverlag Strauß: Köln, 91–7.

Geyer, H., Henze, M.K., Mareck-Engelke, U., *et al.* (2000). Positive doping cases with norandosterone after application of contaminated nutritional supplements. *Dtsch J Sportmed* 51: 378–82.

Geyer, H., Mareck, U., Köhler, K., Parr, M.K., Schänzer, W. (2006). Cross contaminations of vitamin- and mineral-tablets with metandienone and stanozolol. In *Recent Advances in Doping Analysis* (14), Schanzer, W., Geyer, H., Gotzmann, A., Mareck, U. (eds). Sportverlag Strauß: Köln, 11.

Geyer, H., Parr, M.K., Koehler, K., *et al.* (2008). Nutritional supplements cross-contaminated and faked with doping substances. *J Mass Spectrom* 43: 892–902.

Geyer, H., Parr, M.K., Mareck, U., *et al.* (2004b). Analysis of non-hormonal nutritional supplements for anabolic-androgenic steroids – results of an international study. *Int J Sport Med* 25: 124–9.

Gharib, H., Cook, D.M., Saenger, P.H., *et al.* (2003). American Association of Clinical Endocrinologists medical guidelines for clinical practice for growth hormone use in adults and children – 2003 update. *Endocr Pract* 9: 64–76.

Ghezzi, P. (2005). Oxidoreduction of protein thiols in redox regulation. *Biochem Soc Trans* 33: 1378–81.

Ghigo, E., Arvat, E., Gianotti, L., *et al.* (1994). Growth hormone-releasing activity of hexarelin, a new synthetic hexapeptide, after intravenous, subcutaneous, intranasal, and oral administration in man. *J Clin Endocrinol Metab* 78: 693–8.

Gibala, M.J. (2001). Regulation of skeletal muscle amino acid metabolism during exercise. *Int J Sport Nutr Exerc Metabolism* 11: 87–108.

Gibala, M.J., *et al.* (1999). Low glycogen and branched-chain amino acid ingestion do not impair anaplerosis during exercise in humans. *J Appl Physiol* 87: 1662–7.

Gibala, M.J., Peirce, N., Constantin-Teodosiu, D., *et al.* (2002). Exercise with low muscle glycogen augments TCA cycle anaplerosis but impairs oxidative energy provision in humans. *J Physiol* 540: 1079–86.

Girandola, R.N., Wiswell, R.A., Bulbulian, R. (1980). Effects of pangamic acid (B-15) ingestion on metabolic responses to exercise. *Biochem Med* 24: 218–22.

Glaister, M., Pattison, J., Muniz-Pumares, D., Patterson, D., Foley, P. (2014). Effects of dietary nitrate, caffeine and their combination on 20km cycling time-trial performance. *J Strength Cond Res* [Epub ahead of print].

Gleeson, M., Bishop, N.C., Oliveira, M., Tauler, P. (2011). Daily probiotic's (*Lactobacillus casei* Shirota) reduction of infection incidence in athletes. *Int J Sport Nutr Exerc Metab* 21: 55–64.

Gleeson, M., Siegler, J.C., Burke, L.M., Stear, S.J., Castell, L.M. (2012). BJSM reviews: A–Z of nutritional supplements: dietary supplements, sports nutrition foods and ergogenic aids for health and performance Part 31: Probiotics and Pycnogenol. *Br J Sports Med* 46: 377–8.

Gleeson, M., Thomas, L. (2008). Exercise and immune function. Is there any evidence for probiotic benefit for sports people? *Complete Nutr* 8: 3–37.

Glynn, E.L., Fry, C.S., Drummond, M.J., Timmerman, K.L., Dhanani, S., Volpi, E., Rasmussen, B.B. (2010). Excess leucine intake enhances muscle anabolic signalling but not net protein anabolism in young men and women. *J Nutr* 140: 1970–6.

Godfrey, R.J., Laupheimer, M., Stear, S.J., Burke, L.M., Castell, L.M. (2013). BJSM reviews: A–Z of nutritional supplements: dietary supplements, sports nutrition foods and ergogenic aids for health and performance Part 45: Yerba maté, Yohimbine and Yucca. *Br J Sports Med* 47: 659–60.

Goedecke, J.H., Elmer-English, R., Dennis, S.C., Schloss, I., Noakes, T.D., Lambert, E.V. (1999). Effects of medium-chain triacylglycerol ingested with carbohydrate on metabolism and exercise performance. *Int J Sport Nutr* 9: 35–47.

Golbidi, S., Badran, M., Laher, I. (2011). Diabetes and alpha lipoic acid. *Front Pharmacol* 17: 69.

Goldfarb, A.H., Bloomer, R.J. Mckenzie, M.J. (2005). Combined antioxidant treatment effects on blood oxidative stress after eccentric exercise. *Med Sci Sports Exerc* 37: 234–9.

Goldfinch, J., McNaughton, L.R., Davies, P. (1988). Bicarbonate ingestion and its effects upon 400-m. *Eur J Appl Physiol Occup Physiol* 57: 45–8.

Golf, S.W., Happel, O., Graef, V., *et al.* (1984). Plasma aldosterone, cortisol and electrolyte concentrations in physical exercise after magnesium supplementation. *J Clin Chem Clin Biochem* 22: 717–21.

Gomes, E.C., Allgrove, J.E., Florida-James, G., *et al.* (2011). Effect of vitamin supplementation on lung injury and running performance in a hot, humid, and ozone-polluted environment. *Scand J Med Sci Sports* 21: e452–60.

Gómez-Bernal, S., Rodríguez-Pazos, L., Martínez, F.J.G., *et al.* (2011). Systemic photosensitivity due to Goji berries. *Photodermatol Photoimmunol Photomed* 27: 245–7.

Gomez-Cabrera, M.C., Domenech, E., Romagnoli, M., *et al.* (2008). Oral administration of vitamin C decreases muscle mitochondrial biogenesis and hampers training-induced adaptations in endurance performance. *Am J Clin Nutr* 87: 142–9.

Gomez-Merino, D., *et al.* (2001). Evidence that the branched-chain amino acid L-valine prevents exercise-induced release of 5-HT in rat hippocampus. *Int J Sport Med* 22: 317–22.

Goodman, C.A., Horvath, D., Stathis, C., *et al.* (2009). Taurine supplementation increases skeletal muscle force production and protects muscle function during and after high-frequency in vitro stimulation. *J Appl Physiol* 107: 144–54.

Goodman, C., Peeling, P., Ranchordas, M.K., Burke, L.M., Stear, S.J., Castell, L.M. (2011). BJSM reviews: A–Z of nutritional supplements: dietary supplements, sports nutrition foods and ergogenic aids for health and performance Part 21: Iron, α-Ketoisocaproate and α-Ketoisocaproate. *Br J Sports Med* 45: 677–9.

Gorsline, R.T., Kaeding, C.C. (2005). The use of NSAIDs and nutritional supplements in athletes with osteoarthritis: prevalence, benefits, and consequences. *Clin Sports Med* 24: 71–82.

Goss, F., Robertson, R., Riechman, S., *et al.* (2001). Effect of potassium phosphate supplementation on perceptual and physiological responses to maximal graded exercise. *Int J Sport Nutr Exerc Metab* 11: 53–62.

Goulet, E.D., Aubertin-Leheudre, M., Plante, G.E., Dionne, I.J. (2007). A meta-analysis of the effects of glycerol-induced hyperhydration on fluid retention and endurance performance. *Int J Sport Nutr Exerc Metab* 17: 391–410.

Graber, C.D., Goust, J.M., Glassman, A.D., *et al.* (1981). Immunomodulating properties of dimethylglycine in humans. *J Infect Dis* 143: 101–5.

Graham, B.S., Bunton, L.A., Wright, P.F., Karzon, D.T. (1991). Role of T lymphocyte subsets in the pathogenesis of primary infection and rechallenge with respiratory syncytial virus in mice. *J Clin Invest* 88: 1026–33.

Graham, T.E. (2001). Caffeine and exercise: metabolism, endurance and performance. *Sports Med* 31: 765–85.

Graham, T.E., Battram, D.S., Dela, F., El-Sohemy, A., Thong, F.S. (2008). Does caffeine alter muscle carbohydrate and fat metabolism during exercise? *Appl Physiol Nutr Metab* 33: 1311–18.

Graham, T.E., Hibbert, E., Sathasivam, P. (1998). Metabolic and exercise endurance effects of coffee and caffeine ingestion. *J Appl Physiol* 85: 883–9.

Graham, T.E., Spriet, L.L. (1991). Performance and metabolic responses to a high caffeine dose during prolonged exercise. *J Appl Physiol* 71: 2292–8.

Graham, T.E., Spriet, L.L. (1995). Metabolic, catecholamine, and exercise performance responses to various doses of caffeine. *J Appl Physiol* 78: 867–74.

Graham, T.E., Turcotte, L.P., Kiens, B., *et al.* (1995). Training and muscle ammonia and amino acid metabolism in humans during prolonged exercise. *J Appl Physiol* 78: 725–35.

Granados, J., Gillum, T.L., Christmas, K.M., Kuennen, M.R. (1985). Prohormone supplement 3β-hydroxy-5α androst-1-en-17-one enhances resistance training gains but impairs user health. *J Appl Physiol* 116: 560–9.

Gray, M.E., Titlow, L.W. (1982). The effect of pangamic acid on maximal treadmill performance. *Med Sci Sports Exerc* 14: 424–7.

Gray, P., Chappell, A., Jenkinson, A.M., Thies, F., Gray, S.R. (2014). Fish oil supplementation reduces markers of oxidative stress but not muscle soreness after eccentric exercise. *Int J Sport Nutr Exerc Metab* 24: 206–14.

Gray, P., Gabriel, B., Thies, F., Gray, S.R. (2012). Fish oil supplementation augments post-exercise immune function in young males. *Brain Behav Immun* 26: 1265–72.

Greenberg, J.A., Boozer, C.N., Geliebter, A. (2006). Coffee, diabetes, and weight control. *Am J Clin Nutr* 84: 682–93.

Greenwood, M.H., Lader, M.H., Kantameneni, B.D., Curzon, G. (1975). The acute effects of oral tryptophan in human subjects. *Brit J Clin Pharmacol* 2: 165–72.

Greer, F., Friars, D., Graham, T.E. (2000). Comparison of caffeine and theophylline ingestion: exercise metabolism and endurance. *J Appl Physiol Bethesda Md (1985)* 89: 1837–44.

Greiner, C., Röhl, J.E., Ali-Gorji, A., *et al.* (2003). Different actions of γ-hydroxybutyrate: a critical outlook. *Neurol Res* 25: 759–63.

Greiwe, J.S., Kwon, G., McDaniel, M.L., Semenkovich, C.F. (2001). Leucine and insulin activate p70 S6 kinase through different pathways in human skeletal muscle. *Am J Physiol Endocrinol Metab* 281: E466–E471.

Greyling, A., De Witt, C., Oosthuizen, W., Jerling, J.C. (2006). Effects of a policosanol supplement on serum lipid concentrations in hypercholesterolaemic and heterozygous familial hypercholesterolaemic subjects. *Br J Nutr* 95: 968–75.

Griffith, O.W. (1999). Biologic and pharmacologic regulation of mammalian glutathione synthesis. *Free Radic Biol Med* 27: 922–35.

Grimm, T., Schaefer, A., Hogger, P. (2004). Antioxidant activity and inhibition of matrix metalloproteinases by metabolites of maritime pine bark extract. *Free Radic Biol Med* 36: 811–22.

Gropper, S.S., Sorrels, M. and Blessing, D. (2003) Copper status of collegiate female athletes involved in different sports. *International Journal of Sports Nutrition and Exercise Metabolism.* 13: 343–357.

Grunewald, K.K., Bailey, R.S. (1993). Commercially marketed supplements for bodybuilding athletes. *Sports Med Auckl NZ* 15: 90–103.

Gualano, B., Artioli, G.G., Poortmans, J.R., *et al.* (2010). Exploring the therapeutic role of creatine supplementation. *Amino Acids* 38: 31–44.

Guerra, B., Fuentes, T., Delgado-Guerra, S., Guadalupe-Grau, A., Olmedillas, H., Santana, A., Ponce-Gonzalez, J.G., Dorado, C., Calbet, J.A. (2008). Gender dimorphism in skeletal muscle leptin receptors, serum leptin and insulin sensitivity. *PLoS ONE* 3: e3466.

Guerra, B., Olmedillas, H., Guadalupe-Grau, A., Ponce-Gonzalez, J.G., Morales-Alamo, D., Fuentes, T., Chapinal, E., Fernandez-Perez, L., De Pablos-Velasco, P., Santana, A., Calbet, J.A. (2011). Is sprint exercise a leptin signaling mimetic in human skeletal muscle? *J Appl Physiol* 111: 715–25.

Guerra, B., Santana, A., Fuentes, T., Delgado-Guerra, S., Cabrera-Socorro, A., Dorado, C., Calbet, J.A. (2007). Leptin receptors in human skeletal muscle. *J Appl Physiol* 102: 1786–92.

Guerrera, M.P., Volpe, S.L., Mao, J.J. (2009). Therapeutic uses of magnesium. *Am Fam Physician* 80: 157–62.

Guillemard, E., Tanguy, J., Flavigny, A., *et al.* (2010). Effects of consumption of a fermented dairy product containing the probiotic Lactobacillus casei DN-114 001 on common respiratory and gastrointestinal infections in shift workers in a randomized controlled trial. *J Am Coll Nutr* 29: 455–68.

Guo, H., Saiga, A., Sato, M., Miyazawa, I., Shibata, M., Takahata, Y., Morimatsu, F. (2007). Royal jelly supplementation improves lipoprotein metabolism in humans. *J Nutr Sci Vitaminol* (Tokyo) 53: 345–8.

Gurr, M.I., Harwood, J.L., Frayn, K.N. (2002). *Lipid Biochemistry* (Fifth Edition). Blackwell Science: Oxford.

Gwacham, N., Wagner, D.R. (2012). Acute effects of a caffeine-taurine energy drink on repeated sprint performance of American college football players. *Int J Sport Nutr Exerc Metab* 19: 45–56.

Hafiez, A.A., el-Kirdassy, Z.H., Mansour, M.M., *et al.* (1989). Role of zinc in regulating the testicular function. Part 1. Effect of dietary zinc deficiency on serum levels of gonadotropins, prolactin and testosterone in male albino rats. *Die Nahrung* 33: 935–40.

Halestrap, A.P., Meredith, D. (2004). The SLC16 gene family – from monocarboxylate transporters (MCTs) to aromatic amino acid transporters and beyond. *Pflug Archiv Eur J Physiol.* 444: 619–28.

Hall, H., Fahlman, M.M., Engels, H.J. (2007). Echinacea purpurea and mucosal immunity. *Int J Sport Med* 28: 792–7.

Hall, W.L., Millward, D.J., Long, S.J., Morgan, L.M. (2003). Casein and whey exert different effects on plasma amino acid profiles, gastrointestinal hormone secretion and appetite. *Br J Nutr* 89: 239–48.

Halliday, T., Peterson, N., Thomas, J., Kleppinger, K., Hollis, B., Larson-Meyer, D. (2011). Vitamin D status relative to diet, lifestyle, injury and illness in college athletes. *Med Sci Sports Exerc* 42: 335–43.

Halliwell, B., Gutteridge, J. (2007). *Free Radicals in Biology and Medicine*. Oxford Press: Oxford.

Halsey, L.G., Stroud, M.A. (2012). 100 years since Scott reached the pole: a century of learning about the physiological demands of Antarctica. *Physiol Rev* 92: 521–36.

Hamilton, B., Grantham, J., Racinais, S., Chalabi, H. (2010). Vitamin D deficiency is endemic in Middle Eastern sportsmen. *Public Health Nutr* 13: 1528–34.

Hamilton, E.J., Berg, H.M., Easton, C.J., *et al.* (2006). The effect of taurine depletion on the contractile properties and fatigue in fast-twitch skeletal muscle of the mouse. *Amino Acids* 31: 273–8.

Hampson, N., Pollock, N., Piantandosi, C. (2003). Oxygenated water and athletic performance. *JAMA* 290: 2408–9.

Hamza, R.T., Hamed, A.I., Sallam, M.T. (2012). Effect of zinc supplementation on growth hormone insulin growth factor axis in short Egyptian children with zinc deficiency. *Ital J Pediatr* 38: 21.

Hao, Q., Lu, Z., Dong, B.R., Huang, C.Q., Wu, T. (2011). Probiotics for preventing acute upper respiratory tract infections. *Cochrane Database Syst Rev* 9: CD006895.

Harma, M., Laitinen, J., Partinen, M., *et al.* (1994). The effect of four-day round trips over 10 time zones on the circadian variation of salivary melatonin and cortisol in air-time flight attendants. *Ergonomics* 37: 1479–89.

Harmsen, E., de Tombe, P.P., de Jong, J., Achterberg, P.W. (1984). Enhanced ATP and GTP synthesis from hypoxanthine or inosine after myocardial ischaemia. *Am J Physiol* 246: H37–43.

Harpaz, M., Otto, R.M., Smith, T.K. (1985). The effect of N' N'-dimethylglycine ingestion upon aerobic performance. *Med Sci Sports Exerc* 17: 287.

Harris, R.C., Jones, G., Hill, C.H., Kendrick, I.P., Boobis, L., Kim, C.K., Kim, H.J., Dang, V.H., Edge, J., Wise, J.A. (2007). The carnosine content of V Lateralis in vegetarians and omnivores. *FASEB J.* 21: 769.20.

Harris, R.C., Jones, G.A., Kim, H.J., Kim, C.K., Price, K.A., Wise, J.A. (2009). Changes in muscle carnosine of subjects with 4 weeks supplementation with a controlled release formulation of beta-alanine (Carnosyn™), and for 6 weeks post. *FASEB J* 23: 599.4.

Harris, R.C., Söderlund, K., Hultman, E. (1992). Elevation of creatine in resting and exercised muscle of normal subjects by creatine supplementation. *Clin Sci* 83: 367–74.

Harris, R.C., Tallon, M.J., Dunnett, M., Boobis, L.H., Coakley, J., Kim, H.J., Fallowfield, J.L., Chester, C.A., Sale, C., Wise, J.A. (2006). The absorption of orally supplied β-alanine and its effect on muscle carnosine synthesis in human vastus lateralis. *Amino Acids* 30: 279–89.

Hartman, J.W., Tang, J.E., Wilkinson, S.B., *et al.* (2007). Consumption of fat-free fluid milk after resistance exercise promotes greater lean mass accretion than does consumption of soy or carbohydrate in young, novice, male weightlifters. *Am J Clin Nutr* 86: 373–81.

Hasani-Ranjbar, S., Nayebi, N., Larijani, B., *et al.* (2009). A systematic review of the efficacy and safety of herbal medicines used in the treatment of obesity. *World J Gastroenterol* 15: 3073–85.

Hashim, S.A., van Itallie, T.B. (2014). Ketone body therapy: from ketogenic diet to oral administration of ketone ester. *J Lipid Res*: R046599.

Hashimoto, A., Nishikawa, T., Hayashi, T., Fujii, N., Harada, K., *et al.* (1992). The presence of free D-serine in rat brain. *FEBS Lett* 296: 33–6.

Hathcock, J.N., Shao, A. (2006). Risk assessment for carnitine. *Regul Toxicol Pharmacol* 46: 23–8.

Hau, A.K., Kwan, T.H., Li, P.K. (2009). Melamine toxicity and the kidney. *J Am Soc Nephrol* 20: 245–50.

Haub, M.D., Potteiger, J.A., Nau, K.L., Webster, M.J., Zebas, C.J. (1998). Acute L-glutamine ingestion does not improve maximal effort exercise. *J Sports Med Phys Fitness* 38: 240–4.

Hawley, J.A., Brouns, F., Jeukendrup, A. (1998). Strategies to enhance fat utilisation during exercise. *Sports Med* 25: 241–57.

Hawley, J.A., Dennis, S.C., Lindsay, F.H., *et al.* (1995). Nutritional practices of athletes: are they sub-optimal? *J Sport Sci* 13: S75–S87.

Hawley, J.A., Morton, J.P. (2014). Ramping up the signal: promoting endurance training adaptation in skeletal muscle by nutritional manipulation. *Clin Exp Pharmacol Physiol* 41: 608–13.

Haywood, B.A., Black, K.E., Baker, D., *et al.* (2014). Probiotic supplementation reduces the duration and incidence of infections but not severity in elite rugby union players. *J Sci Med Sport* 17: 356–60.

He, C.S., Handzlik, M., Fraser, W.D., Muhamad, A., Preston, H., Richardson, A., *et al.* (2013). Influence of vitamin D status on respiratory infection incidence and immune function during 4 months of winter training in endurance sport athletes. *Exerc Immunol Rev* 19: 86–101.

Heaney, R.P. (2011). Assessing vitamin D status. *Curr Opin Clin Nutr Metab Care* 14: 440–4.

Heaney, R.P., Dowell, M.S. (1994). Absorbability of the calcium in a high calcium mineral water. *Osteoporosis Int* 4: 232–4.

Heaney, R.P., McCarron, D.A., Dawson-Hughes, B., Oparil, S., Berga, S.L., Stern, J.S., Barr, S.I., Rosen, C.J. (1999). Dietary changes favorably affect bone remodeling in older adults. *J Am Diet Assoc* 99: 1228–33.

Heaney, R.P., Recker, R.R., Grote, J., Horst, R.L., Armas, L.A. (2011). Vitamin D(3) is more potent than vitamin D(2) in humans. *J Clin Endocrinol Metab* 96: E447–E452.

Heaney, S., O'Connor, H., Gifford, J., Naughton, G. (2010). Comparison of strategies for assessing nutrition adequacy in elite female athletes' dietary intake. *Int J Sport Nutr Exerc Metab* 20: 245–56.

Heck, C.I., de Mejia, E.G. (2007). Yerba Mate Tea (Ilex paraguariensis): a comprehensive review on chemistry, health implications, and technological considerations. *J Food Sci* 72: R138–R151.

Hedner, T., Edgar, B., Edvinsson, L., Hedner, J., Persson, B., Pettersson, A. (1992). Yohimbine pharmacokinetics and interaction with the sympathetic nervous system in normal volunteers. *Eur J Clin Pharmacol* 43: 651–6.

Heikkinen, A., Alaranta, A., Helenius, I., *et al.* (2011). Use of dietary supplements in Olympic athletes is decreasing: a follow-up study between 2002 and 2009. *J Int Soc Sports Nutr* 8: 1.

Helle, C., Bjerkan, K. (2011). [Vitamin D status blant norske toppidrettsutøvere-OG Faktorer AV Betydning for vitamin D-status.] *Idrettsmedisinsk Høstkongress*: 38.

Heller, J.E., Thomas, J.J., Hollis, B.W., Larson-Meyer, D.E. (2014). Relation between vitamin D status and body composition in collegiate athletes. *Int J Sport Nutr Exerc Metab* [Epub ahead of print].

Hellsten, Y., Nielsen, J., Lykkesfeldt, J., *et al.* (2007). Antioxidant supplementation enhances the exercise-induced increase in mitochondrial uncoupling protein 3 and endothelial nitric oxide synthase mRNA content in human skeletal muscle. *Free Radic Biol Med* 43: 353–61.

Hellsten, Y., Skadhauge, L., Bangsbo, J. (2004). Effect of ribose supplementation on resynthesis of adenine nucleotides after intense intermittent training in humans. *Am J Physiol Regul Integr Comp Physiol* 286: R182–8.

Hemila, H. (2011). Zinc lozenges may shorten the duration of colds: a systematic review. *Open Resp Med J* 5: 51–8.

Henderson, L., Gregory, J., Irving, K., Swan, G. (2003). *The National Diet & Nutrition Survey: Adults aged 19 to 64 years, energy, protein, carbohydrate, fat and alcohol intake.* London: TSO.

Henderson, S., Magu, B., Rasmussen, C., *et al.* (2005). Effects of coleus forskohlii supplementation on body composition and hematological profiles in mildly overweight women. *J Int Soc Sports Nutr* 2: 54–62.

Herbert, V. (1979). Pangamic acid ('vitamin B15'). *Am J Clin Nutr* 32: 1534–40.

Herda, T.J., Ryan, E.D., Stout, J.R., Cramer, J.T. (2008). Effects of a supplement designed to increase ATP levels on muscle strength, power output and endurance. *J Int Soc Sports Nutr* 5: 3.

Herrmann, M., Obeid, R., Scharhag, J. (2005). Altered vitamin B-12 status in recreational endurance athletes. *Int J Sport Nutr Exerc Metab* 15: 433–41.

Hew-Butler, T., Almond, C., Ayus, J.C., *et al.* (2005). Consensus statement of the 1st International Exercise-Associated Hyponatremia Consensus Development Conference, Cape Town, South Africa 2005. *Clin J Sport Med* 15: 208–13.

Hickner, R.C., Tanner, C.J., Evans, C.A., *et al.* (2006). L-citrulline reduces time to exhaustion and insulin response to a graded exercise test. *Med Sci Sports Exerc* 38: 660–6.

Higgins, J.P., Tuttle, T.D., Higgins, C.L. (2010). Energy beverages: content and safety. *Mayo Clin Proc* 85: 1033–41.

Hill, C.A., Harris, R.C., Kim, H.J., Harris, B.D., Sale, C., Boobis, L.H., Kim, C.K., Wise, J.A. (2007). Influence of β-alanine supplementation on skeletal muscle carnosine concentrations and high intensity cycling capacity. *Amino Acids* 32: 225–33.

Hinton, P.S., Giordano, C., Brownlie, T., *et al.* (2000). Iron supplementation improves endurance after training in iron-depleted, nonanemic women. *J Appl Physiol* 88: 1103–11.

Hiscock, N., Petersen, E., Krzywkowski, K., Boza, J., Halkjaer-Kristensen, J., Pedersen, B.K. (2003). Glutamine supplementation further enhances exercise-induced plasma IL-6. *J Appl Physiol* 95: 145–8

Hixt, U., Müller, H.J. (1996). A glutamine dipeptide for parenteral nutrition. *Environ Health Perspect* 2: 72–6.

Hobson, R., Harris, R., Martin, D., Smith, P., Macklin, B., Gualano, B., Sale, C. (2013). Effect of beta-alanine with and without sodium bicarbonate on 2,000-m rowing performance. *Int J Sport Nutr Exerc Metab* 23: 480–7.

Hobson, R.M., Saunders, B., Ball, G., Harris, R.C., Sale, C. (2012). Effects of beta-alanine supplementation on exercise performance: a meta-analysis. *Amino Acids* 43: 25–37.

Hoch, A.Z., Lynch, S.L., Jurva, J.W., *et al.* (2010). Folic acid supplementation improves vascular function in amenorrheic runners. *Clin J Sport Med* 20: 205–10.

Hoch, A.Z., Pajewski, N.M., Hoffmann R.G., *et al.* (2009b). Possible relationship of folic acid supplementation and improved flow-mediated dilation in premenopausal, eumenorrheic athletic women. *Am J Sports Med* 8: 123–9.

Hoch, A.Z., Papanek, P., Havlik H.S., *et al.* (2009a). Prevalence of the female athlete triad/tetrad in professional ballet dancers. *Med Sci Sports Exerc* 41: 524.

Hodgson, A.B., Baskerville, R., Burke, L.M., Stear, S.J., Castell, L.M. (2013a). BJSM reviews: A–Z of nutritional supplements: dietary supplements, sports nutrition foods and ergogenic aids for health and performance Part 42: Valine, Vanadium and Water(oxygenated). *Br J Sports Med* 47: 247–8.

Hodgson, A.B., Randell, R.K., Jeukendrup, A.E. (2013b). The metabolic and performance effects of caffeine compared to coffee during endurance exercise. *PLoS One* 8: e59561.

Hoffman, J.R., Ratamess, N.A., Kang, J., Rashti, S.L., Kelly, N., Gonzalez, A.M., Stec, M., Anderson, S., Bailey, B.L., Yamamoto, L.M., Hom, L.L., Kupchak, B.R., Faigenbaum, A.D., Maresh, C.M. (2010). Examination of the efficacy of acute L-alanyl-L-glutamine ingestion during hydration stress in endurance exercise. *J Int Soc Sports Nutr* 7: 1–12.

Hoffman, P.R., Reeves, M.A. (2009). The human selenoproteome: recent insights into functions and regulation. *Cellular Molec Life Sci* 66: 2457–78.

Holick, M.F. (2007). Vitamin D deficiency. *New Engl J Med* 357: 266–81.

Holick, M.F., Binkley, N.C., Bischoff-Ferrari, H.A., Gordon, C.M., Hanley, D.A., Heaney, R.P., *et al.* (2011). Evaluation, treatment, and prevention of vitamin D deficiency: an endocrine society clinical practice guideline. *J Clin Endocrinol Metab* 96: 1911–30.

Hollis, B.W. (2005). Circulating 25-hydroxyvitamin D levels indicative of vitamin D sufficiency: implications for establishing a new effective dietary intake recommendation for vitamin D. *J Nutr* 135: 317–22.

Hollmann, W. (1998). Efficacy and safety of hydrolytic enzymes and rutin in patients with distortions of the ankle joint. Clinical study report MU-694411, Idv-Datenanalyse und Versuchsplanung Gauting.

Holloszy, J.O., Coyle, E.F. (1984). Adaptations of skeletal muscle to endurance exercise and their metabolic consequences. *J Appl Physiol* 56: 831–8.

Holmay, M.J., Terpstra, M., Coles, L.D., Mishra, U., Ahlskog, M., Oz, G., Cloyd, J.C., Tuite, P.J. (2013). N-Acetylcysteine boosts brain and blood glutathione in Gaucher and Parkinson diseases. *Clin Neuropharmacol* 36: 103–6.

Hoon, M.W., Hopkins, W.G., Jones, A.M., Martin, D.T., Halson, S.L., West, N.P., Johnson, N.A., Burke, L.M. (2014a). Nitrate supplementation and high-intensity performance in competitive cyclists. *Appl Physiol Nutr Metab* 39: 1043–9.

Hoon, M.W., Johnson, N.A., Chapman, P.G., Burke, L.M. (2013). The effect of nitrate supplementation on exercise performance in healthy individuals: a systematic review and meta-analysis. *Int J Sport Nutr Exerc Metab* 23: 522–32.

Hoon, M.W., Jones, A.M., Johnson, N.A., Blackwell, J.R., Broad, E.M., Lundy, B., Rice, A.J., Burke, L.M. (2014b). The effect of variable doses of inorganic nitrate-rich beetroot juice on simulated 2,000-m rowing performance in trained athletes. *Int J Sport Physiol Perform* 9: 615–20.

Hooper, L., Kroon, P.A., Rimm, E.B., *et al.* (2008). Flavonoids, flavonoid-rich foods, and cardiovascular risk: a meta-analysis of randomized controlled trials. *Am J Clin Nutr* 88: 38–50.

Hopkins, W.G., Hawley, J.A., Burke, L.M. (1991). Design and analysis of research on sport performance enhancement. *Med Sci Sports Exerc* 31: 472–85.

Hopkins, W.G., Marshall, S.W., Batterham, A.M., Hanin, J. (2009). Progressive statistics for studies in sports medicine and exercise science. *Med Sci Sports Exerc* 41: 3–13.

Hoseini, S.M., Khosravi-Darani, K., Mozafari, M.R. (2013). Nutritional and medical applications of spirulina microalgae. *Mini Rev Med Chem* 13: 1231–7.

Hossein-Nezhad, A., Holick, M.F. (2013). Vitamin D for health: a global perspective. *Mayo Clin Proc* 88: 720–55.

Houtkooper, L., Manore, M., Senchina, D., Stear, S.J., Burke, L.M., Castell, L.M. (2010). BJSM reviews: A–Z of nutritional supplements: dietary supplements, sports nutrition foods and ergogenic aids for health and performance Part 7: calcium and bone health, Vitamin D, and Chinese herbs. *Br J Sports Med* 44: 389–91.

Howarth, K.R., Phillips, S.M., MacDonald, M.J., Richards, D., Moreau, N.A., Gibala, M.J. (2010). Effect of glycogen availability on human skeletal muscle protein turnover during exercise and recovery. *J Appl Physiol* 109: 431–8.

Huffman, D.M., Altena, T.S., Mawhinney, T.P., Thomas, T.R. (2004). Effect of n-3 fatty acids on free tryptophan and exercise fatigue. *Eur J Appl Physiol* 92: 584–91.

Hurst, R.D., Wells, R.W., Hurst, S.M., *et al.* (2010). Blueberry fruit polyphenolics suppress oxidative stress-induced skeletal muscle cell damage in vitro. *Mol Nutr Food Res* 54: 353–63.

Huxtable, R.J. (1992). Physiological actions of taurine. *Physiol Rev* 72: 101–63.

Hwang, J.C., Khine, K.T., Lee, J.C., *et al.* (2013). Methyl-sulfonyl-methane (MSM)-induced acute angle closure. *J Glaucoma* 2013 [EPub].

Ichihara, A., Noda, C., Ogawa, K. (1973). Control of leucine metabolism with special reference to branched-chain amino acid transaminase isozymes. *Adv Enzyme Regul* 11: 155–66.

IOM Institute of Medicine: Food and Nutrition Board (1998). *Dietary Reference Intakes: Thiamin, Riboflavin, Niacin, Vitamin B-6, Folate, Vitamin B-12, Pantothenic Acid, Biotin, and Choline.* Washington, DC: National Academy Press, 196–305.

IOM Institute of Medicine: Food and Nutrition Board (2011). *Dietary Reference Intakes for Calcium and Vitamin D.* Washington, DC: National Academy Press.

Irwin, C., Desbrow, B., Ellis, A., O'Keeffe, B., Grant, G., Leveritt, M. (2011). Caffeine withdrawal and high-intensity endurance cycling performance. *J Sports Sci* 29: 509–15.

Ivy, J.L. (1998). Effect of puruvate and dihydroxyacetone on metabolism and aerobic endurance capacity. *Med Sci Sports Exerc* 30: 837–43.

Ivy, J.L., Kammer, L., Ding, Z., et al. (2009). Improved cycling time-trial performance after ingestion of a caffeine energy drink. *Int J Sport Nutr Exerc Metab* 19: 61–78.

Iwamoto, J., Takeda, T., Uenishi, K., Ishida, H., Sato, Y., Matsumoto, H. (2010). Urinary levels of cross-linked N-terminal telopeptide of type I collagen and nutritional status in Japanese professional baseball players. *J Bone Miner Metab* 28: 540–6.

Jacobs, P.L., Goldstein, E.R. (2010). Long-term glycine propionyl-l-carnitine supplemention and paradoxical effects on repeated anaerobic sprint performance. *J Int Soc Sports Nutr* 7: 35.

Jäger, R., Purpura, M., Kingsley, M. (2007). Phospholipids and sports performance. *J Int Soc Sports Nutr* 4: 5.

Jain, S., Yadav, H., Sinha, P.R., Marotta, F. (2009). Modulation of cytokine gene expression in spleen and Peyer's patches by feeding dahi containing probiotic Lactobacillus casei in mice. *J Dig Dis* 10: 49–54.

James, J.E., Rogers, P.J. (2005). Effects of caffeine on performance and mood: withdrawal reversal is the most plausible explanation. *Psychopharmacology* 182: 1–8.

Javierre, C., Segura, R., Ventura, J.L. et al. (2010). L-tryptophan supplementation can decrease fatigue perception during an aerobic exercise with supramaximal intercalated anaerobic bouts in young healthy men. *Int J Neurosci* 120: 319–27.

Jeacocke, N., Ekblom, B., Shing, C., Calder, P.C., Lewis, N., Stear, S.J., Burke, L.M., Castell, L.M. (2010). BJSM reviews: A–Z of nutritional supplements: dietary supplements, sports nutrition foods and ergogenic aids for health and performance Part 10: Citrulline, Coenzyme Q10, Colostrum, Conjugated linoleic acid, Copper. *Br J Sports Med* 44: 688–90.

Jeejeebhoy, K.N., Chu, R.C., Marliss, E.B., Greenberg, G.R., Bruce-Robertson, A. (1977). Chromium deficiency, glucose intolerance, and neuropathy reversed by chromium supplementation, in a patient receiving long-term total parenteral nutrition. *Am J Clin Nutr* 30: 531–8.

Jenkinson, D.M., Harbert, A.J. (2008). Supplements and sports. *Am Fam Physician* 78: 1039–46.

Jentjens, R.L., Jeukendrup, A.E. (2005). High rates of exogenous carbohydrate oxidation from a mixture of glucose and fructose ingested during prolonged cycling exercise. *Br J Nutr* 93: 485–92.

Jentjens, R.L., Moseley, L., Waring, R.H., et al. (2004) Oxidation of combined ingestion of glucose and fructose during exercise. *J Appl Physiol* 96: 1277–84.

Jeukendrup, A. (2004). Carbohydrate intake during exercise and performance. *Nutr* 20: 669–77.

Jeukendrup, A. (2008). Carbohydrate feeding during exercise. *Eur J Sport Sci* 8: 77–86.

Jeukendrup, A.E. (2010). Carbohydrate and exercise performance: the role of multiple transportable carbohydrates. *Curr Opin Clin Nutr Metab Care* 13: 452–7.

Jeukendrup, A.E. (2011). Nutrition for endurance sports: marathon, triathlon, and road cycling. *J Sports Sci* 29: S91–9.

Jeukendrup, A. (2013). The new carbohydrate intake recommendations. *Nestlé Nutrition Institute Workshop Series* 75: 63–71.

Jeukendrup, A. (2014). A step towards personalized sports nutrition: carbohydrate intake during exercise. *Sports Med* 44: 25–33.

Jeukendrup, A.E., McLaughlin, J. (2011). Carbohydrate ingestion during exercise: effects on performance, training adaptations and trainability of the gut. In: Maughan, R.J., Burke, L.M. (eds) *Sports Nutrition: More Than Just Calories – Triggers for Adaptation.* Nestlé Nutrition Institute Workshop Series 69: 1–17.

Jeukendrup, A.E., Moseley, L. (2010). Multiple transportable carbohydrates enhance gastric emptying and fluid delivery. *Scand J Med Sci Sports* 20: 112–21.

Jeukendrup, A.E., Saris, W.H.M., Schrauwen, P., Brouns, F., Wagenmakers, A.J.M. (1995). Metabolic availability of medium-chain triglycerides coingested with carbohydrates during prolonged exercise. *J Appl Physiol* 79: 756–62.

Jezova, D., Duncko, R., Lassanova, M., *et al.* (2002). Reduction of rise in blood pressure and cortisol release during stress by Ginkgo biloba extract (EGb 761) in healthy volunteers. *J Physiol Pharmacol* 53: 337–48.

Ji, L.L. (2008). Modulation of skeletal muscle antioxidant defense by exercise: role of redox signaling. *Free Radic Biol Med* 44: 142–52.

Johnson, R., Walton J.L., Krebs, H.A., Williamson, D.H. (1969). Metabolic fuels during and after severe exercise in athletes and non-athletes. *Lancet* 294: 452–5.

Joksimovic, N., Spasovski, G., Joksimovic, V., *et al.* (2012). Efficacy and tolerability of hyaluronic acid, tea tree oil and methyl-sulfonyl-methane in a new gel medical device for treatment of haemorrhoids in a double-blind, placebo-controlled clinical trial. *Updates Surg* 64: 195–201.

Jones, A.W., Cameron, S.J., Thatcher, R., Beecroft, M.S., Mur, L.A., Davison, G. (2013). Effects of bovine colostrum supplementation on upper respiratory illness in active males. *Brain Behav Immun* 39: 194–203.

Jones, A.M., Haramizu, S., Ranchordas, M.K., Burke, L.M., Stear, S.J., Castell, L.M. (2011). BJSM reviews: A–Z of nutritional supplements: dietary supplements, sports nutrition foods and ergogenic aids for health and performance Part 27: Nitrates, Nootkatone, Octacosanol and Policosanol. *Br J Sports Med* 45: 1246–8.

Jorissen, B.L., Brouns, F., Van Boxtel, M.P., Riedel, W.J. (2002). Safety of soy-derived phosphatidylserine in elderly people. *Nutr Neurosci* 5: 337–43.

Joubert, L.M., Manore, M.M. (2008). The role of physical activity level and B-vitamin status on blood homocysteine levels. *Med Sci Sports Exerc* 40: 1923–31.

Jówko, E., Sacharuk, J., Balasinska, B., *et al.* (2012). Effect of a single dose of green tea polyphenols on the blood markers of exercise-induced oxidative stress in soccer players. *Int J Sport Nutr Exerc Metab* 22: 486–96.

Juan, M.E., Vinardell, M.P., Planas, J.M. (2002) The daily oral administration of high doses of trans-resveratrol to rats for 28 days is not harmful. *J Nutr* 132: 257–60.

Juhn, M. (2003). Popular sports supplements and ergogenic aids. *Sports Med* 33: 921–39.

Jung, J., Hermanns-Clausen, M., Weinmann, W. (2006). Anorectic sibutramine detected in a Chinese herbal drug for weight loss. *Forensic Sci Int* 161: 221–2.

Kakigi, R., Yoshihara, T., Ozaki, H., Ogura, Y., Ichinoseki-Sekine, N., Kobayashi, H., Naito, H. (2014). Whey protein intake after resistance exercise activates mTOR signaling in a dose-dependent manner in human skeletal muscle. *Eur J Appl Physiol* 114: 735–42.

Kalafati, M., Jamurtas, A.Z., Nikolaidis, M.G., *et al.* (2010). Ergogenic and antioxidant effects of spirulina supplementation in humans. *Med Sci Sports Exerc* 42: 142–51.

Kale, A., Gawande, S., Kotwal, S., *et al.* (2010). Studies on the effects of oral administration of nutrient mixture, quercetin and red onions on the bioavailability of epigallocatechin gallate from green tea extract. *Phytother Res* 24: S48–55.

Kamakura, M. (2011). Royalactin induces queen differentiation in honeybees. *Nature* 473: 478–83.

Kang, M.-J., Kim, J.-I., Yoon, S.-Y., Kim, J.C., Cha, I.-J. (2006). Pinitol from soybeans reduces postprandial blood glucose in patients with type 2 diabetes mellitus. *J Med Food* 9: 182–6.

Karelis, A.D., Smith, J.W., Passe, D.H., Péronnet, F. (2010). Carbohydrate administration and exercise performance: what are the potential mechanisms involved? *Sports Med* 40: 747–63.

Karlsson, H.K.R., Nilsson, P.-A., Nilsson, J., Chibalin, A.V., Zierath, J.R., Blomstrand, E. (2004). Branched-chain amino acids increase p70^{S6k}phosphorylation in human skeletal muscle after resistance exercise. *Am J Physiol Endocrinol Metab* 287: E1–E7.

Karow, J.H., Abt, H.P., Fröhling, M., Ackermann, H. (2008). Efficacy of Arnica montana D4 for healing of wounds after Hallux valgus surgery compared to diclofenac. *J Altern Complement Med* 14: 17–25.

Karsch-Völk, M., Barrett, B., Kiefer, D., *et al.* (2014). Echinacea for preventing and treating the common cold. *Cochrane Database Syst Rev* 2: CD000530.

Kashiwaya, Y., King, M.T., Veech, R.L. (1997). Substrate signalling by insulin: a ketone bodies ratio mimics insulin action in heart. *Am J Cardiol* 80: 50A–64A.

Kaswala, D.H., Shah, S., Patel, N., Raisoni, S., *et al.* (2014). Hydroxycut-induced liver toxicity. *Ann Med Health Sci Res* 4: 143–5.

Katayama, M., Aoki, M., Kawana, S. (2008). Case of anaphylaxis caused by ingestion of royal jelly. *J Dermatol* 35: 222–4.

Kato, S., Karino, K., Hasegawa, J., *et al.* (1995). Octasanol affects lipid metabolism in rats fed on a high fat diet. *Br J Nutr* 73: 433.

Katz, A., Hernandez, A., Caballero, D.M., Briceno, J.F., Amezquita, L.V., Kosterina, N., Bruton, J.D., Westerblad, H. (2014). Effects of N-acetylcysteine on isolated mouse skeletal muscle: contractile properties, temperature dependence, and metabolism. *Pflugers Arch* 466: 577–85.

Katz, M.H. (2013). How can we know if supplements are safe if we do not know what is in them? Comment on the frequency and characteristics of dietary supplement recalls in the United States. *JAMA Intern Med* 173: 928.

Kekkonen, R.A., Vasankari, T.J., Vuorimaa, T., *et al.* (2007). The effect of probiotics on respiratory infections and gastrointestinal symptoms during training in marathon runners. *Int J Sport Nutr Exerc Metab* 17: 352–83.

Kendrick, I.P., Kim, H.J., Harris, R.C., Kim, C.K., Dang, V.H., Bui, T.T., Wise, J.A. (2009). The effect of 4 weeks β-alanine supplementation and isokinetic training on carnosine concentrations in type I and II human skeletal muscle fibres. *Eur J Appl Physiol* 106: 131–8.

Kendrick, I.P., Kim, H.J., Harris, R.C., Kim, C.K., Dang, V.H., Lam, T.Q., Bui, T.T., Smith, M., Wise, J.A. (2008). The effects of 10 weeks of resistance training combined with β-alanine supplementation on whole body strength, force production, muscular endurance and body composition. *Amino Acids* 34: 547–54.

Kennedy, D.O., Wightman, E.L., Ready, J.L., Lietz, G., Okello, E.J., Wilde, A., Haskell, C.F. (2010). Effects of resveratrol on cerebral blood flow variables and cognitive performance in humans: a double-blind, placebo-controlled, crossover investigation. *Am J Clin Nutr* 91: 1590–7.

Kerkhoffs, G.M.M.J., Struijs, P.A.A., de Wit, C., *et al.* (2004). A double blind, randomised, parallel group study on the efficacy and safety of treating acute lateral ankle sprain with oral hydrolytic enzymes. *Br J Sports Med* 38: 431–5.

Kerksick, C., Rasmussen, C., Bowden, R., Leutholtz, B., Harvey, T., *et al.* (2005). Effects of ribose supplementation prior to and during intense exercise on anaerobic capacity and metabolic markers. *Int J Sport Nutr Exerc Metab* 15: 653–64.

Kerksick, C.M., Wilborn, C.D., Campbell, W.I., Harvey, T.M., Marcello, B.M., Roberts, M.D., *et al.* (2009). The effects of creatine monohydrate supplementation with and without D-pinitol on resistance training adaptations. *J Strength Cond Res* 23: 2673–82.

Kern, M., Lagomarcino, N.D., Misell, L.M., Schuster, V. (2000). The effect of medium-chain triacylglycerols on the blood lipid profile of male endurance runners. *J Nutr Biochem* 11: 288–92.

Khaled, S., Brun, J.F., Cassanas, G., *et al.* (1999). Effects of zinc supplementation on blood rheology during exercise. *Clin Hemorheol Microcirc* 20: 1–10.

Khaled, S., Brun, J.F., Micallel, J.P., *et al.* (1997). Serum zinc and blood rheology in sportsmen (football players). *Clin Hemorheol Microcirc* 17: 47–58.

Kidd, P.M. (2009). Bioavailability and activity of phytosome complexes from botanical polyphenols: the silymarin, curcumin, green tea, and grape seed extracts. *Altern Med Rev J Clin Ther* 14: 226–46.

Kilic, M. (2007). Effect of fatiguing bicycle exercise on thyroid hormone and testosterone levels in sedentary males supplemented with oral zinc. *Neuro Endocrinol Lett* 28: 681–5.

Kilic, M., Baltaci, A.K., Gunay, M., *et al.* (2006). The effect of exhaustion exercise on thyroid hormones and testosterone levels of elite athletes receiving oral zinc. *Neuro Endocrinol Lett* 27: 247–52.

Kim, J., Chun, Y.-S., Kang, S.-K., *et al.* (2010). The use of herbal/traditional products supplementation and doping tests in elite athletes. *Int J Appl Sports Sci* 22: 137–49.

Kim, J.-I., Kim, J.C., Kang, M.-J., Lee, M.-S., Kim, J.-J., Cha, I.-J. (2004). Effects of pinitol isolated from soybeans on glycaemic control and cardiovascular risk factors in Korean patients with type II diabetes mellitus: a randomized controlled study. *Eur J Clin Nutr* 59: 456–8.

Kim, L.S., Axelrod, L.J., Howard, P., *et al.* (2006). Efficacy of methylsulfonylmethane (MSM) in osteoarthritis pain of the knee: a pilot clinical trial. *Osteoarthritis Cartilage* 14: 286–94.

Kimball, S.R., Jefferson, L.S. (2001). Regulation of protein synthesis by branched-chain amino acids. *Curr Opin Clin Nutr Metabolic Care* 4: 39–43.

Kimball, S.R., Jefferson, L.S. (2010). Control of translation initiation through integration of signals generated by hormones, nutrients, and exercise. *J Biol Chem* 285: 29027–32.

King, D.S., Baskerville, R., Hellsten, Y., Senchina, D.S., Burke, L.M., Stear, S.J., Castell, L.M. (2012). BJSM reviews: A–Z of nutritional supplements: dietary supplements, sports nutrition foods and ergogenic aids for health and performance Part 34: Prohormones, Ribose, Royal Jelly and Similax. *Br J Sports Med* 46: 689–90.

King, D.S., Sharp, R.L., Vukovich, M.D., Brown, G.A., Reifenrath, T.A., Uhl, N.L., Parsons, K.A. (1999). Effect of oral androstenedione on serum testosterone and adaptations to resistance training in young men. *JAMA* 281: 2020–8.

Kingsley, M. (2006). Effects of phosphatidylserine supplementation on exercising humans. *Sports Med* 36: 657–69.

Klingshirn, L.A., Pate, R.R., Bourque, S.P., *et al.* (1992). Effect of iron supplementation on endurance capacity in iron-depleted female runners. *Med Sci Sport Exerc* 24: 819–24.

Koehler, K., Geyer, H., Guddat, S., *et al.* (2007). Sibutramine found in Chinese herbal slimming tea and capsules. In: *Recent Advances in Doping Analysis* (15), Schänzer, W., Geyer, H., Gotzmann, A., Mareck, U. (eds). Sportverlag Strauß: Köln, 367–70.

Koehler, K., Parr, M.K., Geyer, H., *et al.* (2009). Serum testosterone and urinary excretion of steroid hormone metabolites after administration of a high-dose zinc supplement. *Eur J Clin Nutr* 63: 65–70.

Koehler, K., Thevis, M., Schaenzer, W. (2013). Meta-analysis: effects of glycerol administration on plasma volume, haemoglobin, and haematocrit. *Drug Test Anal* 5: 896–9.

Kohler, M., Thomas, A., Geyer, H., *et al.* (2010). Confiscated black market products and nutritional supplements with non-approved ingredients analyzed in the Cologne doping control laboratory 2009. *Drug Test Anal* 2: 533–7.

Kok, L., Kreijkamp-Kaspers, S., Grobbee, D.E., *et al.* (2005). Soy isoflavones, body composition, and physical performance. *Maturitas* 52: 102–10.

Konig, D., Weinstock, C., Keul, J., *et al.* (1998). Zinc, iron, and magnesium status in athletes – influence on the regulation of exercise-induced stress and immune function. *Exerc Immunol Rev* 4: 2–21.

Koopman, R., Verdijk, L., Manders, R.J., Gijsen, A.P., Gorselink, M., Pijpers, E., Wagenmakers, A.J., van Loon, L.J. (2006). Co-ingestion of protein and leucine stimulates muscle protein synthesis rates to the same extent in young and elderly lean men. *Am J Clin Nutr* 84: 623–32.

Kopp-Hoolihan, L. (2001). Prophylactic and therapeutic uses of probiotics: a review. *J Am Dietetic Assoc* 101: 229–38.

Kornau, H.C. (2006). GABA$_B$ receptors and synaptic modulation. *Cell Tissue Res* 326: 517–33.

Koury, J.C., De Oliveira, A. E.S., Portella, E.S., De Oliveira, C.F., Lopes, G.C. and Donangelo, C.M. (2004) Zinc and copper biochemical indices of antioxidant status in elite athletes of different modalities. *International Journal of Sports Nutrition and Exercise Metabolism.* 14: 358–372.

Kovacs, E.M.R., Stegen, J.H.C.H., Brouns, F. (1998). Effect of caffeinated drinks on substrate metabolism, caffeine excretion, and performance. *J Appl Physiol* 85: 709–15.

Kraemer, W.J., Gordon, S.E., Lynch, J.M., *et al.* (1995). Effects of multi-buffer supplementation on acid-base balance and 2,3-diphosphoglycerate following repetitive anaerobic exercise. *Int J Sport Nutr* 5: 300–14.

Kräuchi, K., Cajochen, C., Pache, M., Flammer, J., Wirz-Justice, A. (2006). Thermoregulatory effects of melatonin in relation to sleepiness. *Chronobiol. Int* 23: 475–84.

Krause, M., Keane, K., Rodrigues-Krause, J., Crognale, D., Egan, B., De Vito, G., Murphy, C., Newsholme, P. (2014a). Elevated levels of extracellular heat-shock protein 72 (eHSP72) are positively correlated with insulin resistance in vivo and cause pancreatic beta-cell dysfunction and death in vitro. *Clin Sci* (Lond) 126: 739–52.

Krause, M., Rodrigues-Krause, J., O'Hagan, C., De Vito, G., Boreham, C., Susta, D., Newsholme, P., Murphy, C. (2012). Differential nitric oxide levels in the blood and skeletal muscle of type 2 diabetic subjects may be consequence of adiposity: a preliminary study. *Metab* 61: 1528–37.

Krause, M., Rodrigues-Krause, J., O'Hagan, C., Medlow, P., Davison, G., Susta, D., Boreham, C., Newsholme, P., O'Donnell, M., *et al.* (2014b). The effects of aerobic exercise training at two different intensities in obesity and type 2 diabetes: implications for oxidative stress, low-grade inflammation and nitric oxide production. *Eur J Appl Physiol* 114: 251–60.

Krause, M.S., de Bittencourt, P.I., Jr. (2008). Type 1 diabetes: can exercise impair the autoimmune event? The L-arginine/glutamine coupling hypothesis. *Cell Biochem Funct* 26: 406–33.

Krause, M.S., Oliveira, L.P., Jr., Silveira, E.M., Vianna, D.R., Rossato, J.S., Almeida, B.S., Rodrigues, M.F., Fernandes, A.J., Costa, J.A., *et al.* (2007). MRP1/GS-X pump ATPase expression: is this the explanation for the cytoprotection of the heart against oxidative stress-induced redox imbalance in comparison to skeletal muscle cells? *Cell Biochem Funct* 25: 23–32.

Kreider, R.B. (1999). Dietary supplements and the promotion of muscle growth with resistance exercise. *Sports Med* 27: 97–110.

Kreider, R.B., Ferreira, M.P., Greenwood, M., Wilson, M., Almada, A.L. (2002). Effects of conjugated linoleic acid supplementation during resistance training on body composition, bone density, strength, and selected hematological markers. *J Strength Cond Res* 16: 325–34.

Kreider, R.B., Melton, C., Greenwood, M., Rasmussen, C., Lundberg, J., *et al.* (2003). Effects of oral D-ribose supplementation on anaerobic capacity and selected metabolic markers in healthy males. *Int J Sport Nutr Exerc Metab* 13: 76–86.

Kreider, R.B., Miller, G.W., Schenck, D., *et al.* (1992). Effects of phosphate loading on metabolic and myocardial responses to maximal and endurance exercise. *Int J Sport Nutr* 2: 20–47.

Kreider, R.B., Miller, G.W., Williams, M.H., *et al.* (1990). Effects of phosphate loading on oxygen uptake, ventilatory anaerobic threshold, and run performance. *Med Sci Sports Exerc* 22: 250–6.

Kreider, R.B., Wilborn, C.D., Taylor, L., *et al.* (2010). ISSN exercise & sport nutrition review: research & recommendations. *J Int Soc Sports Nutr* 7: 7.

Krzywkowski, K., Petersen, E.W., Ostrowski, K., Kristensen, J.H., Boza, J., Pedersen, B.K. (2001) Effect of glutamine supplementation on exercise-induced changes in lymphocyte function. *Am J Physiol Cell Physiol* 281: C1259–65.

Kuipers, H., van Breda, E., Verlaan, G., Smeets, R. (2002). Effects of oral bovine colostrum supplementation on serum insulin-like growth factor-I levels. *Nutr* 18: 566–7.

Kumar, N. and Low, P.A. (2004) Myeloneuropathy and anemia due to copper malabsorption. *Journal of Neurology.* 251: 747–749.

Laaksi, I., Ruohola, J.P., Tuohimaa, P., Auvinen, A., Haataja, R., Pihlajamaki, H., *et al.* (2007). An association of serum vitamin D concentrations < 40 nmol/L with acute respiratory tract infection in young Finnish men. *Am J Clin Nutr* 86: 714–17.

Lagouge, M., Argmann, C., Gerhart-Hines, Z., Meziane, H., Lerin, C., Daussin, F., *et al.* (2006). Resveratrol improves mitochondrial function and protects against metabolic disease by activating SIRT1 and PGC-1alpha. *Cell* 127: 1109–22.

Lambert, E.V., Goedecke, J.H., Bluett, K., Heggie, K., Claassen, A., Rae, D.E., West, S., Dugas, J., Dugas, L., Meltzeri, S., Charlton, K., Mohede, I. (2007). Conjugated linoleic acid versus high-oleic acid sunflower oil: effects on energy metabolism, glucose tolerance, blood lipids, appetite and body composition in regularly exercising individuals. *Br J Nutr* 97: 1001–11.

Lambert, M., Hefer, J., Millar, R., Macfarlane, P. (1993). Failure of commercial oral amino acid supplements to increase serum growth hormone concentrations in male body-builders. *Int J Sport Nutr Exerc Metab* 3: 298–305.

Lamprecht, M., Hofmanan, P., Greilberger, J.F., Schwaberger, G. (2009). Increased lipid peroxidation in trained men after 2 weeks of antioxidant supplementation. *Int J Sport Nut Exerc Metab* 19: 385–99.

Lancha Jr., A.H., Recco, M.B., Abdalla, D.S.P., Curi, R. (1995). Effect of aspartate, asparagine, and carnitine supplementation in the diet on metabolism of skeletal muscle during moderate exercise. *Physiol Behav* 57: 367–71.

Lane, S.C., Hawley, J.A., Desbrow, B., Jones, A.M., Blackwell, J.R., Ross, M.L., Zemski, A.J., Burke, L.M. (2014). Single and combined effects of beetroot juice and caffeine supplementation on cycling time trial performance. *Appl Physiol Nutr Metab* 39: 1050–7.

Lang, C.H., Pruznak, A., Navaratnarajah, M., Rankine, K.A., Deiter, G., Magne, H., Offord, E.A., Breuillé, D. (2013). Chronic α-hydroxy-isocaproic acid treatment improves muscle recovery after immobilization-induced atrophy. *Am J Physiol Endocrinol Metab* 305: E416–E428.

Lange, K.H., Larsson, B., Flyvbjerg, A., *et al.* (2002). Acute growth hormone administration causes exaggerated increases in plasma lactate and glycerol during moderate to high intensity bicycling in trained young men. *J Clin Endocrinol Metab* 87: 4966–75.

Lanham-New, S.A., Stear, S.J., Shirreffs S.M., Collins A.L. (eds) (2011). *The Nutrition Society Textbook Series: Sport and Exercise Nutrition*. Chichester: Wiley-Blackwell.

Lansley, K.E., Winyard, P.G., Bailey, S.J., Vanhatalo, A., Wilkerson, D.P., Blackwell, J.R., Gilchrist, M., Benjamin, N., Jones, A.M. (2011b). Acute dietary nitrate supplementation improves cycling time trial performance. *Med Sci Sports Exerc* 43: 1125–31.

Lansley, K.E., Winyard, P.G., Fulford, J., Vanhatalo, A., Bailey, S.J., Blackwell, J.R., DiMenna, F.J., Gilchrist, M., Benjamin, N., Jones, A.M. (2011a). Dietary nitrate supplementation reduces the O$_2$ cost of walking and running: a placebo-controlled study. *J Appl Physiol* 110: 591–600.

Lappe, J., Cullen, D., Haynatzki, G., Recker, R., Ahlf, R., Thompson, K. (2008). Calcium and vitamin D supplementation decreases incidence of stress fractures in female navy recruits. *J Bone Miner Res* 23: 741–9.

Larsen, F.J., Schiffer, T.A., Borniquel, S., Sahlin, K., Ekblom, B., Lundberg, J.O., Weitzberg, E. (2011). Dietary inorganic nitrate improves mitochondrial efficiency in humans. *Cell Metab* 13: 149–59.

Larsen, F.J., Weitzberg, E., Lundberg, J.O., Ekblom, B. (2007). Effects of dietary nitrate on oxygen cost during exercise. *Acta Physiol (Oxf)* 191: 59–66.

Larson-Meyer, D.E., Burke, L.M., Stear, S.J., Castell, L.M. (2013). BJSM reviews: A–Z of nutritional supplements: dietary supplements, sports nutrition foods and ergogenic aids for health and performance Part 40: Vitamin D. *Br J Sports Med* 47: 118–20.

Larson-Meyer, D.E., Willis, K.S. (2010). Vitamin D and athletes. *Curr Sports Med Rep* 9: 220–6.

Laughlin, M.R., Taylor, J., Chesnick, A.S., Balaban, R.S. (1994). Nonglucose substrates increase glycogen synthesis in vivo in dog heart. *Am J Physiol* 267: H217–H223.

Laupheimer, M.W., Perry, M., Benton, S., Malliaras, P., Maffulli, N.(2014). Resveratrol exerts no effect on inflammatory response and delayed onset muscle soreness after a marathon in male athletes: a randomised, double-blind, placebo-controlled pilot feasibility study. *Transl Med UniSa* 10: 38–42.

Laupheimer, M.W., Perry, M., Malliaris, P., *et al.* (2013). Resveratrol: a review of basic science and potential indications in sports and exercise medicine. *J Sport Health Res* 5(3): 237–50.

Leadbetter, G., Keyes, L.E., Maakestad, K.M., *et al.* (2009). Ginkgo biloba does – and does not – prevent acute mountain sickness. *Wilderness Environ Med* 20: 66–71.

Leder, B.Z., Catlin, D.H., Longcope, C., Ahrens, B., Schoenfeld, D.A., Finkelstein, J.S. (2001). Metabolism of orally administered androstenedione in young men. *J Clin Endocrinol Metab* 86: 3654–8.

Leder, B.Z., Leblanc, K.M, Longcope, C., Lee, H., Catlin, D.H., Finkelstein, J.S. (2002). Effects of oral androstenedione administration on serum testosterone and estradiol levels in postmenopausal women. *J Clin Endocrinol Metab* 87: 5449–54.

Leder, B.Z., Longcope, C., Catlin, D.H., Ahrens, B., Schoenfeld, D.A., Finkelstein, J.S. (2000). Oral androstenedione administration and serum testosterone concentrations in young men. *JAMA* 283: 779–82.

Leenhardt, F., Fardet, A., Lyan, B., Gueux, E., Rock, E., Mazur, A., Chanliaud, E., Demigné, C., Rémésy, C. (2008). Wheat germ supplementation of a low vitamin E diet in rats affords effective antioxidant protection in tissues. *J Am Coll Nutr* 27: 222–8.

Lehtonen-Veromaa, M., Mottonen, T., Irjala, K., Karkkainen, M., Lamberg-Allardt, C., Hakola, P., et al. (1999). Vitamin D intake is low and hypovitaminosis D common in healthy 9- to 15-year-old Finnish girls. *Eur J Clin Nutr* 53: 746–51.

Lehtoranta, L., Pitkäranta, A., Korpela, R. (2014). Probiotics in respiratory virus infections. *Eur J Clin Microbiol Infect Dis* 33: 1289–302.

Leibetseder, V., Strauss-Blasche, G., Marktl, W., Ekmekcioglu, C. (2006). Does oxygenated water support aerobic performance and lactate kinetics? *Int J Sport Med* 27: 232–5.

Leitzmann, M.F., Stampfer, M.J., Wu, K., et al. (2003). Zinc supplement use and risk of prostate cancer. *J Natl Cancer Institute* 95: 1004–7.

Lemon, P.W., Berardi, J.M., Noreen, E.E. (2002). The role of protein and amino acid supplements in the athlete's diet: does type or timing of ingestion matter? *Curr Sports Med Reports* 1: 214–21.

Lemon, P.W., Nagle, F.J. (1981). Effects of exercise on protein and amino acid metabolism. *Med Sci Sports Exerc* 13: 141–9.

Lenn, J., Uhl, T., Mattacola, C., Boissonneault, G., Yates, J., Ibrahim, W., Bruckner, G. (2002). The effects of fish oil and isoflavones on delayed onset muscle soreness. *Med Sci Sports Exerc* 34: 1605–13.

Leu, S., Havey, J., White, L.E., Martin, N., Yoo, S.S., Rademaker, A.W., Alam, M. (2010). Accelerated resolution of laser-induced bruising with topical 20% arnica: a rater-blinded randomized controlled trial. *Br J Dermatol* 163: 557–63.

Levenhagen, D.K., Carr, C., Carlson, M.G., Maron, D.J., Borel, M.J., Flakoll, P.J. (2002). Postexercise protein intake enhances whole-body and leg protein accretion in humans. *Med Sci Sports Exerc* 34: 828–37.

Levenson, D.I., Brockman, R.S. (1994) A review of calcium preparations. *Nutr Rev* 52: 221–32.

Lewis, N., Keil, M., Ranchordas, M.K., Burke, L.M., Stear, S.J., Castell, L.M. (2012). BJSM reviews: A–Z of nutritional supplements: dietary supplements, sports nutrition foods and ergogenic aids for health and performance Part 35: Selenium, Serine and Sibutramine. *Br J Sports Med* 46: 767–8.

Lewis, N.A., Moore, P. and Cunningham, P. (2010) Serum copper and neutropenia in elite athletes. Abstract accepted at ACSM 2010.

Lewis, R.M., Redzic, M., Thomas, D.T. (2013). The effects of season-long vitamin D supplementation on collegiate swimmers and divers. *Int J Sport Nutr Exerc Metab* 23: 431–40.

Li, J.S., Chen, M., Li, Z.C. (2012). Identification and quantification of dimethylamylamine in geranium by liquid chromatography tandem mass spectrometry. *Anal Chem Insights* 7: 47–58.

Li, P., Yin, Y.L., Li, D., Kim, S.W., Wu, G. (2007). Amino acids and immune function. *Br J Nutr* 98: 237–52.

Lieber, L., Friden, J. (2002). Morphologic and mechanical basis of delayed-onset muscle soreness. *J Am Acad Orthop Surg* 10: 67–73.

Lieberman, H.R., Corkin, S., Spring, B.J., Growdon, J.H., Wurtman, R.J. (1983). Mood, performance, and pain sensitivity: changes induced by food constituents. *J Psychiatr Res* 17: 135–45.

Lila, M.A. (2007). From beans to berries and beyond: teamwork between plant chemicals for protection of optimal human health. *Ann N Y Acad Sci* 1114: 372–80.

Lin, S.-P., Li, C.-Y., Suzuki, K., et al. (2014). Green tea consumption after intense taekwondo training enhances salivary defense factors and antibacterial capacity. *PloS One* 9: e87580.

Lindh, A.M., Peyrebrune, M.C., Ingham, S.A., Bailey, D.M., Folland, J.P. (2007). Sodium bicarbonate improves swimming performance. *Int J Sport Med* 29: 519–23.

Lippiello, L. (2003). Glucosamine and chondroitin sulfate: biological response modifiers of chondrocytes under simulated conditions of joint stress. *Osteoarthritis Cartilage* 11: 335–42.

Lisi, A., Hasick, N., Kazlauskas, R., et al. (2011). Studies of new stimulants. Lecture held at 29th Cologne Workshop on Dope Analysis, Cologne.

Little, J.P., Forbes, S.C., Candow, D.G., et al. (2008). Creatine, arginine α-ketoglutarate, amino acids, and medium-chain triglycerides and endurance performance. *Int J Sport Nutr Exerc Met* 18: 493–508.

Liu, T.H., Wu, C.L., Chiang, C.W., et al. (2009). No effect of short-term arginine supplementation on nitric oxide production, metabolism and performance in intermittent exercise in athletes. *J Nutr Biochem* 20: 462–8.

Liu, Y., Lange, R., Langanky, J., Hamma, T., Yang, B., Steinacker, J.M. (2012). Improved training tolerance by supplementation with α-Keto acids in untrained young adults: a randomized, double blind, placebo-controlled trial. *J Int Soc Sports Nutr* 9: 37.

Lobb, A. (2009). Hepatoxicity associated with weight-loss supplements: a case for better post-marketing surveillance. *World J Gastroenterol* 15: 1786–7.

Lobb, A. (2010). Science of weight loss supplements: compromised by conflicts of interest? *World J Gastroenterol* 16: 4880–2.

Lobb, A. (2012). Science in liquid dietary supplement promotion: the misleading case of mangosteen juice. *Hawaii J Med Pub Health* 71: 46–8.

Lobb, A., Ellison, M., Burke, L.M., Stear, S.J., Castell, L.M. (2011). BJSM reviews: A–Z of nutritional supplements: dietary supplements, sports nutrition foods and ergogenic aids for health and performance Part 19: Glycerol, Guarana and Hydroxycut. *Br J Sports Med* 45: 456–8.

Louard, R.J., Barrett, E.J., Gelfand, R.A. (1995). Overnight branched-chain amino acid infusion causes sustained suppression of muscle proteolysis. *Metabolism* 44: 424–9.

Louis, M., Poortmans, J.R., Francaux, M., et al. (2003). No effect of creatine supplementation on human myofibrillar and sarcoplasmic protein synthesis after resistance exercise. *Am J Physiol Endocrinol Metab* 285: E1089–94.

Lu, H.-K., Hsieh, C.-C., Hsu, J.-J., et al. (2006). Preventative effects of spirulina plantensis on skeletal muscle damage under exercise-induced oxidative stress. *Eur J Appl Physiol* 98: 220–6.

Lüdtke, R., Hacke, D. (2005). Zur Wirksamkeit des homöopathischen Arzneimittels Arnica montana. *Wien Med Wochenschr* 155: 482–90.

Lukaski, H.C. (1989). Effects of exercise training on human copper and zinc nutriture. *Adv Exper Med Biol* 258: 163–70.

Lukaski, H.C. (2004). Vitamin and mineral status: effects on physical performance. *Nutr Burbank Los Angel Cty Calif* 20: 632–44.

Lukaski, H.C., Bolonchuk, W.W., Siders, W.A., Milne, D.B. (1996). Chromium supplementation and resistance training: effects on body composition, strength, and trace element status of men. *Am J Clin Nutr* 63: 954–65.

Lukaski, H.C., Nielsen, F.H. (2002). Dietary magnesium depletion affects metabolic responses during submaximal exercise in postmenopausal women. *J Nutr* 132: 930–5.

Lundberg, J.O., Govoni, M. (2004). Inorganic nitrate is a possible source for systemic generation of nitric oxide. *Free Radic Biol Med* 37: 395–400.

Lundy, B., Miller, J.C., Jackson, K., Senchina, D.S., Burke, L.M., Stear, S.J., Castell, L.M. (2011). BJSM reviews: A–Z of nutritional supplements: dietary supplements, sports nutrition foods and ergogenic aids for health and performance Part 25: Melamine, Melatonin and Methylsulphonylmethane. *Br J Sports Med* 45: 1077–8.

Lunn, W.R., Pasiakos, S.M., Colletto, M.R., *et al.* (2012). Chocolate milk and endurance exercise recovery: protein balance, glycogen, and performance. *Med Sci Sports Exerc* 44: 682–91.

Luo, H., Kashiwagi, A., Shibahara, T., *et al.* (2007). Decreased bodyweight without rebound and regulated lipoprotein metabolism by gymnemate in genetic multifactor syndrome animal. *Mol Cell Biochem* 299: 93–8.

Luo, Q., Li, Z., Yan, J., *et al.* (2009). Lycium barbarum polysaccharides induce apoptosis in human prostate cancer cells and inhibits prostate cancer growth in a xenograft mouse model of human prostate cancer. *J Med Food* 12: 695–703.

Lyall, K.A., Hurst, S.M., Cooney, J., *et al.* (2009). Short-term blackcurrant extract consumption modulates exercise-induced oxidative stress and lipopolysaccharide-stimulated inflammatory responses. *Am J Physiol Regul Integr Comp Physiol* 297: R70–81.

MacAnulty, S.R., Nieman, D.C., Fox-Rabnovich, M., *et al.* (2010). Effect of n-3 fatty acids and antioxidants on oxidative stress after exercise. *Med Sci Sports Exerc* 42: 1704–11.

Macfarlane, G.T., Macfarlane, S. (2011). Fermentation in the human large intestine: its physiologic consequences and the potential contribution of prebiotics. *J Clin Gastroenterol* 45 Suppl: S120–7.

MacLean, D.A., Graham, T.E., Saltin, B. (1994). Branched-chain amino acids augment ammonia metabolism while attenuating protein breakdown during exercise. *Am J Physiol* 267: E1010–E1022.

MacRae, H.S., Mefford, K.M. (2006). Dietary antioxidant supplementation combined with quercetin improves cycling time trial performance. *Int J Sport Nutr Exerc Metab* 16: 405–19.

Maemura, H., Goto, K., Yoshioka, T., Sato, M., Takahata, Y., Morimatsu, F., Takamatsu, K. (2006). Effects of carnosine and anserine supplementation on relatively high intensity endurance. *Int J Sport Health Sci* 4: 86–94.

Maganaris, C.N., Collins, D., Sharp, M. (2000). Expectancy effects and strength training: do steroids make a difference? *Sport Psychologist* 14: 272–8.

Maggini, S., Beveridge, S., Suter, M. (2012). A combination of high-dose vitamin C plus zinc for the common cold. *J Int Med Res* 40: 28–42.

Magkos, F., Kavouras, S.A. (2004). Caffeine and ephedrine: physiological, metabolic and performance-enhancing effects. *Sports Med Auckl NZ* 34: 871–89.

Magnuson, B.A., Burdock, G.A., Doull, J., Kroes, R.M., Marsh, G.M., Pariza, M.W., Spencer, P.S., Waddell, W.J., Walker, R., Williams, G.M. (2007). Aspartame: a safety evaluation based on current use levels, regulations, and toxicological and epidemiological studies. *Crit Rev Toxicol* 37: 629–727.

Maimoona, A., Naeem, I., Saddiqe, Z., *et al.* (2011). A review on the biological, nutraceutical and clinical aspects of French maritime pine bark extract. *J Ethnopharmacol* 133: 261–77.

Maizels, E.Z., Ruderman, N.B., Goodman, M.N., Lau, D. (1977). Effect of acetoacetate on glucose metabolism in the soleus and extensor digitorum longus muscles of the rat. *Biochem J* 162: 557–68.

Malatesta, F., Antonini, G., Sarti, P., Brunori, M. (1995). Structure and function of molecular machine: cytochrome C oxidase. *Biophys Chem* 54: 1–33.

Malm, C., Svensson, M., Ekblom, B., *et al*. (1997). Effect of ubiquinone-10 supplementation and high intensity training on physical performance in humans. *Acta Physiol Scand* 61: 379–84.

Malm, C., Svensson, M., Sjöberg, B., *et al*. (1996). Supplementation with ubiquinone-10 causes cellular damage during intense exercise. *Acta Physiol Scand* 157: 511–12.

Mamerow, M.M., Mettler, J.A., English, K.L., Casperson, S.L., Arentson-Lantz, E., Sheffield-Moore, M., Layman, D.K., Paddon-Jones, D. (2014). Dietary protein distribution positively influences 24-h muscle protein synthesis in healthy adults. *J Nutr* 144: 876–80.

Manach, C., Scalbert, A., Morand, C., Rémésy, C., Jiménez, L. (2004). Polyphenols: food sources and bioavailability. *Am J Clin Nutr* 79: 727–47.

Manna, S., Das, S., Chatterjee, M., Janarthan, M., Chatterjee, M. (2011). Combined supplementation of vanadium and fish oil suppresses tumor growth, cell proliferation and induces apoptosis in DMBA-induced rat mammary carcinogenesis. *J Cell Biochem* 112: 2327–39.

Mannion, A.F., Jakeman, P.M., Dunnett, M., Harris, R.C., Willan, P.L.T. (1992). Carnosine and anserine concentrations in the quadriceps femoris muscle of healthy humans. *Eur J Appl Physiol* 64: 47–50.

Mannix, E.T., Stager, J.M., Harris, A., *et al*. (1990). Oxygen delivery and cardiac output during exercise following oral phosphate-glucose. *Med Sci Sports Exerc* 22: 341–7.

Manore, M.M. (1994). Vitamin B-6 and exercise. *Int J Sport Nutr Exerc Met* 4: 89–103.

Manore, M.M. (2000). Effect of physical activity on thiamine, riboflavin, and vitamin B-6 requirements. *Am J Clinc Nutr* 72: 598S–606S.

Manore, M.M. (2012). Dietary supplements for improving body composition and reducing body weight: where is the evidence? *Int J Sport Nutr Exerc Metab* 22: 139–54.

Manore, M., Meeusen, R., Roelands, B., Moran, S., Popple, A.D., Naylor, M.J, Burke, L.M., Stear, S.J., Castell, L.M. (2011). BJSM reviews: A–Z of nutritional supplements: dietary supplements, sports nutrition foods and ergogenic aids for health and performance Part 16: Folate, γ-Aminobutyric Acid, Gamma-Oryzanol and Ferulic Acid, γ-Hydroxybutyrate and γ-Butyrolactone. *Br J Sports Med* 45: 73–4.

Mansfield, L.E., Goldstein, G.B. (1981). Anaphylactic reaction after ingestion of local bee pollen. *Ann Allergy* 47: 154–6.

Mansour, M.M., Hafiez, A.A., el-Kirdassy, Z.H., *et al*. (1989). Role of zinc in regulating the testicular function. Part 2. Effect of dietary zinc deficiency on gonadotropins, prolactin and testosterone levels as well as 3 beta-hydroxysteroid dehydrogenase activity in testes of male albino rats. *Die Nahrung* 33: 941–7.

Mao, X., Zeng, X., Huang, Z., Wang, J., Qiao, S. (2013). Leptin and leucine synergistically regulate protein metabolism in c2c12 myotubes and mouse skeletal muscles. *Br J Nutr* 110: 256–64.

Marchbank, T., Davison, G., Oakes, J.R., Ghatei, M.A., Patterson, M., Moyer, M.P., Playford, R.J. (2011). The nutriceutical bovine colostrum truncates the increase in gut permeability caused by heavy exercise in athletes. *Am J Physiol Gastrointest Liver Physiol* 300: G477–84.

Maresh, C.M., Armstrong, L.E., Hoffman, J.R., Hannon, D.R., Gabaree, C.L., Bergeron, M.F., Whittlesey, M.J., Deschenes, M.R. (1994). Dietary supplementation and improved anaerobic performance. *Int J Sport Nutr* 4: 387–97.

Margaritis, I., Rosseau, A.S., Hinger, I., *et al*. (2003). Antioxidant supplementation and tapering exercise improve exercise-induced antioxidant response. *J Am Coll Nutr* 22: 147–56.

Margaritis, I., Rosseau, A.S., Hinger, I., Palazzeti, S., Arnaud, J. and Roussel, A.M. (2005). Increase in selenium requirements with physical activity loads in well-trained athletes is not linear. *Biofactors* 23: 45–55.

Margaritis, I., Tessier, F., Prou, E., Marconnet, P., Marini, J.F. (1997). Effects of endurance training on skeletal muscle oxidative capacities with and without selenium supplementation. *J Trace Elements Med Biol* 11: 37–43.

Markus, A., Morris, B.J. (2008). Resveratrol in prevention and treatment of common clinical conditions of aging. *Clin Interven Aging* 2: 331–9.

Marquezi, M.L., Roschel, H.A., Santos-Costa, A., Sawada, L.A., Lancha Jr., A.H. (2003). Effect of aspartate and asparagine supplementation on fatigue determinants in intense exercise. *Int J Sport Nutr Exerc Metab* 13: 65–75.

Marranzino, G., Villena, J., Salva, S., Alvarez, S. (2012). Stimulation of macrophages by immunobiotic *Lactobacillus* strains: influence beyond the intestinal tract. *Microbiol Immunol* 56: 771–81.

Martin, B.J., Tan, R.B., Gillen, J.B., *et al.* (2014). No effect of short-term green tea extract supplementation on metabolism at rest or during exercise in the fed state. *Int J Sport Nutr Exerc Metab* 24: 656–64.

Martineau, M., Parpura, V., Mothet, J.P. (2014). Cell-type specific mechanisms of D-serine uptake and release in the brain. *Front Synaptic Neurosci* 6: 12.

Martinez, S., Pasquerelli , M.N., Romaguera, D., *et al.* (2011). Anthropometric characteristics and nutritional profile of young amateur swimmers. *J Stength Cond Res:* 25: 1126–33.

Martinovic, J., Dopsaj, V., Kotur-Stevuljevic, J., *et al.* (2011). Oxidative stress biomarker monitoring in elite women volleyball athletes during a 6-week training period. *J Strength Conditioning Res* 25: 1360–7.

Marwood, S., Bowtell, J. (2008). No effect of glutamine supplementation and hyperoxia on oxidative metabolism and performance during high-intensity exercise. *J Sports Sci* 26: 1081–90.

Mashhadi, N.S., Ghiasvand, R., Askari, G., *et al.* (2013). Influence of ginger and cinnamon intake on inflammation and muscle soreness endured by exercise in Iranian female athletes. *Int J Prev Med* 4: S11–15.

Maslova, L.V., Kondrat'ev, B., Maslov, L.N., *et al.* (1994). The cardioprotective and antiadrenergic activity of an extract of Rhodiola rosea in stress. *Eksp Klin Farmakol* 57: 61–3.

Mathes, A. (2010). Hepatoprotective actions of melatonin: possible mediation by melatonin receptors. *World J Gastroenterol* 16: 6087–97.

Matsuzaki, T. (1998). Immunomodulation by treatment with *Lactobacillus casei* strain Shirota. *Int J Food Microbiol* 41: 133–40.

Matsuzaki, Y., Miyazaki, T., Miyakawa, S., *et al.* (2002). Decreased taurine concentration in skeletal muscle after exercise of various durations. *Med Sci Sports Exerc* 34: 793–7.

Matter, M., Stittfall, T., Graves, K., *et al.* (1987). The effect of iron and folate therapy on maximal exercise performance in female marathon runers with iron and folate deficiency. *Clin Sci* 72: 415–22.

Mattes, R.D., Popkin, B.M. (2009). Nonnutritive sweetener consumption in humans: effects on appetite and food intake and their putative mechanisms. *Am J Clin Nutr* 89: 1–14.

Matuszczak, Y., Farid, M., Jones, J., Lansdowne, S., Smith, M.A., Taylor, A.A., Reid, M.B. (2005). Effects of Nacetylcysteine on glutathione oxidation and fatigue during handgrip exercise. *Muscle Nerve* 32: 633–8.

Maughan, R.J. (2005). Contamination of dietary supplements and positive drug tests in sport. *J Sports Sci* 23: 883–9.

Maughan, R.J., Burke, L.M., Stear, S.J., Castell, L.M. (2010). BJSM reviews: A–Z of nutritional supplements: dietary supplements, sports nutrition foods and ergogenic aids for health and performance Part 8: Carbohydrate. *Br J Sports Med* 44: 468–70.

Maughan, R.J., Depiesse, F., Geyer, H. (2007). The use of dietary supplements by athletes. *J Sports Sci* 25: S103–13.

Maughan, R.J., Evans, S.P. (1982) Effects of pollen extract upon adolescent swimmers. *Br J Sports Med* 16: 142–5.

Maughan, R.J., Gleeson, M. (2010). *The biochemical basis of sports performance*, 2nd edition. Chapter 4. Oxford: Oxford University Press.

Maughan, R.J., Greenhaff, P.L., Hespel, P. (2011). Dietary supplements for athletes: emerging trends and recurring themes. *J Sports Sci* 29(Suppl 1): S57–66.

Maughan, R.J., Owen, J.H., Shirreffs, S.M., Leiper, J.B. (1994). Post exercise rehydration in man: effects of electrolyte addition to ingested fluids. *Eur J Appl Physiol* 69: 209–15.

McAlindon, T.E., Bannuru, R.R., Sullivan, M.C., Arden, N.K., Berenbaum, F., BiermA–Zeinstra, S.M., *et al.* (2014). OARSI guidelines for the non-surgical management of knee osteoarthritis. *Osteoarthritis and Cartilage* 22: 363–88.

McAnulty, S.R., McAnulty, L.S., Nieman, D.C., *et al.* (2004). Consumption of blueberry polyphenols reduces exercise-induced oxidative stress compared to vitamin C. *Nutr Res* 24: 209–21.

McCarthy, C.G., Canale, R.E., Alleman, R.J., *et al.* (2012). Biochemical and anthropometric effects of a weight loss dietary supplement in healthy men and women. *Nutr Metabolic Insights* 5: 13–22.

McCarty, M.F. (2002). Policosanol safely down-regulates HMG-CoA reductase – potential as a component of the Esselstyn regimen. *Med Hypotheses* 59: 268–79.

McClung, J.P., Martini, S., Murphy, N.E., *et al.* (2013). Effects of a 7-day military training exercise on inflammatory biomarkers, serum hepcidin, and iron status. *Nutr J* 12: 141.

McCrorie, T.A., Keaveney, E.M., Wallace, J.M., Binns, N., Livingstone, M.B. (2011). Human health effects of conjugated linoleic acid from milk and supplements. *Nutr Res Rev* 24: 206–27.

McGinley, C., Shafat, A., Donnelly, A.E. (2009). Does antioxidant vitamin supplementation protect against muscle damage. *Sports Med* 39: 1101–32.

McKenna, M.J. (1992). The role of ionic processes in muscular fatigue during intensive exercise. *Med Sci Sports Exerc* 13: 134–45.

McLellan, T., Gannon, G., Zamecnik, J., Gil, V., Brown, G. (1999). Low doses of melatonin and diurnal effects of thermoregulation and tolerance to uncompensable heat stress. *J App Physiol* 87: 308–16.

McLellan, T.M., Lieberman, H.R. (2012). Do energy drinks contain active components other than caffeine? *Nutr Rev* 70: 730–44.

McLellan, T., Smith, I., Gannon, G., Zamecnik, J. (2000). Melatonin has no effect on tolerance to uncompensable heat stress in man. *Eur J App Physiol* 83: 336–43.

McMorris, T., Mielcarz, G., Harris, R.C., *et al.* (2007). Creatine supplementation and cognitive performance in elderly individuals. *Neuropsychol Dev Cogn B Aging Neuropsychol Cogn* 14: 517–28.

McNaughton, L., Dalton, B., Tarr, J. (1999a). Inosine supplementation has no effect on aerobic or anaerobic cycling performance. *Int J Sport Nutr* 9: 333–44.

McNaughton, L.R., Dalton, B., Palmer, G. (1999b). Sodium bicarbonate can be used as an ergogenic aid in high-intensity, competitive cycle ergometry of 1 h duration. *Eur J Appl Physiol Occup Physiol* 80: 64–9.

McNaughton, L.R., Harris, R.C., Burke, L.M., Stear, S.J., Castell, L.M. (2010). BJSM reviews: A–Z of nutritional supplements: dietary supplements, sports nutrition foods and ergogenic aids for health and performance Part 5: Buffers: Sodium Bicarbonate and Sodium Citrate; β-Alanine and Carnosine. *Br J Sports Med* 44: 77–8.

McNaughton, L.R., Kenney, S., Siegler, J., Midgley, A.W., Lovell, R.J., Bentley, D.J. (2007). The effect of superoxygenated water on blood gases, lactate, and aerobic cycling performance. *Int J Sport Physiol Perform* 2: 377–85.

McNaughton, L.R., Siegler, J., Midgley, A.W. (2008). The ergogenic effects of sodium bicarbonate, *Curr Sports Med Reports* 7: 230–6.

Meacham, S.L., Taper, L.J., Volpe, S.L. (1995). Effect of boron supplementation on blood and urinary calcium, magnesium, and phosphorous, and urinary boron in athletic and sedentary women. *Am J Clin Nutr* 61: 341–5.

Medved, I., Brown, M.J., Bjorksten, A.R. (2003). N-aceytlcysteine infusion alters blood redox status but not time to fatigue in humans. *J Appl Physiol.* 94: 1572–82.

Medved, I., Brown, M.J., Bjorksten, A.R., *et al.* (2004a). Effects of intravenous N-aceytlcysteine infusion on time to fatigue and potassium regulation during prolonged exercise. *J Appl Physiol* 96: 211–17.

Medved, M.J., Brown, A.R., Bjorksten, *et al.* (2004b). N-acetylcysteine enhances muscle cysteine and glutathione availability and attenuates fatigue during prolonged exercise in endurance-trained individuals. *J Appl Physiol* 97: 1477–85.

Meeusen, R., Watson, P., Hasegawa, H., Roelands, B., Piacentini, M.F. (2006). Central fatigue: the serotonin hypothesis and beyond. *Sports Med.* 36: 881–909.

Mekkes, M.C., Weenen, T.C., Brummer, R.J., Claassen, E. (2014). The development of probiotic treatment in obesity: a review. *Benef Microbes* 5: 19–28.

Melnik, B.C., John, S.M., Schmitz, G. (2013). Milk is not just food but most likely a genetic transfection system activating mTORC1 signaling for postnatal growth. *Nutr J* 12: 103.

Mengheri, E. (2008). Health, probiotics and inflammation. *J Clin Gastroenterol* 42: S177–8.

Mero, A., Miikkulainen, H., Riski, J., Pakkanen, R., Aalto, J., Takala, T. (1997). Effects of bovine colostrum supplementation on serum IGF-I, IgG, hormone, and saliva IgA during training. *J Appl Physiol* 83: 1144–51.

Mero, A., Ojala, T., Hulmi, J., Puurtinen, R., Karila, T., Seppälä, T. (2010). Effects of alfa-hydroxy-isocaproic acid on body composition, DOMS and performance in athletes. *J Int Soc Sports Nutr* 7: 1–8.

Meyer-Hoffert, U., Wiedow, O. (2011). Neutrophil serine proteases: mediators of innate immune responses. *Curr Opin Hematol* 18: 19–24.

Michailidis, Y., Karagounis, L.G., Terzis, G., Jamurtas, A.Z., Spengos, K., Tsoukas, D., Chatzinikolaou, A., Mandalidis, D., Stefanetti, R.J., *et al.* (2013). Thiol-based antioxidant supplementation alters human skeletal muscle signaling and attenuates its inflammatory response and recovery after intense eccentric exercise. *Am J Clin Nutr* 98: 233–45.

Mickleborough, T.D., Ionescu, A.A., Lindley, M.R., Fly, A.D. (2006). Protective effect of fish oil supplementation on exercise-induced bronchoconstriction in asthma. *Chest* 29: 39–49.

Mickleborough, T.D., Murray, R., Ionescu, A.A., Lindley, M.R. (2003). Fish oil supplementation reduces the severity of exercise-induced bronchoconstriction in elite athletes. *Am J Resp Crit Care Med* 168: 1181–9.

Miller, P.C., Bailey, S.P., Barnes, M.E., Derr, S.J., Hall, E.E. (2004). The effects of protease supplementation on skeletal muscle function and DOMS following downhill running. *J Sports Sci* 22: 365–72.

Minocha, A. (2009). Probiotics for preventive health. *Nutr Clin Prac* 24: 227–41.

Misell, L.M., Lagomarcino, N.D., Schuster, V., Kern, M. (2001). Chronic medium-chain triacylglycerol consumption and endurance performance in trained runners. *J Sports Med Phys Fitness* 41: 210–15.

Mitchell, C.J., Churchward-Venne, T.A., Parise, G., Bellamy, L., Baker, S.K., Smith, K., et al. (2014). Acute post-exercise myofibrillar protein synthesis is not correlated with resistance training-induced muscle hypertrophy in young men. *PloSOne* 9: e89431.

Mizuno, K., Tanaka, M., Nozaki, S., et al. (2008). Antifatigue effects of coenzyme Q10 during physical fatigue. *Nutrition* 24: 293–9.

Moberg, M., Apró, W., Ohlsson, I., Pontén, M., Villanueva, A., Ekblom, B., Blomstrand, E. (2014). Absence of leucine in an amino acid supplement reduces activation of mTORC1 signalling following resistance exercise in young females. *Appl Physiol Nutr Metab* 39: 183–94.

Möhler, H. (2006). GABA$_A$ receptor diversity and pharmacology. *Cell Tissue Res* 326: 505–16.

Moncada, S., Higgs, A. (1993). The L-arginine-nitric oxide pathway. *N Engl J Med* 329: 2002–12.

Monzón Ballarín, S., López-Matas, M.A., Sáenz Abad, D., et al. (2011). Anaphylaxis associated with the ingestion of Goji berries (Lycium barbarum). *J Investig Allergol Clin Immunol* 21: 567–70.

Moore, D.R., Areta, J., Coffey, V.G., Stellingwerff, T., Phillips, S.M., Burke, L.M., Cléroux, M., Godin, J.P., Hawley, J.A. (2012). Daytime pattern of post-exercise protein intake affects whole-body protein turnover in resistance-trained males. *Nutr Metab (Lond)* 9: 91.

Moore, D.R., Camera, D.M., Areta, J.L., Hawley, J.A. (2014). Beyond muscle hypertrophy: why dietary protein is important for endurance athletes. *Appl Physiol Nutr Metab* 39: 987–97.

Moore, D.R., Robinson, M.J., Fry, J.L., et al. (2009). Ingested protein dose response of muscle and albumin protein synthesis after resistance exercise in young men. *Am J Clin Nutr* 89: 161–8.

Mooren, F.C., Golf, S.W., Lechtermann, A., et al. (2005). Alterations of ionized Mg2+ in human blood after exercise. *Life Sci* 77: 1211–25.

Mooren, F.C., Krüger, K., Völker, K., et al. (2011). Oral magnesium supplementation reduces insulin resistance in non-diabetic subjects – a double-blind, placebo-controlled, randomized trial. *Diabetes Obes Metab* 13: 281–4.

Morihara, N., Nishihama, T., Ushijima, M., et al. (2007). Garlic as an anti-fatigue agent. *Mol Nutr Food* Res 51: 1329–34.

Morillas-Ruiz, J.M., Villegas García, J.A., López, F.J., et al. (2006). Effects of polyphenolic antioxidants on exercise-induced oxidative stress. *Clin Nutr* 25: 444–53.

Morillas-Ruiz, J., Zafrilla, P., Almar, M., et al. (2005). The effects of an antioxidant-supplemented beverage on exercise-induced oxidative stress: results from a placebo-controlled double-blind study in cyclists. *Eur J Appl Physiol* 95: 543–9.

Morita, H., Ikeda, T., Kajita, K., Fujioka, K., Mori, I., Okada, H., et al. (2012). Effect of royal jelly ingestion for six months on healthy volunteers. *Nutr J* 11: 77.

Morris, D.M., Beloni, R.K., Wheeler, H.E. (2013). Effects of garlic consumption on physiological variables and performance during exercise in hypoxia. *Appl Physiol Nutr Metab* 38: 363–7.

Morrison, M.A., Spriet, L.L., Dyck, D.J. (2000). Pyruvate ingestion for 7 days does not improve aerobic performance in well-trained individuals. *J Appl Physiol* 89: 549–56.

Mortenson, L., Charles, P. (1996). Bioavailability of calcium supplements and the effect of vitamin D: comparisons between milk, calcium carbonate, and calcium carbonate plus vitamin D. *Am J Clin Nutr* b63: 354–7.

Morton, A.R., Scott, C.A., Fitch, K.D. (1989). The effects of theophylline on the physical performance and work capacity of well-trained athletes. *J Allergy Clin Immunol* 83: 55–61.

Moukarzel, A.A., Goulet, O., Salas, J.S., *et al.* (1994). Growth retardation in children receiving long-term total parenteral nutrition: Effects of ornithine alpha-ketoglutarate. *Am J Clin Nutr* 60: 408–13.

Mountjoy, M., Sundgot-Borgen, J., Burke, L., Carter, S., Constantini, N., Lebrun, C., Meyer, N., Sherman, R., Steffen, K., Budgett, R., Ljungqvist, A. (2014). The IOC consensus statement: beyond the female athlete triad-relative energy deficiency in sport (RED-S). *Br J Sports Med* 48: 491–7.

Murakami, S., Kurihara, S., Koikawa, N., *et al.* (2009). Effects of oral supplementation with cystine and theanine on the immune function of athletes in endurance athletes: randomised, double blind placebo controlled trial. *Biosci Biotechnol. Biochem* 73: 817–21.

Murase, T., Haramizu, S., Ota, N., Hase, T. (2009). Suppression of the aging-associated decline in physical performance by a combination of resveratrol intake and habitual exercise in senescence-accelerated mice. *Biogerontology* 10: 423–34.

Murase, T., Haramizu, S., Shimotoyodome, A., *et al.* (2006). Green tea extract improves running endurance in mice by stimulating lipid utilization during exercise. *Am J Physiol Regul Integr Comp Physiol* 290: R1550–6.

Murase, T., Misawa, K., Haramizu, S., *et al.* (2010). Nootkatone, a characteristic constituent of grapefruit, stimulates energy metabolism and prevents diet-induced obesity by activating AMPK. *Am J Physiol Endocrinol Metab* 299: E266–E275.

Murphy, C.H., Hector, A.J., Phillips, S.M. (2014). Considerations for protein intake in managing weight loss in athletes. *Eu J Sport Sci* 11: 1–8.

Muthusami, S., Ramachandran, I., Krishnamoorthy, S., Govindan, R., Narasimhan, S. (2011). Cissus quadrangularis augments IGF system components in human osteoblast like SaOS-2 cells. *Growth Horm IGF Res* 21: 343–8.

NADA (2013). Germany. Nutritional supplements adulterated with oxilofrine. Available at: www.nada.de/fileadmin/user_upload/nada/Presse/130912_Warning_Oxilofrine. pdf. Accessed 14 September 2013.

Nagaya, N., Uematsu, M., Oya, H., *et al.* (2001). Short-term oral administration of L-arginine improves hemodynamics and exercise capacity in patients with precapillary pulmonary hypertension. *Am J Respir Crit Care Med* 163: 887–91.

Naghii, M.R. (1999). The significance of dietary boron, with particular reference to athletes. *Nutr Health* 13: 31–7.

Nagpal, R., Behare, P., Rana, R., *et al.* (2011). Bioactive peptides derived from milk proteins and their health beneficial potentials: an update. *Food Funct* 2: 18–27.

Nair, K.S., Schwartz, R.G., Welle, S. (1992). Leucine as a regulator of whole body and skeletal muscle protein metabolism in humans. *Am J Physiol Endocrinol Metab* 263: E928–E934.

Nakazato, K., Ochi, E., Waga, T. (2010). Dietary apple polyphenols have preventive effects against lengthening contraction-induced muscle injuries. *Mol Nutr Food Res* 54: 364–72.

Nakazato, K., Song, H., Waga, T. (2007). Dietary apple polyphenols enhance gastrocnemius function in Wistar rats. *Med Sci Sports Exerc* 39: 934–40.

Narasimh, A., Shetty, P.H., Nanjundaswamy, M.H., *et al.* (2013). Hydroxycut-dietary supplements for weight loss: can they induce mania? *Aust N Z J Psychiatry* 47: 1205.

National Academy of Sciences (2004). Institute of Medicine, Food and Nutrition Board. *Dietary Reference Intakes for Water, Potassium, Sodium, Chloride, and Sulfate*: 186–268.

National Academy of Sciences (2014). Thiamin, riboflavin, niacin, vitamin B6, folate, vitamin B12, pantothenic acid, biotin, and choline. http://fnic.nal.usda.gov/dietary-guidance/dri-reports/thiamin-riboflavin-niacin-vitamin-b6-folate-vitamin-b12-pantothenic. Accessed 18 February 2015.

National Academies Press (2001). *Dietary Reference Intakes for Vitamin A, Vitamin K, Arsenic, Boron, Chromium, Copper, Iodine, Iron, Manganese, Molybdenum, Nickel, Silicon, Vanadium, and Zinc*. Washington, DC: National Academies Press.

Nattiv, A., Loucks, A.B., Manore, M.M., Sanborn, C.F., Sundgot-Borgen, J., Warren, M.P. (2007). American College of Sports Medicine (ACSM) Position Stand. Female Athlete Triad. *Med Sci Sports Exerc* 39: 1867–82.

Navarro, V., Fernández-Quintela, A., Churruca, I., Portillo, M.P. (2006). The body fat-lowering effect of conjugated linoleic acid: a comparison between animal and human studies. *J Physiol Biochem* 62: 137–47.

Naziroğlu, M., Kilinç, F., Uğuz, A.C., *et al.* (2010). Oral vitamin C and E combination modulates blood lipid peroxidation and antioxidant vitamin levels in maximal exercising basketball players. *Cell Biochem Funct* 28: 300–5.

Negro, M., Giardina, S., Marzani, B., Marzatico, F. (2008). Branched-chain amino acid supplementation does not enhance athletic performance but affects muscle recovery and the immune system. *J Sports Med Phys Fitness* 48: 347–51.

Nelson, A.E., Allen, K.D., Golightly, Y.M., Goode, A.P., Jordan, J.M. (2014a). A systematic review of recommendations and guidelines for the management of osteoarthritis: the chronic osteoarthritis management initiative of the U.S. bone and joint initiative. *Semin Arthritis Rheum* 43: 701–12.

Nelson, M.T., Biltz, G.R., Dengel, D.R. (2014b). Cardiovascular and ride time-to-exhaustion effects of an energy drink. *J Int Soc Sports Nutr* 11: 2.

Neumayer, C., Fugl, A., Nanobashvili, J., *et al.* (2006). Combined enzymatic and antioxidative treatment reduces ischemia-reperfusion injury in rabbit skeletal muscle. *J Surg Res* 133: 150–8.

Newhouse, I.J., Finstad, E.W. (2000). The effects of magnesium supplementation on exercise performance. *Clin J Sport Med* 10: 195–200.

Newnham, R.E. (1994). Essentiality of boron for healthy bones and joints. *Environ Health Perspec* 102: 83–5.

Newsholme, E.A., Blomstrand, E., Ekblom, B. (1992). Physical and mental fatigue: metabolic mechanisms and importance of plasma amino acids. *Br Med Bull* 48: 477–95.

Newsholme, E.A., Leech, A.R. (2010). *Functional Biochemistry in Health and Disease*. Chichester: Wiley Blackwell.

Newsholme, P., Homem De Bittencourt, P.I., O'Hagan, C., De Vito, G., Murphy, C., Krause, M.S. (2009). Exercise and possible molecular mechanisms of protection from vascular disease and diabetes: the central role of ROS and nitric oxide. *Clin Sci (Lond)* 118: 341–9.

Newsholme, P., Krause, M., Newsholme, E.A., Burke, L.M., Stear, S.J., Castell, L.M. (2011). BJSM reviews: A–Z of nutritional supplements: dietary supplements, sports nutrition foods and ergogenic aids for health and performance Part 18: Glutamine, Glutathione and Glutamate. *Br J Sports Med* 45: 230–2.

Nguyen, D., Hsu, J.W., Jahoor, F., Sekhar, R.V. (2014). Effect of increasing glutathione with cysteine and glycine supplementation on mitochondrial fuel oxidation, insulin sensitivity, and body composition in older HIV-infected patients. *J Clin Endocrinol Metab* 99: 169–77.

NH & MRC and Ministry of Health (2006). *Nutrient Reference Values for Australia and New Zealand.* Available at: www.moh.govt.nz/publications. Accessed 29 January 2015.

Nicolaï, S.P.A., Kruidenier, L.M., Bendermacher, B.L.W., *et al.* (2013). Ginkgo biloba for intermittent claudication. *Cochrane Database Syst Rev* 6: CD006888.

Nielsen, F.H. (2008). Is boron nutritionally relevant? *Nutr Rev* 66: 183–91.

Nielsen, F.H., Hunt, C.D., Mullen, L.M., Hunt, J.R. (1987). Effect of dietary boron on mineral, estrogen, and testosterone metabolism in postmenopausal women. *FASEB J* 1: 394–7.

Nielsen, F.H., Lukaski, H.C. (2006). Update on the relationship between magnesium and exercise. *Magnes Res* 19: 180–9.

Nieman, D.C. (2008). Immunonutrition support for athletes. *Nutr Rev* 66: 310–20.

Nieman, D.C. (2010). Quercetin's bioactive effects in human athletes. *Curr Topic Nutraceut Res* 8: 33–44.

Nieman, D.C., Gillitt, N.D., Knab, A.M., *et al.* (2013). Influence of a polyphenol-enriched protein powder on exercise-induced inflammation and oxidative stress in athletes: a randomized trial using a metabolomics approach. *PLoS One* 8: e72215.

Nieman, D.C., Gillitt, N.D., Shanely, R.A., Dew, D., Meaney, M.P., Luo, B. (2014). Vitamin D2 supplementation amplifies eccentric exercise-induced muscle damage in NASCAR pit crew athletes. *Nutrients* 6: 63–75.

Nieman, D.C., Henson, D.A., Davis, J.M., *et al.* (2007b). Quercetin ingestion does not alter cytokine changes in athletes competing in the Western States Endurance Run. *J Interferon Cytokine Res* 27: 1003–11.

Nieman, D.C., Henson, D.A., Gross, S.J., *et al.* (2007a). Quercetin reduces illness but not immune perturbations after intensive exercise. *Med Sci Sports Exerc* 39: 1561–9.

Nieman, D.C., Henson, D.A., Maxwell, K.R., *et al.* (2009a). Effects of quercetin and EGCG on mitochondrial biogenesis and immunity. *Med Sci Sports Exerc* 41: 1467–5.

Nieman, D.C., Henson, D.A., McAnulty, S.R., Jin, F., Maxwell, K.R. (2009b). n-3 polyunsaturated fatty acids do not alter immune and inflammation measures in endurance athletes. *Int J Sport Nutr Exerc Metab* 19: 536–46.

Nieman, D.C., Laupheimer, M.W., Ranchordas, M.K., Burke, L.M., Stear, S.J., Castell, L.M. (2012). BJSM reviews: A–Z of nutritional supplements: dietary supplements, sports nutrition foods and ergogenic aids for health and performance Part 33: Querceitin, Resveratrol and Rhodiola rosea. *Br J Sports Med* 46: 618–20.

Nieman, D.C., Stear, S.J., Burke, L.M., Castell, L.M. (2010a). BJSM reviews: A–Z of nutritional supplements: dietary supplements, sports nutrition foods and ergogenic aids for health and performance Part 15: Flavonoids. *Br J Sports Med* 44: 1202–5.

Nieman, D.C., Williams, A.S., Shanely, R.A., *et al.* (2010b). Quercetin's influence on exercise performance and muscle mitochondrial biogenesis. *Med Sci Sports Exerc* 42: 338–45.

Nieper, A. (2005). Nutritional supplement practices in UK junior national track and field athletes. *Br J Sports Med* 39: 645–9.

NIH (2014). National Institutes of Health. Office of Dietary Supplements. *Calcium Dietary Supplements Health Professionals Fact Sheet.*

Nikolaidis, M.G., Kerksick, C.M., Lamprecht, M., *et al.* (2012). Does vitamin C and E supplementation impair the favorable adaptations of regular exercise? *Oxid Med Cell Longev* 2012: 707941.

Nishikawa, T. (2011). Analysis of free D-serine in mammals and its biological relevance. *J Chromatogr B Analyt Technol Biomed Life Sci* 879: 3169–83.

Nissen, S.L., Sharp, R.L. (2003). Effect of dietary supplements on lean mass and strength gains with resistance exercise: a meta-analysis. *J Appl Physiol* 94: 651–9.

Nissen, S., Sharp, R., Ray, M., *et al.* (1996). Effect of leucine metabolite beta-hydroxy-beta-methylbutyrate on muscle metabolism during resistance-exercise training. *J Appl Physiol* 81: 2095–104.

Nogusa, Y., Mizugaki, A., Hirabayashi-Osada, Y., Furuta, C., Ohyama, K., Suzuki, K., Kobayashi, H. (2014). Combined supplementation of carbohydrate, alanine and proline is effective in maintaining blood glucose and increasing endurance performance during long-term exercise in mice. *J Nutr Sci Vitaminol* (Tokyo) 60: 188–93.

Noreen, E.E., Buckley, J.G., Lewis, S.L., *et al.* (2013). The effects of an acute dose of Rhodiola rosea on endurance exercise performance. *J Strength Cond Res Natl Strength Cond Assoc* 27: 839–47.

Norton, L.E., Wilson, G.J., Layman, D.K., Moulton, C.J., Garlick, P.J. (2012). Leucine content of dietary proteins is a determinant of postprandial skeletal muscle protein synthesis in adult rats. *Nutr Metab (Lond)* 9: 67.

Notarnicola, A., Pesce, V., Vicenti, G., *et al.* (2012). SWAAT study: extracorporeal shock wave therapy and arginine supplementation and other nutraceuticals for insertional Achilles tendinopathy. *Adv Ther* 29: 799–814.

Nunan, D., Howatson, G., van Someren, K.A. (2010). Exercise-induced muscle damage is not attenuated by beta-hydroxy-beta-methylbutyrate and alpha-ketoisocaproic acid supplementation. *J Strength Cond Res* 24: 531–7.

Nuviala, R., Lapieza, M.G., Bernal, E. (1999) Magnesium, zinc, and copper status in women involved in different sports. *International Journal of Sports Nutrition.* 9: 295–309.

Oben, J.E., Enyegue, D.M., Fomekong, G.I., *et al.* (2007). The effect of *Cissus quadrangularis* (CQR-300) and a Cissus formulation (CORE) on obesity and obesity-induced oxidative stress. *Lipids Health Dis* 6: 4.

Oegema Jr., T.R., Deloria, L.B., Sandy, J.D., Hart, D.A. (2002). Effect of oral glucosamine on cartilage and meniscus in normal and chymopapain-injected knees of young rabbits. *Arthritis Rheum* 46: 2495–503.

Ohtani, M., Sugita, M., Maruyama, K. (2006). Amino acid mixture improves training efficiency in athletes. *J Nutr* 136: 538S–543S.

Olmedillas, H., Guerra, B., Guadalupe-Grau, A., Santana, A., Fuentes, T., Dorado, C., Serrano-Sanchez, J.A., Calbet, J.A. (2011). Training, leptin receptors and socs3 in human muscle. *Int J Sport Med* 32: 319–26.

Olmedillas, H., Sanchis-Moysi, J., Fuentes, T., Guadalupe-Grau, A., Ponce-Gonzalez, J.G., Morales-Alamo, D., Santana, A., Dorado, C., Calbet, J.A., Guerra, B. (2010). Muscle hypertrophy and increased expression of leptin receptors in the musculus triceps brachii of the dominant arm in professional tennis players. *Eur J Appl Physiol* 108: 749–58.

Om, A.S., Chung, K.W. (1996). Dietary zinc deficiency alters 5 alpha-reduction and aromatization of testosterone and androgen and estrogen receptors in rat liver. *J Nutr* 126: 842–8.

Onakpoya, I.J., Posadzki, P.P., Watson, L.K., Davies, L.A. Ernst, E. (2012). The efficacy of long-term conjugated linoleic acid (CLA) supplementation on body composition in overweight and obese individuals: a systematic review and meta-analysis of randomized clinical trials. *Eur J Nutr* 51: 127–34.

Onakpoya, I., Terry, R., Ernst, E. (2011). The use of green coffee extract as a weight loss supplement: a systematic review and meta-analysis of randomised clinical trials. *Gastroenterol Res Pract* 2011: 382852. Published online 31 August 2010. doi: 10.1155/2011/382852

Oostenbrug, G.S., Mensink, R.P., Hardeman, M.R., de Vries, T., Brouns, F., Hornstra, G. (1997). Exercise performance, red blood cell deformability, and lipid peroxidation: effects of fish oil and vitamin. *Eur J Appl Physiol* 83: 746–52.

Ostler, T., Davidson, W., Ehl, S. (2002). Virus clearance and immunopathology by CD8(+) T cells during infection with respiratory syncytial virus are mediated by IFN-gamma. *Eur J Immunol* 32: 2117–23.

Ostojic, S.M. (2006). Yohimbine: the effects on body composition and exercise performance in soccer players. *Res Sports Med* 14: 289–99.

Ostuland, R.E., Racete, S.B., Stenson, W.F. (2003). Inhibition of cholesterol absorption by phytosterol-replete wheatgerm compared with phytosterol-depleted wheat germ. *Am J Clin Nutr* 77: 1385–9.

Outlaw, J., Wilborn, C., Smith, A., Urbina, S., Hayward, S., Foster, C., Wells, S., Wildman, R., Taylor, L. (2013). Effects of ingestion of a commercially available thermogenic dietary supplement on resting energy expenditure, mood state and cardiovascular measures. *J Int Soc Sports Nutr* 10: 25.

Palacios, C. (2006). The role of nutrients in bone health, from A to Z. *Critical Rev Food Sci Nutr* 46: 621–8.

Panza, V.S., Wazlawik, E., Ricardo Schütz, G., *et al.* (2008). Consumption of green tea favorably affects oxidative stress markers in weight-trained men. *Nutr* 24: 433–42.

Papagelopoulos, P.J., Mavrogenis, A.F., Soucacos, P.N. (2004). Doping in ancient and modern Olympic Games. *Orthopedics* 27: 1226–31.

Parise, G., Mihic, S., MacLennan, D., *et al.* (2001). Effects of acute creatine monohydrate supplementation on leucine kinetics and mixed-muscle protein synthesis. *J Appl Physiol* 91: 1041–7.

Parisi, A., Quaranta, F., Masala, D., Fagnani, F., Di Salvo, V., Casasco, M., Pigozzi, F. (2007). Do aspartate and asparagine acute supplementation influence the onset of fatigue in intense exercise? *J Sports Med Phys Fitness* 47: 422–6.

Parisi, A., Tranchita, E., Duranti, G., *et al.* (2010). Effects of chronic Rhodiola rosea supplementation on sport performance and antioxidant capacity in trained male: preliminary results. *J Sports Med Phys Fitness* 50: 57–63.

Pariza, M.W., Park, Y., Cook, M.E. (2001). The biologically active isomers of conjugated linoleic acid. *Prog Lipid Res* 40: 283–98.

Parr, M.K., Koehler, K., Geyer, H., *et al.* (2008). Clenbuterol marketed as dietary supplement. *Biomed Chromatogr* 22: 298–300.

Parry-Billings, M., Budgett, R., Koutedakis, Y., Blomstrand, E., Brooks, S., Williams, C.V., Calder, P.C., Pilling, S., Baigrie, R., Newsholme, E.A. (1992). Plasma amino acid concentrations in the overtraining syndrome: possible effects on the immune system. *Med Sci Sports Exerc* 24: 1353–8.

Patel, S. (2012). Yucca: a medicinally significant genus with manifold therapeutic attributes. *Natural Prod Bioprospecting* 2: 231–4.

Paul, M.A., Miller, J.C., Gray, G.W., Love, R.J., Lieberman, H.R., Arendt, J. (2010). Melatonin treatment for eastward and westward travel preparation. *Psychopharmacology (Berl.)* 208: 377–86.

Paulsen, G., Cumming, K.T., Holden, G., Hallen, J., Ronnestad, B.R., Sveen, O., Skaug, A., Paur, I., Bastani, N.E., Ostgaard, H.N., Buer, C., Midttun, M., Freuchen, F., Wiig, H., Ulseth, E.T., Garthe, I., Blomhoff, R., Benestad, H.B., Raastad, T. (2014). Vitamin C and E supplementation hampers cellular adaptation to endurance training in humans: a double-blind randomized controlled trial. *J Physiol* 592: 1887–901.

Pavelka, K., Gatterova, J., Olejarova, M., Machacek, S., Giacovelli, G., Rovati, L.C. (2002). Glucosamine sulfate use and delay of progression of knee osteoarthritis: a 3-year, randomized, placebo-controlled, double-blind study. *Arch Intern Med* 162: 2113–23.

Pearce, J., Borchers, J.R., Kaeding, C.C., Rawson, E.S., Shaw, G., Burke, L.M., Stear, S.J., Castell, L.M. (2010). BJSM reviews: A–Z of nutritional supplements: dietary supplements, sports nutrition foods and ergogenic aids for health and performance Part 9: Choline Bitartrate plus Acetylcholine, Chondroitin/Glucosamine, Chromium Picolinate and Cissus Quadrangularis. *Br J Sports Med* 44: 609–11.

Pearce, J., Norton, L., Senchina, D.S., Spriet, L.L., Burke, L.M., Stear, S.J., Castell, L.M. (2012). BJSM reviews: A–Z of nutritional supplements: dietary supplements, sports nutrition foods and ergogenic aids for health and performance Part 37: Stacking, Taurine, Theobromine and Theophylline. *Br J Sports Med* 46: 954–6.

Peart, D.J., Siegler, J.C., Vince, R.V. (2012). Practical recommendations for coaches and athletes: a meta-analysis of sodium bicarbonate use for athletic performance. *J Strength Cond Res* 26: 1975–83.

Pedersen, B.K. (2006). The anti-inflammatory effect of exercise: its role in diabetes and cardiovascular disease control. *Essays Biochem* 42: 105–17.

Pedersen, B.K. (2007). IL-6 signalling in exercise and disease. *Biochem Soc Trans* 35: 1295–7.

Peeling, P. (2010). Exercise as a mediator of hepcidin activity in athletes. *Eur J Appl Physiol* 110: 877–83.

Peeling, P., Blee, T., Goodman, C., *et al.* (2007). Effect of iron injections on aerobic exercise performance of iron depleted female athletes. *Int J Sport Nutr Exerc Metab* 17: 221–31.

Peeling, P., Dawson, B., Goodman, C., *et al.* (2008). Athletic induced iron deficiency: new insights into the role of inflammation, cytokines and hormones. *Eur J Appl Physiol* 103: 381–91.

Peeling, P., Sim, M., Badenhorst, C.E., *et al.* (2014). Iron status and the acute post-exercise hepcidin response in athletes. *PLoS One* 9: e93002.

Pennings, B., Boirie, Y., Senden, J.M., Gijsen, A.P., Kuipers, H., van Loon, L.J. (2011). Whey protein stimulates postprandial muscle protein accretion more effectively than do casein and casein hydrolysate in older men. *Am J Clin Nutr* 93: 997–1005.

Pennings, B., Groen, B., de Lange, A., Gijsen, A.P., Zorenc, A.H., Senden, J.M., *et al.* (2012). Amino acid absorption and subsequent muscle protein accretion following graded intakes of whey protein in elderly men. *Am J Physiol Endocrinol Metab* 302: E992–E999.

Penry, J., Manore, M. (2008). Choline: an important micronutrient for maximal endurance-exercise performance. *Int J Sport Nutr Exerc Metab* 18: 191–203.

Peoples, G.E., McLennan, P.L., Howe, P.R., Groeller, H. (2008). Fish oil reduces heart rate and oxygen consumption during exercise. *J Cardiovasc Pharmacol* 52: 540–7.

Pérez-Guisado, J., Jakeman, P.M. (2010). Citrulline malate enhances athletic anaerobic performance and relieves muscle soreness. *J Strength Condit Res* 24: 1215–22.

Persky, A.M., Rawson, E.S. (2007). Safety of creatine supplementation in health and disease. In: Salomons, G.J., Wyss, M. (eds) *Creatine and Creatine Kinase in Health and Disease*. Springer: Dordrecht, 275–89.

Peternelj, T.T., Coombes, J.S. (2011). Antioxidant supplementation during exercise training: beneficial or detrimental? *Sports Med* 41: 1043–69.

Petersen, A.C., McKenna, M.J., Medved, I., Murphy, K.Y., Brown, M.J., Della Gatta, P., Cameron-Smith, D. (2012). Infusion with the antioxidant N-acetylcysteine attenuates early adaptive responses to exercise in human skeletal muscle. *Acta Physiol (Oxf)* 204: 382–92.

Petroczi, A., Naughton, D.P. (2008). The age-gender-status profile of high performing athletes in the UK taking nutritional supplements: lessons for the future. *J Int Soc Sports Nutr* 5: 2.

Pfeiffer, B., Stellingwerff, T., Zaltas, E., Jeukendrup, A.E. (2010a). CHO oxidation from a CHO gel compared with a drink during exercise. *Med Sci Sports Exerc* 42: 2038–45.

Pfeiffer, B., Stellingwerff, T., Zaltas, E., Jeukendrup, A.E. (2010b). Oxidation of solid versus liquid CHO sources during exercise. *Med Sci Sports Exerc* 42: 2030–7.

Pham, C.T. (2008). Neutrophil serine proteases fine-tune the inflammatory response. *Int J Biochem Cell Biol* 40: 1317–33.

Phillips, S.M. (2012a). Dietary protein requirements and adaptive advantages in athletes. *Br J Nutr* 108s: S158–67.

Phillips, S.M. (2012b). Nutrient-rich meat proteins in offsetting age-related muscle loss. *Meat Sci* 92: 174–8.

Phillips, S.M., Tipton, K.D., Aarsland, A., Wolf, S.E., Wolfe, R.R. (1997). Mixed muscle protein synthesis and breakdown after resistance exercise in humans. *Am J Physiol* 273: E99–107.

Phillips, S.M., Tipton, K.D., Ferrando, A.A., *et al.* (1999). Resistance training reduces the acute exercise-induced increase in muscle protein turnover. *Am J Physiol* 276: E118–24.

Phillips, S.M., van Loon, L.J. (2011). Dietary protein for athletes: from requirements to optimum adaptation. *J Sports Sci* 29: S29–38.

Phillips, T., Childs, A.C., Dreon, D.M., Phinney, S., Leeuwenburgh, C. (2003). A dietary supplement attenuates IL-6 and CRP after eccentric exercise in untrained males. *Med Sci Sports Exerc* 35: 2032–7.

Piantadosi, C.A. (2006). 'Oxygenated' water and athletic performance. *Br J Sports Med* 40: 740.

Pigozzi, F., Sacchetti, M., di Salvo, V., *et al.* (2003). Oral theophylline supplementation and high-intensity intermittent exercise. *J Sports Med Phys Fitness* 43: 535–8.

Pilaczynska-Szczesniak, L., Skarpanska-Steinborn, A., Deskur, E., *et al.* (2005). The influence of chokeberry juice supplementation on the reduction of oxidative stress resulting from an incremental rowing ergometer exercise. *Int J Sport Nutr Exerc Metab* 15: 48–58.

Pittler, M.H., Schmidt, K., Ernst, E. (2005). Adverse events of herbal food supplements for body weight reduction: systematic review. *Obes Rev* 6: 93–111.

Plezbert, J.A., Burke, J.R. (2005). Effects of the homeopathic remedy arnica on attenuating symptoms of exercise-induced muscle soreness. *J Chiropr Med* 4: 152–61.

Plourde, M., Jew, S., Cunnane, S.C., Jones, P.J. (2008). Conjugated linoleic acids: why the discrepancy between animal and human studies? *Nutr Rev* 66: 415–21.

Poddar, K., Kolge, S., Bezman, L., *et al.* (2011). Nutraceutical supplements for weight loss: a systematic review. *Nutr Clin Pract* 26: 539–52.

Pokrywka, A., Obmiński, Z., Malczewska-Lenczowska, J., *et al.* (2014). Insights into Tribulus terrestris supplements used by athletes. *J Hum Kinet* 41: 99–105.

Pollock, N., Dijkstra, P., Chakraverty, R., Hamilton, B. (2012). Low 25(OH) vitamin D concentrations in international UK track and field athletes. *S Afr J SM* 24: 55–9.

Polyviou, T.P., Easton, C., Beis, L., Malkova, D., Takas, P., Hambly, C., Speakman, J.R., Koehler, K., Pitsiladis, Y.P. (2012a). Effects of glycerol and creatine hyperhydration on doping-relevant blood parameters. *Nutrients* 4: 1171–86.

Polyviou, T.P., Pitsiladis, Y.P., Lee, W.C., Pantazis, T., Hambly, C., Speakman, J.R., Malkova, D. (2012b). Thermoregulatory and cardiovascular responses to creatine, glycerol and alpha lipoic acid in trained cyclists. *J Int Soc Sports Nutr* 9: 29.

Poortmans, J.R., Francaux, M. (2000). Adverse effects of creatine supplementation: fact or fiction? *Sports Med* 30: 155–70.

Poortmans, J.R., Francaux, M. (2008). Creatine consumption in health. In: Stout, J., Antonio, J., Kalman, D. (eds) *Essentials of Creatine in Sports and Health*. Totowa, New Jersey, USA: Humana Press, 127–72.

Poortmans, J.R., Kumps, A., Duez, P., *et al.* (2005). Effect of oral creatine supplementation on urinary methylamine, formaldehyde, and formate. *Med Sci Sports Exerc* 37: 1717–20.

Poortmans, J.R., Rawson, E.S., Burke, L.M., Stear, S.J., Castell, L.M. (2010). BJSM reviews: A–Z of nutritional supplements: dietary supplements, sports nutrition foods and ergogenic aids for health and performance Part 11: Creatine. *Br J Sports Med* 44: 765–6.

Porcari, J.P., Otto, J., Felker, H., Mikat, R.P., Foster, C. (2006). The placebo effect on exercise performance. *J Cardiopulmon Rehabil Prev* 26: 269.

Portal, S., Eliakim, A., Nemet, D., *et al.* (2010). Effect of HMB supplementation on body composition, fitness, hormonal profile and muscle damage indices. *J Pediatr Endocrinol Metab* 23: 641–50.

Portier, H., Chatard, J.C., Filaire, E., Jaunet-Devienne, M.F., Robert, A., Guezennec, C.Y. (2008). Effects of branched-chain amino acids supplementation on physiological and psychological performance during an offshore sailing race. *Eur J Appl Physiol* 104: 787–94.

Potterat, O. (2010). Goji (Lycium barbarum and L. chinense): phytochemistry, pharmacology and safety in the perspective of traditional uses and recent popularity. *Planta Med* 76: 7–19.

Potu, B.K., Bhat, K.M., Rao, M.S., Nampurath, G.K., Chamallamudi, M.R., Nayak, S.R., *et al.* (2009). Petroleum ether extract of Cissus quadrangularis (Linn.) enhances bone marrow mesenchymal stem cell proliferation and facilitates osteoblastogenesis. *Clinics* 64: 993–8.

Potu, B.K., Rao, M.S., Nampurath, G.K., Chamallamudi, M.R., Nayak, S.R., Thomas, H. (2010). Anti-osteoporotic activity of the petroleum ether extract of Cissus quadrangularis Linn. in ovariectomized Wistar rats. *Chang Gung Medical Journal* 33: 252–7.

Powers, M.E., Yarrow, J.F., McCoy, S.C., Borst, S.E. (2007). Growth hormone isoform responses to GABA ingestion at rest and after exercise. *Med Sci Sports Exerc* 40: 104–10.

Powers, S.K., DeRuisseau, K.C., Quindry, J., Hamilton, K.L. (2004). Dietary antioxidants and exercise. *J Sports Sci* 22: 81–94.

Powers, S.K., Duarte, J., Kavazis, A.N., Talbert, E.E. (2010a). Reactive oxygen species are signalling molecules for skeletal muscle adaptation. *Exper Physiol* 95: 1–9.

Powers, S.K., Jackson, M.J. (2008). Exercise-induced oxidative stress: cellular mechanisms and impact on muscle force production. *Physiol Rev* 88: 1243–76.

Powers, S.K., Kavazis, A.N., Nelson, W.B., Ernst, E., Stear, S.J., Burke, L.M., Castell, L.M. (2009). BJSM reviews: A–Z of nutritional supplements: dietary supplements, sports nutrition foods and ergogenic aids for health and performance Part 3: Antioxidants and Arnica. *Br J Sports Med* 43: 890–2.

Powers, S.K., Lennon, S.L. (1999). Analysis of cellular responses to free radicals: focus on exercise and skeletal muscle. *Proc Nutr Soc* 58: 1025–33.

Powers, S.K., Smuder, A.J., Kavazis, A.N., *et al.* (2010b). Experimental guidelines for studies designed to investigate the impact of antioxidant supplementation on exercise performance. *Int J Sport Nutr Exerc Metab* 20: 2–14.

Prasad, A.S. (2009). Impact of the discovery of human zinc deficiency on health. *J Am Coll Nutr* 28: 257–65.

Prasad, A.S., Abbasi, A.A., Rabbani, P., *et al.* (1981). Effect of zinc supplementation on serum testosterone level in adult male sickle cell anemia subjects. *Am J Hematol* 10: 119–27.

Prentice, A. (1997). Is nutrition important in osteoporosis? *Proc Nutr Soc* 56: 357–67.

Prentice, A., Bates, C.J. (1994). Adequacy of dietary mineral supply for human bone growth and mineralisation. *Eur J Clin Nutr* 48: S161–77.

Preuss, H.G., Bagchi, D., Bagchi, M., *et al.* (2004). Efficacy of a novel, natural extract of (−)-hydroxycitric acid (HCA-SX) and a combination of HCA-SX, niacin-bound chromium and *Gymnema sylvestre* extract in weight management in human volunteers: a pilot study. *Nutr Res* 24: 45–58.

Price, M., Moss, P., Rance, S. (2003). Effects of sodium bicarbonate ingestion on prolonged intermittent exercise. *Med Sci Sports Exerc* 35: 1303–8.

Pumpa, K.L., Fallon, K.E., Bensoussan, A., Papalia, S. (2014). The effects of topical Arnica on performance, pain and muscle damage after intense eccentric exercise. *Eur J Sport Sci* 14: 294–300.

Pyne, D.B., Hopkins, W.G., Batterham, A.M., Gleeson, M., Fricker, P.A. (2005). Characterising the individual performance responses to mild illness in international swimmers. *Br J Sports Med* 39: 752–6.

Qureshi, N.A., Al-Bedah, A.M. (2013). Mood disorders and complementary and alternative medicine: a literature review. *Neuropsychiatr Dis Treat* 9: 639–58.

Raastad, T., Høstmark, A.T., Strømme, S.B. (1997). Omega-3 fatty acid supplementation does not improve maximal aerobic power, anaerobic threshold and running performance in well-trained soccer players. *Scand J Med Sci Sports* 7: 25–31.

Rainieri, A., *et al.*, (2009). The use of alpha-lipoic acid (ALA), gamma linolenic acid (GLA) and rehabilitation in the treatment of back pain: effect of health-related quality of life. *Int J Immunopathol Pharmacol* 22: 45–50.

Ramos, S., Almeida, R.M., Moura, J.J., Aureliano, M. (2011). Implications of oxidovanadium(IV) binding to actin. *J Inorg Biochem* 105: 777–83.

Ranchordas, M.K., Blomstrand, E., Calder, P.C., Burke, L.M., Stear, S.J., Castell, L.M. (2011). BJSM reviews: A–Z of nutritional supplements: dietary supplements, sports nutrition foods and ergogenic aids for health and performance Part 23: Leucine, Lecithin, Linoleic and Linolenic acid. *Br J Sports Med* 45: 830–1.

Ranchordas, M.K., Burd, N.A., Senchina, D.S., Burke, L.M., Stear, S.J., Castell, L.M. (2012). BJSM reviews: A–Z of nutritional supplements: dietary supplements, sports nutrition foods and ergogenic aids for health and performance Part 29: Phlogenzym and Wobenzym, Phosphatidylserine and Plant Stanols. *Br J Sports Med* 46: 155–6.

Ranchordas, M.K., Lundy, B., Burke, L.M., Stear, S.J., Castell, L.M. (2013a). BJSM reviews: A–Z of nutritional supplements: dietary supplements, sports nutrition foods and ergogenic aids for health and performance Part 41: Vitamin B and K. *Br J Sports Med* 47: 185–6.

Ranchordas, M.K., Stear, S.J., Burd, N.A., Godfrey, R.J., Senchina, D.S., Burke, L.M., Castell, L.M. (2013b). BJSM reviews: A–Z of nutritional supplements: dietary supplements, sports nutrition foods and ergogenic aids for health and performance Part 43: Wheat Germ Oil, Whey Protein and Wolfberry. *Br J Sports Med* 47: 659–60.

Randell, R.K., Hodgson, A.B., Lotito, S.B., *et al.* (2014). Variable duration of decaffeinated green tea extract ingestion on exercise metabolism. *Med Sci Sports Exerc* 46: 1185–93.

Randle, P.J., Garland, P.B., Hales, C.N., Newsholme, E.A. (1963). The glucose fatty-acid cycle. Its role in insulin sensitivity and the metabolic disturbances of diabetes mellitus. *Lancet* 281: 785–9.

Rawson, E.S., Persky, A.M. (2007). Mechanisms of muscular adaptations to creatine supplementation. *Int SportMed J* 8: 43–53.

Rawson, E.S., Venezia, A.C. (2011). Use of creatine in the elderly and evidence for effects on cognitive function in young and old. *Amino Acids* 40: 1349–62.

Rayman, M.P. (2012). Selenium and human health. *Lancet* 29: 1–13.

Raymer, G.H., Marsh, G.D., Kowalchuk, J.M., Thompson, R.T. (2004). Metabolic effects of induced alkalosis during progressive forearm to fatigue. *J Appl Physiol* 96: 2050–6.

Reap, E.A., Lawson, J.W. (1990). Stimulation of the immune response by dimethylglycine, a nontoxic metabolite. *J Lab Clin Med* 115: 481–6.

Rebouche, C.J., Lombard, K.A., Chenard, C.A. (1993). Renal adaptation to dietary carnitine in humans. *Am J Clin Nutr* 58: 660–5.

Reginster, J.Y., Deroisy, R., Rovati, L.C., Lee, R.L., Lejeune, E., Bruyere, O., *et al.* (2001). Long-term effects of glucosamine sulphate on osteoarthritis progression: a randomised, placebo-controlled clinical trial. *Lancet* 357: 251–6.

Rehder, D. (2012). The potentiality of vanadium in medicinal applications. *Future Med Chem* 4: 1823–37.

Reid, M.B. (2008). Free radicals and muscle fatigue: of ROS, canaries, and the IOC. *Free Radic Biol Med* 44: 169–79.

Reid, M.B., Stokic, D.S., Koch, S.M., *et al.* (1994). N-aceytlcysteine inhibits muscle fatigue in humans. *J Clin Invest* 94: 2468–74.

Rezaee, M.E., Manneh, C.A., Graver, A.M., *et al.* (2012). Global reach of online direct-to-consumer drug advertising. *Am J Health Syst Pharm* 69: 96–7.

Richards, J.C., Lonac, M.C., Johnson, T.K., *et al.* (2010). Epigallocatechin-3-gallate increases maximal oxygen uptake in adult humans. *Med Sci Sports Exerc* 42: 739–44.

Rimaniol, A.C., Mialocq, P., Clayette, P., *et al.* (2001). Role of glutamate transporters in the regulation of glutathione levels in human macrophages. *Am J Physiol Cell Physiol* 281: C1964–70.

Ristow, M., Zarse, K., Oberbach, A., *et al.* (2009). Antioxidants prevent health-promoting effects of physical exercise in humans. *Proc Natl Acad Sci* 106: 8665–70.

Roberts, L.A., Beattie, K., Close, G.L., *et al.* (2011). Vitamin C consumption does not impair training-induced improvements in exercise performance. *Int J Sport Physiol Perform* 6: 58–69.

Robinson, A.M., Williamson, D.H. (1980). Physiological roles of ketone bodies as substrates and signals in mammalian tissues. *Physiol Rev* 60: 143–87.

Roche, H.M., Noone, E., Nugent, A.P., Gibney, M.J. (2001). Conjugated linoleic acid: a novel therapeutic nutrient? *Nutr Res Rev* 14: 173–87.

Rodricks, J.V., Lumpkin, M.H. (2013). DMAA as a dietary ingredient. *JAMA Int Med* 173: 594.

Rodriguez, N.R., DiMarco, N.M., Langley, S. (2009a). American College of Sports Medicine position stand. Nutrition and athletic performance. *Med Sci Sports Exerc* 41: 709–31.

Rodriguez, N.R., DiMarco, N.M., Langley, S. (2009b). Position of the American Dietetic Association, Dietitians of Canada, and the American College of Sports Medicine: Nutrition and athletic performance. *J Am Dietetic Assoc* 109: 509–27.

Rogers, P.J., Blomstrand, E., Gurr, S., Mitchell, N., Stephens, F.B., Greenhaff, P.L., Burke, L.M., Stear, S.J., Castell, L.M. (2009). BJSM reviews: A–Z of nutritional supplements: dietary supplements, sports nutrition foods and ergogenic aids for health and performance Part 4: Aspartame, Branched Chain Amino Acids, Bee Pollen, Boron, Carnitine. *Br J Sports Med* 43: 1088–90.

Rogers, P.J., Pleming, H.C., Blundell, J.E. (1990). Aspartame ingested without tasting inhibits hunger and food intake. *Physiol Behav* 47: 1239–43.

Rogerson, S., Riches, C.J., Jennings, C., *et al.* (2007). The effect of five weeks of Tribulus terrestris supplementation on muscle strength and body composition during preseason training in elite rugby league players. *J Strength Cond Res Natl Strength Cond Assoc* 21: 348–53.

Rohdewald, P. (2002). A review of the French maritime pine bark extract (Pycnogenol), a herbal medication with a diverse clinical pharmacology. *Int J Clin Pharmacol Ther* 40: 158–68.

Rokitzki, L., Sagredos, A.N., Reuss, F. (1994). Acute changes in vitamin B-6 status in endurance athletes before and after a marathon. *Int J Sport Nutr* 4: 154–65.

Romijn, J., Coyle, E.F., Sidossis, L.S., Gastaldelli, A., Horowitz, J.F., Endert, E., Wolfe, R.R. (1993). Regulation of endogenous fat and carbohydrate metabolism in relation to exercise intensity and duration. *Am J Physiol Endocrinol Metabolism* 265: E380–E391.

Romijn, J., Coyle, E.F., Sidossis, L.S., Zhang, X.-J., Wolfe, R.R. (1995). Relationship between fatty acid delivery and fatty acid oxidation during strenuous exercise. *J Appl Physiol* 79: 1939–45.

Rondanelli, M., Opizzi, A., Perna, S., *et al.* (2013). Improvement in insulin resistance and favourable changes in plasma inflammatory adipokines after weight loss associated with two months' consumption of a combination of bioactive food ingredients in overweight subjects. *Endocrine* 44: 391–401.

Ronsen, O., Sundgot-Borgen, J., Maehlum, S. (1999). Supplement use and nutritional habits in Norwegian elite athletes. *Scand J Med Sci Sports* 9: 28–35.

Rossi, A., Hawkins, S., Cornwell, A., DiCaprio, P., Chou, C.Y., Khodiguian, N. (2006). The effects of modified chronic sodium bicarbonate ingestion on short-duration, high-intensity performance in elite middle-distance runners. *Med Sci Sport Exerc* 38: S402.

Rossi, P., Buonocore, D., Altobelli, E., *et al.* (2014). Improving training condition assessment in endurance cyclists: effects of *Ganoderma lucidum* and *Ophiocordyceps sinensis* dietary supplementation. *Evid-Based Complement Altern Med* 2014: 979613.

Rowlands, D.S., Thomson, J.S. (2009). Effects of beta-hydroxy-beta-methylbutyrate supplementation during resistance training on strength, body composition, and muscle damage in trained and untrained young men: a meta-analysis. *J Strength Cond Res* 23: 836–46.

Ruohola, J.P., Laaksi, I., Ylikomi, T., Haataja, R., Mattila, V.M., Sahi, T., *et al.* (2006). Association between serum 25(OH)D concentrations and bone stress fractures in Finnish young men. *J Bone Miner Res* 21: 1483–8.

Rutherford, J.A., Spriet, L.L., Stellingwerff, T. (2010). The effect of acute taurine ingestion on endurance performance and metabolism in trained cyclists. *Int J Sport Nutr Exerc Met* 20: 322–9.

Saad, M.A., Eid, N.I., Adb El-Latif, H.A., Sayed, H.M. (2013). Potential effects of yohimbine and sildenafil on erectile dysfunction in rats. *Eur J Pharmacol* 700: 127–33.

Saint-John, M., McNaughton, L. (1986). Octasanol ingestion and its effects on metabolic responses to submaximal cycle ergometry, reaction time and chest grip strength. *Int Clin Nutr Rev* 6: 81.

Sakko, M., Tjäderhane, L., Sorsa, T., Hietala, P., Järvinen, A., Bowyer, P., Rautemaa, R. (2012). α-Hydroxyisocaproic acid (HICA): a new potential topical antibacterial agent. *Int J Antimicrobial Agents* 39: 539–40.

Salas-Salvadó, J., Márquez-Sandoval, F., Bulló, M. (2006). Conjugated linoleic acid intake in humans: a systematic review focusing on its effect on body composition, glucose, and lipid metabolism. *Crit Rev Food Sci Nutr* 46: 479–88.

Sale, C., Artioli, G.G., Gualano, B., Saunders, B., Hobson, R.M., Harris, R.C. (2013). Carnosine: from exercise performance to health. *Amino Acids* 44: 1477–91.

Sale, C., Harris, R.C., Florance, J., *et al.* (2009). Urinary creatine and methylamine excretion following 4 × 5 g × day−1 or 20 × 1 g × day−1 of creatine monohydrate for 5 days. *J Sports Sci* 27: 759–66.

Sale, C., Saunders, B., Hudson, S., Wise, J.A., Harris, R.C., Sunderland, C.D. (2011). Effect of β-alanine plus sodium bicarbonate on high-intensity cycling capacity. *Med Sci Sports Exerc* 43: 1972–8.

Saliou, C., Rimbach, G., Moini, H., *et al.* (2001). Solar ultraviolet-induced erythema in human skin and nuclear factor=kappa-B-dependent gene expression in keratinocytes are modulated by a French maritime pine bark extract. *Free Radic Biol Med* 30: 154–60.

Salomon, F., Cuneo, R.C., Hesp, R., Sonksen, P.H. (1989). The effects of treatment with recombinant human growth hormone on body composition and metabolism in adults with growth hormone deficiency. *New Engl J Med* 321: 1797–803.

Sandberg, M., Pettersson, U., Henriksnas, J., Jansson, L. (2013). The α2-adrenoceptor antagonist yohimbine normalizes increased Islet blood flow in GK rats: a model of type 2 diabetes. *Horm Metab Res* 45: 252–4.

Santos, D.A., Matias, C.N., Monteiro, C.P., Silva, A.M., Rocha, P.M., Minderico, C.S., Bettencourt Sardinha, L., Laires, M.J. (2011). Magnesium intake is associated with strength performance in elite basketball, handball and volleyball players. *Magnes Res* 24: 215–19.

Sasabe, J., Miyoshi, Y., Suzuki, M., Mita, M., Konno, R., Matsuoka, M., *et al.* (2012). D-amino acid oxidase controls motoneuron degeneration through D-serine. *Proc Natl Acad Sci* 109: 627–32.

Sasaki, S. (2008). Dietary Reference Intakes (DRIs) in Japan. *Asia Pac J Clin Nutr* 17: 420–44.

Sato, A., Shimoyama, Y., Ishikawa, T., *et al.* (2011). Dietary thiamin and riboflavin intake and blood thiamin and riboflavin concentrations in college swimmers undergoing intensive training. *Int J Sport Nutr Exerc Metab* 21: 195–204.

Sato, K., Kashiwaya,Y., Keon, C.A., Tsuchiya, N., King, M.T., et al (1995). Insulin, ketone bodies, and mitochondrial energy transduction. *FASEB J* 9: 651–8.

Saunders, B., Sale, C., Harris, R.C., Sunderland, C. (2014) Sodium bicarbonate and high intensity cycling capacity: variability in responses. *Int J Sport Physiol Perf* 9: 627–32.

Saur, P., Joneleit, M., Tölke, H., *et al.* (2002). Evaluation of the magnesium status in athletes. *German J Sports Med* 53: 72–8.

Sauret, J.M., Marinides, G., Wang, G.K. (2002). Rhabdomyolysis. *Am Fam Physician* 65: 907–12.

Sawka, M.N., Burke, L.M., Eichner, E.R., *et al.* (2007). American College of Sports Medicine position stand. Exercise and fluid replacement. *Med Sci Sports Exerc* 39: 377–90.

Sawka, M.N., Montain, S.J. (2000). Fluid and electrolyte supplementation for exercise heat stress. *Am J Clin Nutr* 72: 564S–72S.

SCF (2003). Opinion of the Scientific Committee on Food on additional information on 'energy' drinks. Available at: http://ec.europa.eu/food/fs/sc/scf/out169_en.pdf. Accessed 20 January 2015.

Schänzer, W. (2002). Analysis of non-hormonal nutritional supplements for anabolic-androgenic steroids—an international study. Institute of Biochemistry German Sport University Cologne, 31 May 2013. www.olympic.org/Documents/Reports/EN/en_report_324.pdf

Schauster, A.C., Geletko, S.M., Mikolich, D.J. (2000). Diabetes mellitus associated with recombinant human growth hormone for HIV wasting syndrome. *Pharmacotherapy* 20: 1129–34.

Scherr, J., Nieman, D.C., Schuster, T., *et al.* (2012b). Nonalcoholic beer reduces inflammation and incidence of respiratory tract illness. *Med Sci Sports Exerc* 44: 18–26.

Scherr, J., Schuster, T., Pressler, A., Roeh, A., Christle, J., Wolfarth, B., Halle, M. (2012). Repolarization perturbation and hypomagnesemia after extreme exercise. *Med Sci Sports Exerc* 44: 1637–43.

Schilling, B.K., Hammond, K.G., Bloomer, R.J., *et al.* (2013). Physiological and pharmacokinetic effects of oral 1,3-dimethylamylamine administration in men. *BMC Pharmacol Toxicol* 14: 52.

Schimpl, F.C., da Silva, J.F., Gonçalves, J.F., Mazzafera, P. (2013). Guarana: revisiting a highly caffeinated plant from the Amazon. *J Ethnopharmacol* 150: 14–31.

Schoenfeld, B.J., Aragon, A.A., Krieger, J.W. (2013). The effect of protein timing on muscle strength and hypertrophy: a meta-analysis. *J Int Soc Sport Nutr* 10: 13.

Schoop, R., Büechi, S., Suter, A. (2006). Open, multicenter study to evaluate the tolerability and efficacy of Echinaforce Forte tablets in athletes. *Adv Ther* 23: 823–33.

Schubert, M.M., Astorino, T.A., Azevedo, J.L. Jr. (2013). The effects of caffeinated 'energy shots' on time trial performance. *Nutrients* 5: 2062–75.

Schwedhelm, E., Maas, R., Freese, R., *et al.* (2008). Pharmacokinetic and pharmacodynamic properties of oral L-citrulline and L-arginine: impact on nitric oxide metabolism. *Br J Clin Pharmacol* 65: 51–9.

Science, M., Johnstone, J., Roth, D.E., *et al.* (2012). Zinc for the treatment of the common cold: a systematic review and meta-analysis of randomized controlled trials. *Can Med Assoc J* 184: E551–61.

Segura, R., Ventura, J.L. (1988). Effect of L-tryptophan supplementation on exercise performance. *Int J Sport Med* 9: 301–5.

Sekhar, R.V., McKay, S.V., Patel, S.G., Guthikonda, A.P., Reddy, V.T., Balasubramanyam, A., Jahoor, F. (2011a). Glutathione synthesis is diminished in patients with uncontrolled diabetes and restored by dietary supplementation with cysteine and glycine. *Diabetes Care* 34: 162–7.

Sekhar, R.V., Patel, S.G., Guthikonda, A.P., Reid, M., Balasubramanyam, A., Taffet, G.E., Jahoor, F. (2011b). Deficient synthesis of glutathione underlies oxidative stress in aging and can be corrected by dietary cysteine and glycine supplementation. *Am J Clin Nutr* 94: 847–53.

Senchina, D.S. (2013). Athletics and herbal supplements. *Am Sci* 101: 134–41.

Senchina, D.S., Bermon, S., Stear, S.J., Burke, L.M., Castell, L.M. (2011). BJSM reviews: A–Z of nutritional supplements: dietary supplements, sports nutrition foods and ergogenic aids for health and performance Part 17: Gingko, Ginseng, Green Tea, Garlic and Glandulars. *Br J Sports Med* 45: 150–1.

Senchina, D.S., Burke, L.M., Stear, S.J., Castell, L.M. (2012a). BJSM reviews: A–Z of nutritional supplements: dietary supplements, sports nutrition foods and ergogenic aids for health and performance Part 39: Vitamins A, C and E. *Br J Sports Med* 46: 1145–6.

Senchina, D.S., Hallam, J.E., Cheney, D.J. (2013a). Multidisciplinary perspectives on mechanisms of activity of popular immune-enhancing herbal supplements used by athletes. *Front Biol* 8: 78–100.

Senchina, D.S., Hallam, J.E., Dias, A.S., Perera, M.A. (2009a) Human blood mononuclear cell in vitro cytokine response before and after two different strenuous exercise bouts in the presence of bloodroot and echinacea extracts. *Blood Cell Mol Dis* 43: 298–303.

Senchina, D.S., Hallam, J.E., Kohut, M.L., *et al.* (2014). Alkaloids and athlete immune function: caffeine, theophylline, gingerol, ephedrine, and their congeners. *Exerc Immunol Rev* 20: 68–93.

Senchina, D.S., Hallam, J.E., Thompson, N.M., *et al.* (2012b). Alkaloids and endurance athletes. *Track Cross Ctry J* 2: 2–18.

Senchina, D.S., Shah, N.B., Doty, D.M., *et al.* (2009b). Herbal supplements and athlete immune function: what's proven, disproven, and unproven? *Exerc Immunol Rev* 15: 66–106.

Senchina, D.S., Stear, S.J., Burke, L.M., Castell, L.M. (2013b). BJSM reviews: A–Z of nutritional supplements: dietary supplements, sports nutrition foods and ergogenic aids for health and performance Part 44: Weight Loss strategies and Herbal Weight Loss Supplements. *Br J Sports Med* 47: 595–8.

Senturk, U.K., Yalcin, O., Gunduz, F., *et al.* (2005). Effect of antioxidant vitamin treatment on the time course of hematological and hemorheological alterations after an exhausting exercise episode in human subjects. *J Appl Physiol Bethesda Md 1985* 98: 1272–9.

Setnikar, I., Palumbo, R., Canali, S., Zanolo, G. (1993). Pharmacokinetics of glucosamine in man. *Arzneimittelforschung* 43: 1109–13.

Setnikar, I., Rovati, L.C. (2001). Absorption, distribution, metabolism and excretion of glucosamine sulfate. A review. *Arzneimittelforschung* 51: 699–725.

Shafiei Neek, L., Gaeini, A.A., Choobineh, S. (2011). Effect of zinc and selenium supplementation on serum testosterone and plasma lactate in cyclist after an exhaustive exercise bout. *Biol Trace Element Res* 144: 454–62.

Shanely, R.A., Knab, A.M., Nieman, D.C., *et al.* (2010). Quercetin supplementation does not alter antioxidant status in humans. *Free Radic Res* 44: 224–31.

Shanely, R.A., Nieman, D.C., Zwetsloot, K.A., *et al.* (2014). Evaluation of Rhodiola rosea supplementation on skeletal muscle damage and inflammation in runners following a competitive marathon. *Brain Behav Immun* 39: 204–10.

Sharma, K., Paradakar, M. (2010). The melamine adulteration scandal. *Food Secur* 2: 97–107.

Sharpe, P.A., Granner, M.L., Conway, J.M., *et al.* (2006). Availability of weight-loss supplements: results of an audit of retail outlets in a southeastern city. *J Am Diet Assoc* 106: 2045–51.

Sharples, A.P., Al-Shanti, N., Hughes, D.C., Lewis, M.P., Stewart, C.E. (2013). The role of insulin-like growth factor binding protein 2 (igfbp2) and phosphatase and tensin homologue (pten) in the regulation of myoblast differentiation and hypertrophy. *Growth Horm IGF Res* 23: 53–61.

Shay, K.P., Moreau, R.F., Smith, E.J., Smith, A.R., Hagen, T.M. (2009). Alpha-lipoic acid as a dietary supplement: molecular mechanisms and therapeutic potential. *Biochim Biophys Acta* 1790: 1149–60.

Sheffield-Moore, M., Yeckel, C.W., Volpi, E., *et al.* (2004). Postexercise protein metabolism in older and younger men following moderate-intensity aerobic exercise. *Am J Physiol Endocrinol Metab* 287: E513–E522.

Sherid, M., Samo, S., Sulaiman, S., *et al.* (2013). Ischemic colitis induced by the newly reformulated multicomponent weight-loss supplement Hydroxycut. *World J Gastrointest Endosc* 5: 180–5.

Shevtsov, V.A., Zholus, B.I., Shervarly, V.I., *et al.* (2003). A randomized trial of two different doses of a SHR-5 Rhodiola rosea extract versus placebo and control of capacity for mental work. *Phytomedicine* 10: 95–105.

Shi, X., Summers, R.W., Schedl, H.P., *et al.* (1995). Effects of carbohydrate type and concentration and solution osmolality on water absorption. *Med Sci Sports Exerc* 27: 1607–15.

Shi, X., Summers, R.W., Schedl, H.P., Flanagan, S.W., Chang, R., Gisolfi, C.V. (1997). Effects of carbohydrate type and concentration and solution osmolality on water absorption. *Med Sci Sports Exerc* 27: 1607–15.

Shikhman, A.R., Amiel, D., D'Lima, D., Hwang, S.B., Hu, C., Xu, A., *et al.* (2005). Chondroprotective activity of N-acetylglucosamine in rabbits with experimental osteoarthritis. *Ann Rheum Dis* 64: 89–94.

Shimoda, H., Seki, E., Aitani, M. (2006). Inhibitory effect of green coffee bean extract on fat accumulation and body weight gain in mice. *BMC Complement Altern Med* 6: 9.

Shindle, M., Voos, J., Gulotta, L., Weiss, L., Roder, S., Kelly, G., *et al.* (2011). Vitamin D status in a professional American football team. *Med Sci Sports Exerc* 43: S340–1.

Shing, C.M., Hunter, D.C., Stevenson, L.M. (2009). Bovine colostrum supplementation and exercise performance: potential mechanisms. *Sports Med* 39: 1033–54.

Shing, C.M., Jenkins, D.G., Stevenson, L., Coombes, J.S. (2006). The influence of bovine colostrum supplementation on exercise performance in highly-trained cyclists. *Br J Sports Med* 40: 797–801.

Shing, C.M., Peake, J.M., Suzuki, K., Jenkins, D.G., Coombes, J.S. (2013). A pilot study: bovine colostrum supplementation and hormonal and autonomic responses to competitive cycling. *J Sports Med Phys Fitness* 53: 490–501.

Shirreffs, S.M., Armstrong, L.E., Cheuvront, S.N. (2004). Fluid and electrolyte needs for preparation and recovery from training and competition. *J Sports Sci* 22: 57–63.

Shirreffs, S.M., Maughan, R.J. (1998). Volume repletion after exercise-induced volume depletion in humans: replacement of water and sodium losses. *Am J Physiol* 274: F868–F875.

Shirreffs, S.M., Sawka, M.N., Stone, M. (2006). Water and electrolyte needs for football training and match-play. *J Sports Sci* 24: 699–707.

Shneir, A.B. (2001). Acute gamma-hydroxybutyrate toxicity. *Cal J Emerg Med* 2: 7–8.

Siegel, A.J., Januzzi, J., Sluss, P., Lee-Lewandrowski, E., Wood, M., Shirey, T., Lewandrowski, K.B. (2008). Cardiac biomarkers, electrolytes, and other analytes in collapsed marathon runners: implications for the evaluation of runners following competition. *Am J Clin Pathol* 129: 948–51.

Siegler, J.C., Hirscher, K. (2010). Sodium bicarbonate ingestion and boxing performance. *J Strength Cond Res* 24: 103–8.

Siegler, J.C., Keatley, S., Midgley, A.W., Nevill, A.M., McNaughton, L.R. (2007) Influence of pre-exercise alkalosis and recovery mode on the kinetics of acid-based recovery following intense exercise. *Int J Sport Med* 28: 1–7.

Siegler, J.C., Marshall, P.W.M., Bray, J., Towlson, C. (2012). Sodium bicarbonate supplementation and ingestion timing, does it matter? *J Strength Cond Res* 26: 1953–8.

Sim, M., Dawson, B., Landers, G.J., *et al.* (2014). A seven day running training period increases basal urinary hepcidin levels as compared to cycling. *Int Soc Sports Nutr* 11: 14.

Singer, F., Singer, C., Oberleitner, H. (2001). Phlogenzym versus Diclofenac in the treatment of activated osteoarthritis of the knee. A double blind prospective randomized study. *Int J Immunotherapy* XVII: 135–41.

Singer, N., Lattman, P. (2013). A workout booster, and a lawsuit. *New York Times*, 13 February 2013. Available at: www.nytimes.com/2013/02/14/business/death-after-use-of-jack3d-shows-gap-in-regulation.html?_r=0. Accessed 29 January 2015.

Singh, B.K., Mehta, J.L. (2002). Management of dyslipidemia in the primary prevention of coronary heart disease. *Curr Opin Cardiol* 17: 503–11.

Singh, M., Das, R.R. (2013). Zinc for the common cold. *Cochrane Database Syst Rev* 6: CD001364.

Singh, V., Singh, N., Pal, U.S., Dhasmana, S., Mohammad, S., Singh, N. (2011). Clinical evaluation of cissus quadrangularis and moringa oleifera and osteoseal as osteogenic agents in mandibular fracture. *Natl J maxillofacial Surgery* 2: 132–6.

Skarpanska-Stejnborn, A., Pilaczynska-Szczesniak, L., Basta, P., *et al.* (2008). The influence of supplementation with artichoke (Cynara scolymus L.) extract on selected redox parameters in rowers. *Int J Sport Nutr Exerc Metab* 18: 313–27.

Skarpanska-Stejnborn, A., Pilaczynska-Szczesniak, L., Basta, P., *et al.* (2009). The influence of supplementation with Rhodiola rosea L. extract on selected redox parameters in professional rowers. *Int J Sport Nutr Exerc Metab* 19: 186–99.

Small, E. (2011). 37. Spirulina – food for the universe. *Biodiversity* 12: 255–65.

Smith, A.E., Fukuda, D.H., Kendall, K.L., *et al.* (2010a). The effects of a pre-workout supplement containing caffeine, creatine, and amino acids during three weeks of high-intensity exercise on aerobic and anaerobic performance. *J Int Soc Sports Nutr* 7: 10.

Smith, D.M., Pickering, R.M., Lewith, G.T. (2008a). A systematic review of vanadium oral supplements for glycaemic control in type 2 diabetes mellitus. *QJM* 101: 351–8.

Smith, J.W., Pascoe, D.D., Passe, D.H., *et al.* (2013). Curvilinear dose-response relationship of carbohydrate (0-120 g.h(-1)) and performance. *Med Sci Sports Exerc* 45: 336–41.

Smith, J.W., Zachwieja, J.J., Peronnet, F., *et al.* (2010b). Fuel selection and cycling endurance performance with ingestion of [13C]glucose: evidence for a carbohydrate dose response. *J Appl Physiol* 108: 1520–9.

Smith, K., Reynolds, N., Downie, S., Patel, A., Rennie, M.J. (1998). Effects of flooding amino acids on incorporation of labeled amino acids into human muscle protein. *Am J Physiol* 275: E73–E78.

Smith, N., Atroch, A.L. (2007). Guaraná's journey from regional tonic to aphrodisiac and global energy drink. *Evid Based Complement Alternat Med* 5: 5.

Smith, T.B., Staub, B.A., Natarajan, G.M., *et al.* (2014). Acute myocardial infarction associated with dietary supplements containing 1,3-dimythlamylamine and citrus aurantium. *Tex Heart Inst J* 41: 70–2.

Smith, W.A., Fry, A.C., Tschume L.C., *et al.* (2008b). Effect of glycine propionyl-L-carnitine on aerobic and anaerobic exercise performance. *Int J Sport Nutr Exerc Metab* 18: 19–36.

Snider, I.P., Bazzarre, T.L., Murdoch, S.D., Goldfarb, A. (1992). Effects of coenzyme athletic performance system as an ergogenic aid on endurance performance to exhaustion. *Int J Sport Nutr* 2: 272–86.

Sobal, J., Marquart, L.F. (1994). Vitamin/mineral supplement use among athletes: a review of the literature. *Int J Sport Nutr* 4: 320–34.

Song, M.K., Roufogalis, B.D., Huang, T.H.W. (2012). Reversal of the Caspase-dependent Apoptotic Cytotoxicity pathway by taurine from Lycium barbarum (Goji berry) in human retinal pigment epithelial cells: potential benefit in diabetic retinopathy. *J Evid-Based Complement Altern Med* 2012: 323784.

Sonneville, K.R., *et al.* (2012). Vitamin D, calcium, and dairy intakes and stress fractures among female adolescents. *Arch Pediatr Adolesc Med* 166: 595–600.

Souci, S.W., Fachmann, W., Kraut, H. (2008). *Food Composition and Nutrition Tables*. 7th edn. Stuttgart, Germany: MedPharm Scientific Publishers.

Spasov, A.A., Wikman, G., Mandrikov, V.B., *et al.* (2000). A double-blind, placebo-controlled pilot study of the stimulating and adaptogenic effect of Rhodiola rosea SHR-5 extract on the fatigue of students caused by stress during an examination period with repeated low-dose regimen. *Phytomedicine* 7: 85–9.

Spector, S., Jackman, M., Sabounjian, L., *et al.* (1995). Effect of choline supplementation on fatigue in trained cyclists. *Med Sci Sports Exerc* 27: 668–73.

Spellerberg, A.E. (1952). Increase of athletic effectiveness by systematic ultraviolet irradiation. *Strahlentherapie* 88: 567–70.

Spriet, L.L. (1997). Ergogenic aids: recent advances and retreats. In: Lamb, D.R., Murray, R. (eds) *Perspectives in Exercise Science and Sports Medicine*. Carmel, IN: Cooper, 185–238.

Spriet, L.L., Stear, S.J., Burke, L.M., Castell, L.M. (2010). BJSM reviews: A–Z of nutritional supplements: dietary supplements, sports nutrition foods and ergogenic aids for health and performance Part 6: Caffeine. *Br J Sports Med* 44: 297–8.

Stachenfeld, N.S. (2008). Acute effects of sodium ingestion on thirst and cardiovascular function. *Curr Sports Med Rep* 7: S7–13.

Stadheim, H.K., Spencer, M., Olsen, R., Jensen, J. (2014). Caffeine and performance over consecutive days of simulated competition. *Med Sci Sports Exerc* 46: 1787–96.

Stamler, J.S., Meissner, G. (2001). Physiology of nitric oxide in skeletal muscle. *Physiol Rev* 81: 209–37.

Stankiewicz, A. (1981). AMP-deaminase from human skeletal muscle. subunit structure, amino-acid composition and metal content of the homogenous enzyme. *Int J Biochem* 13: 1177–83.

Stanko, R.T., Robertson, R.J., Galbreath, R.W., *et al.* (1990b). Enhanced leg exercise endurance with a high-carbohydrate diet and dihydroxyacetone and pyruvate. *J Appl Physiol* 69: 1651–6.

Stanko, R.T., Robertson, R.J., Spina, R.J., *et al.* (1990a). Enhancement of arm exercise endurance capacity with dihydroxyacetone and pyruvate. *J Appl Physiol* 68: 119–24.

Starling, R.D., Trappe, T.A., Short, K.R., Sheffield-Moore, M., Jozosi A.C., Fink, W.J., Costill, D.L. (1996). Effect of inosine supplementation on aerobic and anaerobic cycling performance. *Med Sci Sports Exerc* 28: 1193–8.

Staton, W. (1951). The influence of soya lecithin on muscular strength. *Res Quart Am Assoc Health Physic Educ* 22: 201–7.

Stear, S. (2004). *Fuelling Fitness for Sports Performance*. London: The British Olympic Association and The Sugar Bureau.

Stear, S.J., Whyte, G.P., Budgett, R. (2006). Declared dietary supplement usage by British Olympians. *Med Sci Sports Exerc* 38: S409.

Steben, R.E., Boudreaux, P. (1978). The effects of pollen and protein extracts on selected blood factors and performance of athletes. *J Sports Med Phys Fitness* 18: 221–6.

Stefanidou, M., Maravelias, C., Dona, A., *et al.* (2006). Zinc: a multipurpose trace element. *Archives of Toxicology* 80: 1–9.

Stegen, S., Bex, T., Vervaet, C., Vanhee, L., Achten, E., Derave, W. (2014). β-Alanine dose for maintaining moderately elevated muscle carnosine levels. *Med Sci Sports Exerc* 46: 1426–32.

Stegen, S., Blancquaert, L., Everaert, I., Bex, T., Taes, Y., Calders, P., Achten, E., Derave, W. (2013). Meal and beta-alanine coingestion enhances muscle carnosine loading. *Med Sci Sports Exerc* 45: 1478–85.

Stellingwerff, T. (2013). Contemporary nutrition approaches to optimize elite marathon performance. *Int J Sport Physiol Perform* 8: 573–8.

Stellingwerff, T., Cox, G.R. (2014). Systematic review: carbohydrate supplementation on exercise performance or capacity of varying durations. *Appl Physiol Nutr Metab* 39: 998–1011.

Stensrud, T., Ingjer, F., Holm, H., Stromme, S.B. (1992). L-tryptophan does not improve running performance. *Int J Sport Med* 13: 481–5.

Stephens, F.B., Constantin-Teodosiu, D., Greenhaff, P.L. (2007a). New insights concerning the role of carnitine in the regulation of fuel metabolism in skeletal muscle. *J Physiol* 581: 431–44.

Stephens, F.B., Evans, C.E., Constantin-Teodosiu, D., Greenhaff, P.L. (2007b). Carbohydrate ingestion augments L-carnitine retention in humans. *J Appl Physiol* 102: 1065–70.

Stephens, F.B., Wall, B.T., Marimuthu, K., Shannon, C.E., Constantin-Teodosiu, D., Macdonald, I.A., Greenhaff, P.L. (2013). Skeletal muscle carnitine loading increases energy expenditure, modulates fuel metabolism gene networks and prevents body fat accumulation in humans. *J Physiol* 591: 4655–66.

Stephens, T.J., McKenna, M.J., Canny, B.J., Snow, R.J., McConnell, G.K. (2002). Effect of sodium bicarbonate on muscle metabolism during intense endurance cycling. *Med Sci Sports Exerc* 34: 614–21.

Stepto, N.K., Shipperd, B.B., Hyman, G., McInerney, B., Pyne, D.B. (2011) Effects of high-dose large neutral amino acid supplementation on exercise, motor skills, and mental performance in Australian Rules football players. *Appl Physiol Nutr Metab* 36: 671–6.

Stevinson, C., Devaraj, V.S., Fountain-Barber, A., Hawkins, S., Ernst, E. (2003). Homeopathic arnica for prevention of pain and bruising: randomized placebo-controlled trial in hand surgery. *J R Soc Med* 96: 60–5.

Stipanuk, M.H. (1986). Metabolism of sulfur-containing amino acids. *Ann Rev Nutr* 6: 179–209.

Stohs, S.J., Ray, S.D. (2013). A review and evaluation of the efficacy and safety of Cissus quadrangularis extracts. *Phytother Res* 27: 1107–14.

Stone, M.H., Sanborn, K., Smith, L.L., *et al.* (1999). Effects of in-season (5 weeks) creatine and pyruvate supplementation on anaerobic performance and body composition in American football players. *Int J Sport Nutr* 9: 146–65.

Strüder, H.K., Hollmann, W., Platen, P., Donike, M., Gotzmann, A., Weber, K. (1998). Influence of paroxetine, branched-chain amino acids and tyrosine on neuroendocrine system responses and fatigue in humans. *Horm Metab Res* 30: 188–94.

Sukala, W.R. (1998). Pyruvate: beyond the marketing hype. *Int J Sport Nutr* 8: 241–9.

Suksomboon, N., Poolsup, N., Yuwanakorn, A. (2014). Systematic review and meta-analysis of the efficacy and safety of chromium supplementation in diabetes. *J Clin Pharm Ther* 39: 292–306.

Sulzer, N.U., Schwellnus, M.P., Noakes, T.D. (2005). Serum electrolytes in ironman triathletes with exercise-associated muscle cramping. *Med Sci Sports Exerc* 37: 1081–5.

Sureda, A., Córdova, A., Ferrer, M.D., *et al.* (2010). L-citrulline-malate influence over branched chain amino acid utilization during exercise. *Eur J Appl Physiol* 110: 341–51.

Sureda, A., Córdova, A., Ferrer, M.D., Tauler, P., Pérez, G., Tur, J.A., Pons, A. (2009). Effects of L-citrulline oral supplementation on polymorphonuclear neutrophils oxidative burst and nitric oxide production after exercise. *Free Radic Res* 43: 828–35.

Sureda, A., Pons, A. (2013). Arginine and citrulline supplementation in sports and exercise: ergogenic nutrients? In: Lamprecht, M. (ed.) *Acute Topics in Sports Nutrition*. Med Sport Sci. Basel, Karger 59: 18–28.

Suzic Lazic, J., Dikic, N., Radivojevic, N., *et al.* (2011). Dietary supplements and medications in elite sport – polypharmacy or real need? *Scand J Med Sci Sports* 21: 260–7.

Suzuki, Y., Nakao, T., Maemura, H., Sato, M., Kamahara, K., Morimatsu, F., Takamatsu, K. (2006). Carnosine and anserine ingestion enhances contribution of nonbicarbonate buffering. *Med Sci Sports Exerc* 38: 334–8.

Svingen, G.F., Schartum-Hansen, H., Ueland, P.M., Pedersen, E.R., Seifert, R., Ebbing, M., *et al.* (2014). Elevated plasma dimethylglycine is a risk marker of mortality in patients with coronary heart disease. *Eur J Prev Cardiol* [Epub ahead of print].

Swanston-Flatt, S.K., Day, C., Bailey, C.J., *et al.* (1989a). Evaluation of traditional plant treatments for diabetes: studies in streptozotocin diabetic mice. *Acta Diabetol Lat* 26: 51–5.

Swanston-Flatt, S.K., Day, C., Flatt, P.R., *et al.* (1989b). Glycaemic effects of traditional European plant treatments for diabetes. Studies in normal and streptozotocin diabetic mice. *Diabetes Res Edinb Scotl* 10: 69–73.

Szczurko, O., Cooley, K., Mills, E.J., *et al.* (2009). Naturopathic treatment of rotator cuff tendinitis among Canadian postal workers: a randomized controlled trial. *Arthritis Rheum* 15: 1037–45.

Taaffe, D.R., Pruitt, L., Reim, J., *et al.* (1994). Effect of recombinant human growth hormone on the muscle strength response to resistance exercise in elderly men. *J Clin Endocrinol Metab* 79: 1361–6.

Tabatabaie, L., Klomp, L.W., Berger, R., de Koning, T.J. (2010). L-serine synthesis in the central nervous system: a review on serine deficiency disorders. *Mol Genet Metab* 99: 256–62.

Takahara, J., Yunoki, S., Yakushiji, W., *et al.* (1977). Stimulatory effects of gamma-hydroxybutyric acid on growth hormone and prolactin release in humans. *J Clin Endocrinol Metab* 44: 1014–17.

Takeda, K., Machida, M., Kohara, A., *et al.* (2011). Effects of citrulline supplementation on fatigue and exercise performance in mice. *J Nutr Sci Vitaminol (Tokyo)* 57: 246–50.

Tang, J.E., Moore, D.R., Kujbida, G.W., Tarnopolsky, M.A., Phillips, S.M. (2009). Ingestion of whey hydrolysate, casein, or soy protein isolate: effects on mixed muscle protein synthesis at rest and following resistance exercise in young men. *J Appl Physiol* 107: 987–92.

Tang, J.E., Phillips, S.M. (2009). Maximizing muscle protein anabolism: the role of protein quality. *Curr Opinion Clin Nutri Metabol Care* 12: 66–71.

Tarazona-Díaz, M.P., Alacid, F., Carrasco, M., *et al.* (2013). Watermelon juice: potential functional drink for sore muscle relief in athletes. *J Agric Food Chem* 61: 7522–8.

Tarnopolsky, M. (2004). Protein requirements for endurance athletes. *Nutr* 20: 662–8.

Tarnopolsky, M., Zimmer, A., Paikin, J., Safdar, A., Aboud, A., Pearce, E., Roy, B., Doherty, T. (2007). Creatine monohydrate and conjugated linoleic acid improve strength and body composition following resistance exercise in older adults. *PLoS One* 22: e991.

Tarnopolsky, M.A. (2007). Clinical use of creatine in neuromuscular and neurometabolic disorders. *Subcell Biochem* 46: 183–204.

Tarnopolsky, M.A., Parise, G., Yardley, N.J., Ballantyne, C.S., Olatinji, S., Phillips, S.M. (2001). Creatine-dextrose and protein-dextrose induce similar strength gains during training. *Med Sci Sports Exerc* 33: 2044–52.

Tartibian, B., Maleki, B.H., Abbasi, A. (2009). The effects of ingestion of omega-3 fatty acids on perceived pain and external symptoms of delayed onset muscle soreness in untrained men. *Clin J Sport Med* 19: 115–19.

Taylor, J.C., Rapport, L., Lockwood, G.B. (2005). Octacosanol in human health. *Nutr* 19: 192–5.

Teichman, S.L., Neale, A., Lawrence, B., Gagnon, C., Castaigne, J.P., Frohman, L.A. (2006). Prolonged stimulation of growth hormone (GH) and insulin-like growth factor I secretion by CJC-1295, a long-acting analog of GH-releasing hormone, in healthy adults. *J Clin Endocrinol Metab* 91: 799–805.

Telford, R.D., Catchpole, E.A., Deakin, V., *et al.* (1992). The effect of 7 to 8 months of vitamin/mineral supplementation on the vitamin and mineral status of athletes. *Int J Sport Nutr* 2: 123–34.

Terao, J., Kawai, Y., Murota, K. (2008). Vegetable flavonoids and cardiovascular disease. *Asia Pac J Clin Nutr* 17: 291–3.

Terry, R., Posadzki, P., Watson, L.K., *et al.* (2011). The use of ginger (Zingiber officinale) for the treatment of pain: a systematic review of clinical trials. *Pain Med* 12: 1808–18.

Theodorou, A.A., Nikolaidis, M.G., Paschalis, V., *et al.* (2011). No effect of antioxidant supplementation on muscle performance and blood redox status adaptations to eccentric training. *Am J Clin Nutr* 93: 1373–83.

Thevis, M., Geyer, H., Thomas, A., Schänzer, W. (2011). Trafficking of drug candidates relevant for sports drug testing: detection of non-approved therapeutics categorized as anabolic and gene doping agents in products distributed via the Internet. *Drug Test Anal* 3: 331–6.

Thevis, M., Sigmund, G., Geyer, H., *et al.* (2010). Stimulants and doping in sports. *Endocrinol Metab Clin N Am* 39: 89–105.

Thien, F.C., Leung, R., Baldo, B.A., Weiner, J.A., Plomley, R., Czarny, D. (1996). Asthma and anaphylaxis induced by royal jelly. *Clin Exp Allergy* 26: 216–22.

Thom, E., Wadstein, J., Gudmundsen, O. (2001). Conjugated linoleic acid reduces body fat in healthy exercising humans. *J Int Med Res* 29: 392–6.

Thomas, A., Kohler, M., Mester, J., *et al.* (2010). Identification of the growth-hormone-releasing peptide-2 (GHRP-2) in a nutritional supplement. *Drug Test Anal* 2: 144–8.

Tian, H., Guo, X., Wang, X., He, Z., Sun, R., Ge, S., Zhang, Z. (2013). Chromium picolinate supplementation for overweight and obese adults. *Cochrane Database Syst Rev* 29: 1–89.

Tilwe, G.H., Beria, S., Turakhia, N.H., *et al.* (2001). Efficacy and tolerability of oral enzyme therapy as compared to diclofenac in active osteoarthritis of knee joint: an open randomized controlled clinical trial. *J Assoc Physicians India* 49: 617–21.

Timmons, B.W., Newhouse, I.J., Thayer, R.E., *et al.* (2000). The efficacy of SPORT as a dietary supplement on performance and recovery in trained athletes. *Can J Appl Physiol* 25: 55–67.

Tiollier, E., Chennaoui, C.D.T.M., Gomez-Merino, D., *et al.* (2007). Effect of a probiotic supplementation on respiratory infections and immune and hormonal parameters during intense military training. *Mil Med* 172: 1006–11.

Tipton, K.D., Elliott, T.A., Cree, M.G., Aarsland, A.A., Sanford, A.P., Wolfe, R.R. (2007). Stimulation of net muscle protein synthesis by whey protein ingestion before and after exercise. *Am J Physiol Endocrinol Metab* 292: E71–6.

Tipton, K.D., Elliott, T.A., Ferrando, A.A., Aarsland, A.A., Wolfe, R.R. (2009). Stimulation of muscle anabolism by resistance exercise and ingestion of leucine plus protein. *Appl Physiol Nutr Metab* 34: 151–61.

Tipton, K.D., Ferrando, A.A., Phillips, S.M., Doyle, D., Wolfe, R.R. (1999). Postexercise net protein synthesis in human muscle from orally administered amino acids. *Am J Physiol Endocrinol Metab* 276: E628–E634.

Tischler, M., Desautels, M., Goldberg, A. (1982). Does leucine, leucyl-tRNA, or some metabolite of leucine regulate protein synthesis and degradation in skeletal and cardiac muscle? *J Biol Chem* 257: 1613–21.

Topo, E., Soricelli, A., D'Aniello, A., Ronsini, S., D'Aniello, G. (2009). The role and molecular mechanism of D-aspartic acid in the release and synthesis of LH and testosterone in humans and rats. *Reprod Biol Endocrinol* 7: 120.

Townsend, D.M., Tew, K.D., Tapiero, H. (2003). The importance of glutathione in human disease. *Biomed Pharmacother* 57: 145–55.

Travaline, J.M., Sudarshan, S., Roy, B.G., *et al.* (1997). Effect of N-acetylcysteine on human diaphragm strength and fatigability. *Am J Respir Crit Care Med* 156: 1567–71.

Trent, L.K., Thieding-Cancel, D. (1995). Effects of chromium picolinate on body composition. *J Sports Med Phys Fitness* 35: 273–80.

Trewin, A.J., Petersen, A.C., Billaut, F., McQuade, L.R., McInerny, B.V., Stepto, N.K. (2013). N-acetylcysteine alters substrate metabolism during high-intensity exercise in well-trained humans. *Appl Physiol Nutr Metab* 38: 1217–27.

Tricon, S., Burdge, G.C., Williams, C.M., Calder, P.C., Yaqoob, P. (2005). The effects of conjugated linoleic acid on human health-related outcomes. *Proc Nutr Soc* 64: 171–82.

Tricon, S., Yaqoob, P. (2006). Conjugated linoleic acid and human health: a critical evaluation of the evidence. *Curr Opin Clin Nutr Metab Care* 9: 105–10.

Triplett, D., Doyle, J.A., Rupp, J.C., *et al.* (2010). An isocaloric glucose-fructose beverage's effect on simulated 100-km cycling performance compared with a glucose-only beverage. *Int J Sport Nutr Exerc Metab* 20: 122–31.

Trombold, J.R., Barnes, J.N., Critchley, L., *et al.* (2010). Ellagitannin consumption improves strength recovery 2-3d after eccentric exercise. *Med Sci Sports Exerc* 42: 493–8.

Trudeau, F. (2008). Aspartate as an ergogenic supplement. *Sports Med* 38: 9–16.

Tse, S.Y. (1992). Cholinomimetic compound distinct from caffeine contained in coffee. II: Muscarinic actions. *J Pharm Sci* 81: 449–52.

Tumilty, L., Davison, G., Beckmann, M., Thatcher, R. (2011). Oral tyrosine supplementation improves exercise capacity in the heat. *Eur J Appl Physiol* 111: 2941–50.

Tumilty, L., Davison, G., Beckmann, M., Thatcher, R. (2013). Acute administration of a tyrosine and phenylalanine-free amino acid mixture reduces the exercise capacity in the heat. *Eur J Appl* 113: 1511–22.

Tumilty, L., Davison, G., Beckmann, M., Thatcher, R. (2014). Failure of oral tyrosine supplementation to improve exercise performance in the heat. *Med Sci Sports Exerc* 46: 1417–25.

Tveiten, D., Bruset, S. (2003). Effect of Arnica D30 in marathon runners. Pooled results from two double-blind placebo controlled studies. *Homeopathy* 92: 187–9.

Tyan, Y.-C., Yang, M.-H., Jong, S.-B., *et al.* (2009). Melamine contamination. *Anal Bioanal Chem* 395: 729–35.

Uauy, R., Olivares, M. and Gonzalez, M. (1998) Essentiality of copper in humans. *American Journal of Clinical Nutrition.* 67: 952S–959S.

Udani, J.K., Singh, B.B., Singh, V.J., Sandoval, E. (2009). BounceBack™ capsules for reduction of DOMS after eccentric exercise: a randomized, double-blind, placebo-controlled, crossover pilot study. *J Int Soc Sports Nutr* 6: 14.

Uebelhart, D., Malaise, M., Marcolongo, R., DeVathaire, F., Piperno, M., Mailleux, E., *et al.* (2004). Intermittent treatment of knee osteoarthritis with oral chondroitin sulfate: a one-year, randomized, double-blind, multicenter study versus placebo. *Osteoarthritis Cartilage* 12: 269–76.

UNESCO (2011). Conference of Parties to the International Convention against Doping in Sport, Third Session. Implementation of Article 10 of the International Convention against Doping in Sport. Paris: UNESCO. Available at: http://unesdoc.unesco.org/images/0021/002140/214047e.pdf. Accessed 29 January 2015.

USDA (2007). USDA Nutrient Data Laboratory: *Database for the Flavonoid Content of Selected Foods*. Beltsville, MD: U.S. Dept. of Agriculture. www.ars.usda.gov/nutrientdata.

USDA (2009). USDA National Nutrient Database for Standard Reference, Release 20: 23 April 2009, www.ars.usda.gov/ba/bhnrc/ndl. Accessed 1 June 2015.

USDA/NAS (2012). *Dietary Reference Intakes*. Available from: http://fnic.nal.usda.gov/dietary-guidance/dietary-reference-intakes/dri-tables. Accessed 1 June 2015.

USDHHS (2004). U.S. Department of Health and Human Services. *Bone Health and Osteoporosis: A Report of the Surgeon General*. Rockville, MD.

USFDA (2011). Health Hazard Evaluation Board. www.fda.gov/downloads/NewsEvents/PublicHealthFocus/UCM160672.pdf. Accessed 2 February 2011.

USFDA (2014a). DMAA in Dietary Supplements. Available at: www.fda.gov/food/dietarysupplements/qadietarysupplements/ucm346576.htm#FAQs. Accessed 30 May 2014.

USFDA (2014b). OxyElite Pro supplements recalled. Available at: www.fda.gov/forconsumers/consumerupdates/ucm374742.htm. Accessed 1 June 2014.

Usha, P.R., Naidu, M.U. (2004). Randomised, double-blind, parallel, placebo-controlled study of oral glucosamine, methylsulfonylmethane and their combination in osteoarthritis. *Clin Drug Investig* 24: 353–63.

Vaananen, H.K., Kumpulainen, T., Korhonen, L.K. (1982). Carbonic anhydrase in the type I skeletal muscle fibers of the rat. An immunohistochemical study. *J Histochem Cytochem* 30: 1109–13.

Valencia, E., Hardy, G., Marin, A. (2002). Glutathione-nutritional and pharmacologic viewpoints: part VI. *Nutr* 18: 291–2.

Valentine, V. (2007). The importance of salt in the athlete's diet. *Curr Sports Med Rep* 6: 237–40.

Valeri, C.R. (1976). *Blood Banking and the Use of Frozen Blood Products*. Cleveland: CRC Press.

van Cauter, E., Plat, L., Scharf, M.B., *et al.* (1997). Simultaneous stimulation of slow-wave sleep and growth hormone secretion by gamma-hydroxybutyrate in normal young men. *J Clin Invest* 100: 745–53.

van Coevorden, A., Mockel, J., Laurent, E., Kerkhofs, M., L'Hermite-Balériaux, M., Decoster, C., *et al.* (1991). Neuroendocrine rhythms and sleep in aging men. *Am J Physiol* 260: E651–61.

van der Beek, E.J., van Dokkum, W., Schrijver, J., *et al.* (1988). Thiamin, riboflavin and vitamins B-6 and C: impact of combined restricted intake on physical performance in man. *Am J Clin Nutr* 48: 1451–62.

van der Beek, E.J., van Dokkum, W., Wedel, M., *et al.* (1994). Thiamin, riboflavin and vitamins B-6: impact of restricted intake on physical performance in man. *J Am Coll Nutr* 13: 629–40.

van Dijk, A.E., Olthof, M.R., Meeuse, J.C., Seebus, E., Heine, R.J., van Dam, R.M. (2009). Acute effects of decaffeinated coffee and the major coffee components chlorogenic acid and trigonelline on glucose tolerance. *Diabetes Care* 32: 1023–5.

van Dijk, C.N. (1994). A double blind comparative study on the efficacy of MU-410 vs. placebo in patients with acute disruption of the anterior fibulotalr ligament. Study Nr. 4903XV, Amsterdam.

van Itallie, T.B., Nufert, T.H. (2003). Ketones: metabolism's ugly duckling. *Nutr Rev* 61: 327–41.

van Loon, L.J., Greenhaff, P.L., Constantin-Teodosiu, D., Saris, W.H.M., Wagenmakers, A.M. (2001). The effects of increasing exercise intensity on muscle fuel utilisation in humans. *J Physiol* 536: 295–304.

van Rosendal, S.P., Coombes, J.S. (2012). Glycerol use in hyperhydration and rehydration: scientific update. *Med Sport Sci* 59: 104–12.

van Rosendal, S.P., Osborne, M.A., Fassett, R.G., Coombes, J.S. (2010). Guidelines for glycerol use in hyperhydration and rehydration associated with exercise. *Sports Med* 40: 113–29.

Van Schuylenbergh, R., Van Leemputte, M., Hespel, P. (2003). Effects of oral creatine-pyruvate supplementation in cycling performance. *Int J Sport Med* 24: 144–50.

van Someren, K.A., Edwards, A.J., Howatson, G. (2005). Supplementation with beta-hydroxyl beta-methylbutyrate (HMB) and alpha-ketoisocaproic acid (KIC) reduces signs and symptoms of exercise-induced muscle damage in man. *Int J Sport Nutr Exerc Metab* 15: 413–24.

Van Zyl, C.G., Lambert, E.V., Hawley, J.A., Noakes, T.D., Dennis, S.C. (1996). The effect of medium-chain triglyceride ingestion on fuel metabolism and cycling performance. *J Appl Physiol* 80: 2217–25.

Vangsness, C.T., Spiker, W., Erickson, J. (2009). A review of evidence-based medicine for glucosamine and chondroitin sulfate use in knee osteoarthritis. *Arthroscopy* 25: 86–94.

Vanhatalo, A., Bailey, S.J., Blackwell, J.R., DiMenna, F.J., Pavey, T.G., Wilkerson, D.P., Benjamin, N., Winyard, P.G., Jones, A.M. (2010). Acute and chronic effects of dietary nitrate supplementation on blood pressure and the physiological responses to moderate-intensity and incremental exercise. *Am J Physiol Regul Integr Comp Physio* 299: R1121–31.

Varady, K.A., Ebine, N., Vanstone, C.A., *et al.* (2004). Plant sterols and endurance training combine to favorably alter plasma lipid profiles in previously sedentary hypercholesterolemic adults after 8 wk. *Am J Clin Nutr* 80: 1159–66.

Varnier, M., Leese, G.P., Thompson, J., Rennie, M.J. (1995). Stimulatory effect of glutamine on glycogen accumulation in human skeletal muscle. *Am J Physiol* 269: E309–E315.

Vayer, P., Mandel, M., Maitre, M. (1987). Gamma-hydroxybutyrate, a possible neurotransmitter. *Life Sci* 41: 1547–57.

Vaz, M., Pauline, M., Unni, U.S., Parikh, P., Thomas, T., *et al.* (2011). Micronutrient supplementation improves physical performance measures in Asian Indian school-age children. *J Nutr* 141: 2017–23.

Veech, R.L. (2004). The therapeutic implications of ketone bodies: the effects of ketone bodies in pathological conditions: ketosis, ketogenic diet, redox states, insulin resistance, and mitochondrial metabolism. *Prostagland Leukotr Essent Fatty Acids* 70: 309–19.

Venkatramani, D.V., Goel, S., Ratra, V., Gandhi, R.A. (2013). Toxic optic neuropathy following ingestion of homeopathic medication Arnica-30. *Cutan Ocul Toxicol* 32: 95–7.

Vernec, A., Stear, S.J., Burke, L.M., Castell, L.M. (2013). BJSM reviews: A–Z of nutritional supplements: dietary supplements, sports nutrition foods and ergogenic aids for health and performance Part 48: The World Anti Doping Agency. *Br J Sports Med* 47: 998–1000.

Vettenniemi, E. (2010). Why was doping banned in 1928? The IAAF, stimulants and the impact of racial beliefs. *Liikunta Tiede* 47: 24–9.

Vidal, C., Quandte, S. (2006). Identification of a sibutramine-metabolite in patient urine after intake of a 'pure herbal' Chinese slimming product. *Therapeutic Drug Monitoring* 28: 690–2.

Vincent, J.B. (2003). The potential value and toxicity of chromium picolinate as a nutritional supplement, weight loss agent and muscle development agent. *Sports Med* 33: 213–30.

Vinciguerra, G., Belcaro, G., Bonanni, E., *et al.* (2013). Evaluation of the effects of supplementation with Pycnogenol® on fitness in normal subjects with the Army Physical Fitness Test and in performances of athletes in the 100-minute triathlon. *J Sports Med Phys Fitness* 53: 644–54.

Vinson, J.A., Burnham, B.R., Nagendran, M.V. (2012). Randomized, double-blind, placebo-controlled, linear dose, crossover study to evaluate the efficacy and safety of a green coffee bean extract in overweight subjects. *Diabetes Metab Syndr Obes* 5: 21–7.

von Allwörden, H.N., Horn, S., Kahl, J., Feldheim, W. (1993). The influence of lecithin on plasma choline concentrations in triathletes and adolescent runners during exercise. *Eur J Appl Physiol* 67: 87–91.

von Mühlen, D., Laughlin, G.A., Kritz-Silverstein, D., Barrett-Connor, E. (2007). The Dehydroepiandrosterone And WellNess (DAWN) study: research design and methods. *Contemp Clin Trials* 28:153–68.

Wächter, S., Vogt, M., Kreis, R., Boesch, C., Bigler, P., Hoppeler, H., Krähenbühl, S. (2002). Long term administration of L-carnitine to humans: effect on skeletal muscle carnitine content and physical performance. *Clin Chim Acta* 318: 51–61.

WADA (2010). Statement of the first worldwide human growth hormone case. Secondary Statement of the first worldwide human growth hormone case. Available at: www.wada-ama.org/en/media-center/archives/articles/wada-statement-on-first-worldwide-human-growth-hormone-case/. Accessed 29 January 2014.

WADA (2014a). Laboratory Testing Figures. Available at: www.wada-ama.org/en/Science-Medicine/Anti-Doping-Laboratories/Laboratory-Testing-Figures. Accessed 5 March 2014.

WADA (2014b). Prohibited List. World Anti-Doping Agency. Available at: www.wada-ama.org/en/World-Anti-Doping-Program/Sports-and-Anti-Doping-Organizations/International-Standards/Prohibited-List/. Accessed 5 March 2014.

Wagenmakers, A.J. (1998). Muscle amino acid metabolism at rest and during exercise: role in human physiology and metabolism. *Exerc Sport Sci Rev* 26: 287–314.

Wagenmakers, A.J. (1999). Amino acid supplements to improve athletic performance. *Curr Opin Nutr Metab Care* 2: 539–44.

Walker, L.S., Bemben, M.G., Bemben, D.A., Knehans, A.W. (1998). Chromium picolinate effects on body composition and muscular performance in wrestlers. *Med Sci Sports Exerc* 30: 1730–7.

Walker, T.B., Roberts, R.A. (2006). Does Rhodiola rosea possess ergogenic properties? *Int J Sport Nutr Exerc Metab* 16: 305–15.

Wall, B.T., Hamer, H.M., de Lange, A., *et al.* (2013). Leucine co-ingestion improves post-prandial muscle protein accretion in elderly men. *Clin Nutr* 32: 412–19.

Wall, B.T., Stephens, F.B., Constantin-Teodosiu, D., Marimuthu, K., Macdonald, I.A., Greenhaff, P.L. (2011). Chronic oral ingestion of L-carnitine and carbohydrate increases muscle carnitine content and alters muscle fuel metabolism during exercise in humans. *J Physiol* 589: 963–73.

Wallis, G.A., Rowlands, D.S., Shaw, C., *et al.* (2005). Oxidation of combined ingestion of maltodextrins and fructose during exercise. *Med Sci Sports Exerc* 37: 426–32.

Walser, B., Stebbins, C.L. (2008). Omega-3 fatty acid supplementation enhances stroke volume and cardiac output during dynamic exercise. *Eur J Appl Physiol* 104: 455–61.

Walsh, N.P., Gleeson, M., Pyne, D.B., Nieman, D.C., Dhabhar, F.S., Shephard, R.J., Oliver, S.J., Bermon, S., Kajeniene, A. (2011a). Position Statement Part Two: maintaining immune health. *Exerc Immunol Rev* 17: 64–103.

Walsh, N.P. *et al.* (2011b). Position Statement Part One: Immune function and exercise. *Exerc Immunol Rev* 17: 6–63.

Wang, L., Lee, I.M., Zhang, S.M., *et al.* (2009). Dietary intake of selected flavonols, flavones, and flavonoid-rich foods and risk of cancer in middle-aged and older women. *Am J Clin Nutr* 89: 905–12.

Wang, X., Qiao, S., Yin, Y., Yue, L., Wang, Z., Wu, G. (2007). A deficiency or excess of dietary threonine reduces protein synthesis in jejunum and skeletal muscle of young pigs. *J Nutr* 137: 1442–6.

Warber, J., Patton, J., Tharion, W., *et al.* (2000). The effects of choline supplementation on physical performance. *Int J Sport Nutr Exerc Metab* 10: 170–81.

Warskulat, U., Flögel, U., Jacoby, C., *et al.* (2004). Taurine transporter knockout depletes muscle taurine levels and results in severe skeletal muscle impairment but leaves cardiac function uncompromised. *FASEB J* 18: 577–9.

Watford, M. (2008). Glutamine metabolism and function in relation to proline synthesis and the safety of glutamine and proline supplementation. *J Nutr* 138: 2003S–2007S.

Watson, P., Enever, S., Page, A., Stockwell, J., Maughan, R. (2012). Tyrosine supplementation does not influence the capacity to perform prolonged exercise in a warm environment. *Int J Sport Nutr Exerc Metab* 22: 363–73.

Watson, P., Hasegawa, H., Roelands, B., Piacentini, M.F., Looverie, R., Meeusen, R. (2005). Acute dopamine/noradrenaline reuptake inhibition enhances human exercise performance in warm, but not temperate conditions. *J Physiol* 565: 873–83.

Watt, K.K., Garnham, A.P., Snow, R.J. (2004). Skeletal muscle total creatine content and creatine transporter gene expression in vegetarians prior to and following creatine supplementation. *Int J Sport Nutr Exerc Metab* 14: 517–31.

Wax, B., Hilton, L., Vickers, B., Gilliland, K., Conrad, M. (2013a). Effects of glycine-arginine-α-ketoisocaproic acid supplementation in college-age trained females during multi-bouts of resistance exercise. *J Diet Suppl* 10: 6–16.

Wax, B., Kavazis, A.N., Brown, S.P., Hilton, L. (2013b). Effects of supplemental GAKIC ingestion on resistance training performance in trained men. *Res Q Exerc Sport* 84: 245–51.

Weaver, C.M. (1994). Age related calcium requirements due to changes in absorption and utilization. *J Nutr* 124: 1418S–1425S.

Webster, M.J., Scheett, T.P., Doyle, M.R. (1997). The effect of a thiamine derivative on exercise performance. *Eur J Appl Physiol Occup Physiol* 75: 520–4.

Weinheimer, E.M., Conley, T.B., Kobza, V.M., *et al.* (2012). Whey protein supplementation does not affect exercise training-induced changes in body composition and indices of metabolic syndrome in middle-aged overweight and obese adults. *J Nutr* 142: 1532–9.

Weiss, R.C. (1992). Immunologic responses in healthy random-source cats fed N,N-dimethylglycine-supplemented diets. *Am J Vet Res* 53: 829–33.

Welbourne, T.C. (1995). Increased plasma bicarbonate and growth hormone after an oral glutamine load. *Am J Clin Nutr* 61: 1058–61.

Welle, S., Jozefowicz, R., Statt, M. (1990). Failure of dehydroepiandrosterone to influence energy and protein metabolism in humans. *J Clin Endocrinol Metab* 71: 1259–64.

Wells, A.J., Hoffman, J.R., Gonzalez, A.M., *et al.* (2013). Phosphatidylserine and caffeine attenuate postexercise mood disturbance and perception of fatigue in humans. *Nutr Res* 33: 464–72.

West, D.W., Burd, N.A., Coffey, V.G., *et al.* (2011a). Rapid aminoacidemia enhances myofibrillar protein synthesis and anabolic intramuscular signaling responses after resistance exercise. *Am J Clin Nutr* 94: 795–803.

West, D.W., Burd, N.A., Tang, J.E., *et al.* (2010). Elevations in ostensibly anabolic hormones with resistance exercise enhance neither training-induced muscle hypertrophy nor strength of the elbow flexors. *J Appl Physiol* 108: 60–7.

West, J.S., Ayton, T., Wallman, K.E., Guelfi, K.J. (2012). The effect of 6 days of sodium phosphate supplementation on appetite, energy intake, and aerobic capacity in trained men and women. *Int J Sport Nutr Exerc Metab* 22: 422–9.

West, N.P., Horn, P.L., Pyne, D.B., *et al.* (2014). Probiotic supplementation for respiratory and gastrointestinal illness symptoms in healthy physically active individuals. *Clin Nutr* 33: 581–7.

West, N.P., Pyne, D.B., Cripps, A.W., *et al.* (2011b). *Lactobacillus fermentum* (PCC®) supplementation and gastrointestinal and respiratory tract illness symptoms: a randomised control trial in athletes. *Nutr J* 10: 30.

West, N.P., Pyne, D.B., Peake, J.M., Cripps, A.W. (2009). Probiotics, immunity and exercise: a review. *Exerc Immunol Rev* 15: 107–26.

Wheeler, K.B., Garleb, K.A. (1991). Gamma oryzanol – plant sterol supplementation: metabolic, endocrine, and physiologic effects. *Int J Sport Nutr* 1: 170–7.

Whelan, A.M., Jurgens, T.M., Szeto, V. (2010). Case report. Efficacy of Hoodia for weight loss: is there evidence to support the efficacy claims? *J Clin Pharm Ther* 35: 609–12.

Whitehead, M.T., Martin, T.D., Scheett, T.P., *et al.* (2007). The effect of 4 wk of oral echinacea supplementation on serum erythropoietin and indices of erythropoietic status. *Int J Sport Nutr Exerc Metab* 17: 378–90.

Whitehead, M.T., Martin, T.D., Scheett, T.P., *et al.* (2012a). Running economy and maximal oxygen consumption after 4 weeks of oral echinacea supplementation. *J Strength Cond Res Natl Strength Cond Assoc* 26: 1928–33.

Whitehead, P.N., Schilling, B.K., Farney, T.M., *et al.* (2012b). Impact of a dietary supplement containing 1,3-dimethylamylamine on blood pressure and bloodborne markers of health: a 10-week intervention study. *Nutr Metabolic Insights* 5: 33–9.

Whiting, P.J., Wafford, K.A., McKernan, R.M. (2001). Pharmacological subtypes of GABAA receptors based upon subunit composition. In: Martin, D.L., Olsen, R.W. (eds) *GABA in the Nervous System*. New York: Lippincott, Williams & Wilkins.

Whiting, S.J., Barabash, W.A. (2006). Dietary Reference Intakes for the micronutrients: considerations for physical activity. *Appl Physiol Nutr Metab* 31: 80–5.

WHO/FAO Joint Working Group (2002). Guidelines for the evaluation of probiotics in food. Available at: www.who.int/foodsafety/fs_management/en/probiotic_guidelines.pdf. Accessed 29 January 2014.

Widrig, R., Suter, A., Saller, R., Melzer, J. (2007). Choosing between NSAID and arnica for topical treatment of hand osteoarthritis in a randomised, double-blind study. *Rheumatol Int* 27: 585–91.

Wijnands, K.A., Vink, H., Briedé, J.J., *et al.* (2012). Citrulline a more suitable substrate than arginine to restore NO production and the microcirculation during endotoxemia. *PLoSOne* 7: e37439.

Wilborn, C.D., Kerksick, C.M., Campbell, B.I., *et al.* (2004). Effects of zinc magnesium aspartate (ZMA) supplementation on training adaptations and markers of anabolism and catabolism. *J Int Soc Sports Nutri* 1: 12–20.

Wiles, J.D., Coleman, D., Tegerdine, M., Swaine, I.L. (2006). The effects of caffeine ingestion on performance time, speed and power during a laboratory-based 1 km cycling time-trial. *J Sports Sci* 24: 1165–71.

Wiles, J.D., *et al.* (1992). Effect of caffeinated coffee on running speed, respiratory factors, blood lactate and perceived exertion during 1500-m treadmill running. *Br J Sports Med* 26: 116–20.

Wilkinson, D.J., Hossain, T., Hill, D.S., *et al.* (2013). Effects of leucine and its metabolite beta-hydroxy-beta-methylbutyrate on human skeletal muscle protein metabolism. *J Physiol* 591: 2911–23.

Wilkinson, S.B., Phillips, S.M., Atherton, P.J., *et al.* (2008). Differential effects of resistance and endurance exercise in the fed state on signalling molecule phosphorylation and protein synthesis in human muscle. *J Physiol* 586: 3701–17.

Wilkinson, S.B., Tarnopolsky, M.A., Macdonald, M.J., Macdonald, J.R., Armstrong, D., Phillips, S.M. (2007). Consumption of fluid skim milk promotes greater muscle protein accretion after resistance exercise than does consumption of an isonitrogenous and isoenergetic soy-protein beverage. *Am J Clin Nutr* 85: 1031–40.

Williams, A.D., Cribb, P.J., Cooke, M.B., *et al.* (2008). The effect of ephedra and caffeine on maximal strength and power in resistance-trained athletes. *J Strength Cond Res* 22: 464–70.

Williams, M.H., Kreider, R.B., Hunter, D.W., Somma, T., Shall, L.M., Woodhouse, M.L., Rokitski, L, (1990). Effect of inosine supplementation on 3 mile treadmill run performance and VO_2 peak. *Med Sci Sports Exerc* 22: 517–22.

WIllis, M.S., Monaghan, S.A., Miller, M.L., Mckenna, R.W., Perkins, W.D., Levinson, B.S., Bhushan, V. and Kroft, S.H. (2005) Zinc induced copper deficiency. *American Journal of Clinical Pathology*. 123: 125–131.

Willis, K.S., Smith, D.T., Broughton, K.S., Larson-Meyer, D.E. (2012). Vitamin D status and biomarkers of inflammation in runners. *J Sports Med* 3: 35–42.

Willoughby, D.S., Leutholtz, B. (2013). D-Aspartic acid supplementation combined with 28 days of heavy resistance training has no effect on body composition, muscle strength, and serum hormones associated with the hypothalamo-pituitary-gonadal axis in resistance-trained men. *Nutr Res* 33: 803–10.

Willsky, G.R., Chi, L.H., Liang, Y., Gaile, D.P., Hu, Z., Crans, D.C. (2006). Diabetes-altered gene expression in rat skeletal muscle corrected by oral administration of vanadyl sulfate. *Physiol Genomics* 26: 192–201.

Wilmert, N., Porcari, J., Foster, C., Doberstien, S., Brice, G. (2002). The effects of oxygenated water on exercise physiology during incremental exercise and recovery. *J Exerc Physiol (online)* 5: 16–21.

Wilund, K.R., Feeney, L.A., Tomayko, E.J., *et al.* (2009). Effects of endurance exercise training on markers of cholesterol absorption and synthesis. *Physiol Res* 58: 545–52.

Winder, W.W., Holloszy, J.O., Baldwin, K.M. (1974). Enzymes involved in ketone utilization in different types of muscle: adaptation to exercise. *Euro J Biochem* 47: 461–7.

Wing-Gaia, S., Subudhi, A., Askew, E. (2005). Effect of purified oxygenated water on exercise performance during acute hypoxic exposure. *Int J Sport Nutr Exerc Metab* 15: 680–8.

Winkler, P., de Vrese, M., Laue, Ch., Schrezenmeir, J. (2005). Effect of a dietary supplement containing probiotic bacteria plus vitamins and minerals on common cold infections and cellular immune parameters. *Int J Clin Pharmacol Ther* 43: 318–26.

Wiswedel, I., Hirsch, D., Kropf, S., *et al.* (2004). Flavanol-rich cocoa drink lowers plasma F(2)-isoprostane concentrations in humans. *Free Radic Biol Med* 37: 411–21.

Witard, O.C., Jackman, S.R., Breen, L., Smith, K., Selby, A., Tipton, K.D. (2014b). Myofibrillar muscle protein synthesis rates subsequent to a meal in response to increasing doses of whey protein at rest and after resistance exercise. *Am J Clin Nutr* 99: 86–95.

Witard, O.C., Tieland, M., Beelen, M., Tipton, K.D., van Loon, L.J., Koopman, R. (2009). Resistance exercise increases postprandial muscle protein synthesis in humans. *Med Sci Sports Exerc* 41: 144–54.

Witard, O.C., Turner, J.E., Jackman, S.R., *et al.* (2014a). High dietary protein restores over-reaching induced impairments in leukocyte trafficking and reduces the incidence of upper respiratory tract infection in elite cyclists. *Brain Behav Immun* 39: 211–19.

Wolfe, R.R. (2002). Regulation of muscle protein by amino acids. *J Nutr* 132: 3219S–24S.

Womack, C.J., Saunders, M.J., Bechtel, M.K., Bolton, D.J., Martin, M., *et al.* (2012). The influence of a CYP1A2 polymorphism on the ergogenic effects of caffeine. *J Int Soc Sports Nutr* 9: 7.

Woodhouse, M.L., Williams, M., Jackson, C. (1987). The effects of varying doses of orally ingested bee pollen extract upon selected performance variables. *J Athletic Training* 22: 22–8.

Woolf, K., Manore, M.M. (2006). B-Vitamins and exercise: does exercise alter requirements? *Int J Sport Nutr Exerc Met* 16: 453–84.

World Anti-Doping Agency (2013a). List of Prohibited Substances and Methods. World Anti-Doping Agency, 2013. Web. 31 May 2013. http://list.wada-ama.org/

World Anti-Doping Agency (2013b). World Anti-Doping Code 2009. World Anti-Doping Agency, 2009. Web. 31 May 2013. www.wada-ama.org/Documents/World_Anti-Doping_Program/WADP-The-Code/WADA_Anti-Doping_CODE_2009_EN.pdf

Wu, G., Bazer, F.W., Burghardt, R.C., Johnston, G.A., Kim, S.W., Knabe, D.A., Li, P., Li, X., McKnight, J.R., Satterfield, M.C., Spencer, T.E. (2011). Proline and hydroxyproline metabolism: implications for animal and human nutrition. *Amino Acids* 40: 10531–63.

Wu, G., Bazer, F.W., Davis, T.A., *et al.* (2009). Arginine metabolism and nutrition in growth, health and disease. *Amino Acids* 37: 153–68.

Wu, G., Fang, Y.Z., Yang, S., Lupton, J.R., Turner, N.D. (2004). Glutathione metabolism and its implications for health. *J Nutr* 134: 489–92.

Wu, G., Morris Jr, S.M. (1998). Arginine metabolism: nitric oxide and beyond. *Biochem J* 336: 1–17.

Wu, R.-R., Huang, W.-C., Liao, C.-C., Chang, Y.-K., Kan, N.-W., Huang, C.-C. (2013). Resveratrol protects against physical fatigue and improves exercise performance in mice. *Molecules* 18: 4689–702.

Wu, X., Wu, H., Xia, L., *et al.* (2010). Socio-technical innovations for total food chain safety during the 2008 Beijing Olympics and Paralympics and beyond. *Trends Food Sci Technol* 21: 44–51.

Wylie, L.J., Kelly, J., Bailey, S.J., Blackwell, J.R., Skiba, P.F., Winyard, P.G., Jeukendrup, A.E., Vanhatalo, A., Jones, A.M. (2013a). Beetroot juice and exercise: pharmacodynamic and dose-response relationships. *J Appl Physiol* 115: 325–36.

Wylie, L.J., Mohr, M., Krustrup, P., Jackman, S.R., Ermidis, G., Kelly, J., Black, M.I., Bailey, S.J., Vanhatalo, A., Jones, A.M. (2013b). Dietary nitrate supplementation improves team sport-specific intense intermittent exercise performance. *Eur J Appl Physiol* 113: 1673–84.

Wyon, M.A., Koutedakis, Y., Wolman, R., Nevill, A.M., Allen, N. (2014). The influence of winter vitamin D supplementation on muscle function and injury occurrence in elite ballet dancers: a controlled study. *J Sci Med Sport* 17: 8–12.

Xu, Z.R., Tan, Z.J., Zhang, Q., Gui, Q.F., Yang, Y.M. (2014). The effectiveness of leucine on muscle protein synthesis, lean body mass and leg lean mass accretion in older people: a systematic review and meta-analysis. *Br J Nutr* 19: 1–10.

Yamamoto, T., Azechi, H., Board, M. (2012). Essential role of excessive tryptophan and its neurometabolites in fatigue. *Can J Neurol Sci* 39: 40–7.

Yamamoto, T., Newsholme, E.A. (2000). Diminished central fatigue by inhibition of the L-system transporter for the uptake of tryptophan. *Brain Res Bull* 52: 35–8.

Yamashita, M., Yamamoto, T. (2014). Tryptophan and kynurenic acid may produce an amplified effect in central fatigue induced by chronic sleep disorder. *Int J Tryptophan Res* 7: 9–14.

Yang, A., Palmer, A.A., de Wit, H. (2010a). Genetics of caffeine consumption and responses to caffeine. *Psychopharmacology (Berl)* 211: 245–57.

Yang, J.H., Wada, A., Yoshida, K., Miyoshi, Y., Sayano, T., *et al.* (2010b). Brain-specific Phgdh deletion reveals a pivotal role for L-serine biosynthesis in controlling the level of D-serine, an N-methyl-D-aspartate receptor co-agonist, in adult brain. *J Biol Chem* 285: 41380–90.

Yang, Y., Breen, L., Burd, N.A., Hector, A.J., Churchward-Venne, T.A., Josse, A.R., *et al.* (2012a). Resistance exercise enhances myofibrillar protein synthesis with graded intakes of whey protein in older men. *Br J Nutr* 108: 1780–8.

Yang, Y., Churchward-Venne, T.A., Burd, N.A., Breen, L., Tarnopolsky, M.A., Phillips, S.M. (2012b). Myofibrillar protein synthesis following ingestion of soy protein isolate at rest and after resistance exercise in elderly men. *Nutr Metab* 9: 57.

Yarasheski, K.E., Zachweija, J.J., Angelopoulos, T.J., Bier, D.M. (1993). Short-term growth hormone treatment does not increase muscle protein synthesis in experienced weight lifters. *J Appl Physiol* 74: 3073–6.

Yarasheski, K.E., Zachwieja, J.J., Campbell, J.A., Bier, D.M. (1995). Effect of growth hormone and resistance exercise on muscle growth and strength in older men. *Am J Physiol* 268: E268–76.

Yarrow, J., Parr, J., White, L., Borsa, P., Stevens, B. (2007). The effects of short-term alpha-ketoisocaproic acid supplementation on exercise performance: a randomized controlled trial. *J Int Soc Sports Nutr* 4: 1–6.

Yary, T., Aazami, S. (2012). Dietary intake of zinc was inversely associated with depression. *Biol Trace Element Res* 145: 286–90.

Yatabe, Y., Miyakawa, S., Miyazaki, T., *et al.* (2003). Effects of taurine administration in rat skeletal muscles on exercise. *J Orthop Sci.* 8: 415–19.

Yau, S.W., Henry, B.A., Russo, V.C., McConell, G.K., Clarke, I.J., Werther, G.A., Sabin, M.A. (2014). Leptin enhances insulin sensitivity by direct and sympathetic nervous system regulation of muscle igfbp-2 expression: evidence from nonrodent models. *Endocrinology* 155: 2133–43.

Yeghiayan, S., Luo, S., Shukitt-Hale, B., Lieberman, H.R. (2001). Tyrosine improves behavioral and neurochemical deficits caused by cold exposure. *Physiol Behav* 72: 311–16.

Yfanti, C., Akerström, T., Nielsen, S., *et al.* (2010). Antioxidant supplementation does not alter endurance training adaptation. *Med Sci Sports Exerc* 42: 1388–95.

Yfanti, C., Fischer, C.P., Nielsen, S., *et al.* (2012). Role of vitamin C and E supplementation on IL-6 in response to training. *J Appl Physiol Bethesda Md 1985* 112: 990–1000.

Ylikoski, T., Piiranen, J., Hanninen, O., Penttinen, J. (1997). The effect of coenzyme Q10 on the exercise performance of cross-country skiers. *Moloc Aspects Med* 18: 283–90.

Yonei, Y., Shibagaki, K., Tsukada, N., Nagasu, N., Inagaki, Y., Miyamoto, K., Suzuki, O., Kiryu, Y. (1997). Case report: haemorrhagic colitis associated with royal jelly intake. *J Gastroenterol Hepatol* 12: 495–9.

Yoshida, K., Furuya, S., Osuka, S., Mitoma, J., Shinoda, Y., *et al.* (2004). Targeted disruption of the mouse 3-phosphoglycerate dehydrogenase gene causes severe neurodevelopmental defects and results in embryonic lethality. *J Biol Chem.* 279: 3573–7.

Young, C., Oladipo, O., Frasier, S., *et al.* (2012). Hemorrhagic stroke in young healthy male following use of sports supplement Jack3d. *Mil Med* 177: 1450–4.

Young, V.R., Borgonha, S. (2000). Nitrogen and amino acid requirements: the Massachusetts Institute of Technology amino acid requirement pattern. *J Nutr* 130: 1841S–9S.

Yuldasheva, N.K., Ul'chenko, N.T., Glushenkova, A.I. (2010). Wheat germ oil. *Chemistry of Natural Compounds* 46: 97–8.

Zamora-Ros, R., Andres-Lacueva, C., Lamuela-Raventós, R.M., *et al.* (2010). Estimation of dietary sources and flavonoid intake in a Spanish adult population (EPIC-Spain). *J Am Diet Assoc* 110: 390–8.

Zanchi, N.E., Gerlinger-Romero, F., Guimaraes-Ferreira, L. *et al.* (2011). HMB supplementation: clinical and athletic performance-related effects and mechanisms of action. *Amino Acids* 40: 1015–25.

Zembron-Lacny, A., Slowinska-Lisowska, M., Szygula, Z., Witkowski, K., Stefaniak, T., Dziubek, W. (2009). Assessment of the antioxidant effectiveness of alpha-lipoic acid in healthy men exposed to muscle-damaging exercise. *J Physiol Pharmacol* 60: 139–43.

Zemski, A.J., Quinlivan, R.M., Gibala, M., Burke, L.M., Stear, S.J., Castell, L.M. (2012). BJSM reviews: A–Z of nutritional supplements: dietary supplements, sports nutrition foods and ergogenic aids for health and performance Part 36: Spirulina, Succinate, Sucrose. *Br J Sports Med* 46: 893–4.

Zhang, L., Zuo, Z., Lin, G. (2007). Intestinal and hepatic glucuronidation of flavonoids. *Mol Pharm* 4: 833–45.

Zhang, X.-J., Chinkes, D.L., Wolfe, R.R. (2008). The anabolic effect of arginine on proteins in skin wound and muscle is independent of nitric oxide production. *Clin Nutr* 27: 649–56.

Zhang, Y., Woods, R.M., Breitbach, Z.S., *et al.* (2012). 1,3-Dimethylamylamine (DMAA) in supplements and geranium products: natural or synthetic? *Drug Test Anal* 4: 986–90.

Zhong, Z., Wheeler, M.D., Li, X., *et al.* (2003). L-Glycine: a novel antinflammatory, immunmodulatory, and cytoprotective agent. *Curr Opinion Clin Nutr Metab Care* 6: 229–40.

Zhou, S., Zhang, Y., Davie, A., *et al.* (2005). Muscle and plasma coenxyme Q10 concentration, aerobic power and exercise economy of healthy men in response to four weeks of supplementation. *J Sports Med Phys Fitness* 45: 337–46.

Ziemann, E., Zembroñ-Lacny, A., Kasperska, A., *et al.* (2013). Exercise training-induced changes in inflammatory mediators and heat shock proteins in young tennis players. *J Sports Sci Med* 12: 282.

Zittermann, A. (2003). Vitamin D in preventive medicine: are we ignoring the evidence? *Br J Nutr* 89: 552–72.

Zuhl, M., Dokladny, K., Memier, C., Schneider, S., Salgado, R., Moseley, P. (2014). The effects of acute oral glutamine supplementation on exercise-induced gastrointestinal permeability and heat-shock protein expression in peripheral blood mononuclear cells. *Cell Stress Chaperones*; 26 July [EPub].

Further reading

Burke, L.M. (2007). *Practical Sports Nutrition*. Champaign, Illinois: Human Kinetics Publishers.

Burke, L.M., Desbrow, B., Spriet, L. (2013). *Caffeine for Sports Performance*. Champaign, Illinois: Human Kinetics Publishers.

Calder, P.C., Burdge, G.C. (2004). Fatty Acids. In: Nicolaou, A., Kafatos, G. (eds) *Bioactive Lipids*. Bridgewater: The Oily Press, 1–36.

Calder, P.C., Yaqoob, P. (2014). *Diet, Immunity and Inflammation*. Cambridge: Woodhead Publishing.

Department of Health (2001). Report 41: *Dietary Reference Values for Food and Energy and Nutrients for the United Kingdom*. London: HMSO.

Frayn, K.N. (2010). *Metabolic Regulation – A Human Perspective* (3rd edition). Chichester: Wiley-Blackwell.

Jeukendrup, A., Gleeson, M. (2009). *Sport Nutrition* (2nd edition). Champaign, Illinois: Human Kinetics Publishers.

Lanham-New, S.A., Stear, S.J., Shirreffs, S.M., Collins A.L. (eds) (2011). *The Nutrition Society Textbook Series: Sport and Exercise Nutrition*. Chichester: Wiley-Blackwell.

Manore, M.M., Meyer, N.L., Thompson, J.L. (2009). *Sport Nutrition for Health and Performance* (2nd Edition). Champaign, Illinois: Human Kinetics Publishers.

Maughan, R.J., Gleeson, M. (2010). *The Biochemical Basis of Sports Performance* (2nd edition). Oxford: Oxford University Press.

Newsholme, E.A., Leech, A.R. (2010). *Functional Biochemistry in Health and Disease*. Chichester: Wiley Blackwell.

Poortmans, J.R., Francaux, M. (2008). Creatine consumption in health. In: Stout, J., Antonio, J., Kalman, D. (eds) *Essentials of Creatine in Sports and Health*. Totowa, NJ: Humana Press, 127–72.

Stear, S.J. (2004). *Fuelling Fitness for Sports Performance*. London: The British Olympic Association and The Sugar Bureau.

WADA (2014). Prohibited List. World Anti-Doping Agency. Available at www.wada-ama.org/en/World-Anti-Doping-Program/Sports-and-Anti-Doping-Organizations/International-Standards/Prohibited-List/.

Williams, M.H. (1985). Ergogenic Aids. In: Williams, M. *Nutritional Aspects of Human Physical and Athletic Performance* (2nd edition). Springfield, IL: Thomas Books, 296–321.

Websites

Australian Institute of Sport (AIS) – Nutrition: www.ausport.gov.au/ais/nutrition
Australian Sports AntiDoping Authority (ASADA): www.asada.gov.au
European Food Safety Authority (EFSA): www.efsa.europa.eu
NIH Office of Dietary Supplements (USA): http://ods.od.nih.gov/
Supplement 411 (USA): www.supplement411.org
UK Anti-Doping: www.ukad.org.uk
United States Anti-Doping Agency: www.usada.org
US Food and Drug Administration (FDA): www.fda.gov
World Anti-Doping Agency (WADA): www.wada-ama.org

INDEX

CPSIA information can be obtained
at www.ICGtesting.com
Printed in the USA
BVHW040432131118
532765BV00009B/4/P